MW01278485

BREATHING DISORDERS OF SLEEP

CONTEMPORARY ISSUES in PULMONARY DISEASE VOLUME 5

SERIES EDITORS

Neil S. Cherniack, M.D.
Professor of Medicine
Chief, Division of Pulmonary Medicine
Case Western Reserve University School of Medicine
Veterans Administration Medical Center
Cleveland, Ohio

Norman H. Edelman, M.D.
Professor of Medicine and Physiology
Chief, Pulmonary Diseases Division
UMDNJ—Rutgers Medical School
New Brunswick, New Jersey

Volumes in the Series

Vol. 1 Chronic Obstructive Pulmonary Disease
Hugo D. Montenegro, M.D., Editor

Vol. 2 Occupational Lung Disease
J. Bernard L. Gee, M.D., Editor

Vol. 3 Noninvasive Respiratory Monitoring
Michael L. Nochomovitz, M.D., and
Neil S. Cherniack, M.D., Editors

Vol. 4 Abnormal Pulmonary Circulation
Edward H. Bergofsky, M.D., Editor

Vol. 5. Breathing Disorders of Sleep
Norman H. Edelman, M.D., and
Teodoro V. Santiago, M.D., Editors

BREATHING DISORDERS OF SLEEP

Edited by

Norman H. Edelman, M.D.

Professor of Medicine and Physiology
Chief, Pulmonary Diseases Division
UMDNJ-Rutgers Medical School
New Brunswick, New Jersey

Teodoro V. Santiago, M.D.

Professor of Medicine
Pulmonary Diseases Division
UMDNJ-Rutgers Medical School
New Brunswick, New Jersey

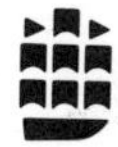

CHURCHILL LIVINGSTONE

NEW YORK, EDINBURGH, LONDON, MELBOURNE

1986

Library of Congress Cataloging-in-Publication Data

Breathing disorders of sleep.

(Contemporary issues in pulmonary disease; v. 5)
Includes bibliographies and index.
1. Sleep apnea syndromes. I. Edelman, Norman H.
II. Santiago, Teodoro V. III. Series. [DNLM:
1. Respiration. 2. Sleep. 3. Sleep Apnea Syndromes.
W1 CO769MRS v.5 / WF 143 B828]
RC737.5.B73 1986 616.2 86-13613
ISBN 0-443-08398-3

Distributed in the United Kingdom by Churchill Livingstone, Robert Stevenson House, 1-3 Baxter's Place, Leith Walk, Edinburgh EH1 3AF and by associated companies, branches and representatives throughout the world.

Accurate indications, adverse reactions, and dosage schedules for drugs are provided in this book, but it is possible that they may change. The reader is urged to review the package information data of the manufacturers of the medications mentioned.

Acquisitions Editor: *Kim Loretucci*
Copy Editor: *Ozzievelt Owens*
Production Supervisor: *Jocelyn Eckstein*

Printed in the United States of America

First published in 1986

Contributors

N. R. Anthonisen, M.D., Ph.D.
Head, Section of Repiratory Medicine, Faculty of Medicine, The University of Manitoba, Winnipeg, Manitoba, Canada

Anne Berssenbrugge, Ph.D.
Research Assistant, John Rankin Laboratory of Pulmonary Medicine, Department of Preventive Medicine, University of Wisconsin Medical School, Madison, Wisconsin

Waldemar A. Carlo, M.D.
Assistant Professor of Pediatrics, Department of Pediatrics, Rainbow Babies and Children's Hospital, Case Western Reserve University, Cleveland, Ohio

Sudhansu Chokroverty, M.D.
Chief, Division of Neurophysiology, UMDNJ-Rutgers Medical School, New Brunswick, New Jersey

Martin A. Cohn, M.D., F.A.C.P., F.C.C.P.
Chief, Sleep Disorders Center; Associate Chief, Division of Pulmonary Disease, Mount Sinai Medical Center, Miami Beach, Florida

Jerome Dempsey, Ph.D.
Professor of Medicine, John Rankin Laboratory of Pulmonary Medicine, Department of Preventive Medicine, University of Wisconsin Medical School, Madison, Wisconsin

Norman H. Edelman, M.D.
Professor of Medicine and Physiology; Chief, Pulmonary Diseases Division, UMDNJ-Rutgers Medical School, New Brunswick, New Jersey

Barbara Gothe, M.D.
Associate Professor of Medicine, Case Western Reserve Univeristy School of Medicine, Cleveland, Ohio

Gabriel G. Haddad, M.D.
Associate Professor of Pediatrics; Director, Sleep Physiology Laboratory, Pediatric Pulmonary Division, Columbia University College of Physicians and Surgeons, New York, New York

Meir Kryger, M.D., F.R.C.P.C.
Director, Sleep Laboratory, Faculty of Medicine, The University of Manitoba, Winnepeg, Manitoba, Canada

Richard J. Martin, M.D.
Associate Professor of Pediatrics, Codirector of Neonatalogy, Department of Pediatrics Rainbow Babies and Children's Hospital, Case Western Reserve University School of Medicine, Cleveland, Ohio

Martha J. Miller, M.D.
Assistant Professor of Pediatrics, Department of Pediatrics, Rainbow Babies and Children's Hospital, Case Western Reserve University School of Medicine, Cleveland, Ohio

Judith A. Neubauer, Ph.D.
Assistant Professor of Medicine, Department of Medicine, UMDNJ-Rutgers Medical School, New Brunswick, New Jersey

John M. Orem, Ph.D.
Professor of Physiology, School of Medicine, Texas Tech University Health Sciences Center, Lubbock, Texas

Richard A. Parisi, M.D.
Assistant Professor of Medicine, Department of Medicine, UMDNJ-Rutgers Medical School, New Brunswick, New Jersey

Marvin A. Sackner, M.D.
Consultant Physician, Sleep Disorders Center, Mount Sinai Medical Center, Miami Beach, Florida

Teodoro V. Santiago, M.D.
Associate Professor of Medicine, Pulmonary Diseases Division, Department of Medicine, UMDNJ-Rutgers Medical School, New Brunswick, New Jersey

Philip L. Schiffman, M.D.
Associate Professor of Medicine, Pulmonary Diseases Division, Department of Medicine, UMDNJ-Rutgers Medical School, New Brunswick, New Jersey

James Skatrud, M.D.
Associate Professor of Medicine; Chief of Pulmonary Medicine, Department of Medicine, University of Wisconsin Medical School, Madison, Wisconsin

Kingman P. Strohl, M.D.
Associate Professor of Medicine, Case Western Reserve University School of Medicine; Director, Pulmonary Function Laboratory, Asthma and Allergic Disease Center, University Hospitals, Cleveland, Ohio

Marie C. Trontell, M.D.
Assistant Professor of Medicine, Pulmonary Diseases Division, Department of Medicine, UMDNJ-Rutgers Medical School, New Brunswick, New Jersey

Preface

He sleeps well who knows not that he sleeps ill.

—Old Latin Proverb

A great source of awe and delight to physiologists and physicians is the continual emergence of new fields of inquiry, often involving the discovery of "new" diseases. Discoveries are most exciting when the uncovered discipline or disorder has been right under our noses—obvious, but ignored because of that wonderful human potential to disregard what we are unable to understand or study.

Such is the case with breathing during sleep. Sleep, with its attendant phenomenon of dreaming, has been a source of wonder to man since the beginning of recorded time. Nevertheless, scientific study of sleep is recent and still embryonic. The discovery of breathing abnormalities during sleep, and the subsequent study of the underlying physiology, is even more recent. The results, however, have been nothing short of explosive. A newly recognized syndrome, obstructive sleep apnea, has been shown to be serious, associated with a high degree of morbidity, and perhaps, mortality. It is common—by some estimates approaching asthma in its incidence. Less typical or milder versions of the syndrome may explain everyday perplexing phenomena, such as hypersomnolence in the elderly.

The importance of respiratory changes during sleep is now recognized to extend far beyond the obstructive sleep apnea syndrome. Important phenomena occur in neonates, patients with chronic lung diseases and a host of neurologic diseases. In addition,the range of sleep disordered breathing transcends the confines of the usual medical concerns, from the mundane, associated with the common cold, to the exotic, such as the cyclic breathing of high altitude explorers.

This is an ambitious volume. We start with history and literature, followed by basic neuroscience. We dwell at some length on the relevant physiology, considering control of breathing during sleep in both adults and children and paying special attention to critical areas such as the control of the upper airway and the complexities of the response to hypoxia. The clinically oriented section explores the various sleep apnea syndromes and devotes considerable attention to diagnostic methodologies, again paying separate attention to the differences between methods and entities in the adult and pediatric populations. We discuss current concepts of therapy from a mechanistic point of view and end with detailed descriptions of breathing abnormalities in chronic lung disease and neuromuscular disorders.

Our goal was not to be encyclopedic or to represent all points of view. Nevertheless, the scope of the work, stature of the contributors, and our encouragement to include as much text and references as "necessary" have resulted in most topics being presented in considerable depth. The addition of a few concise chapters makes the volume of likely interest to a broad segment of the potential audience. It is our expectation that the progress and new developments in this field will necessitate coverage by texts many times the size of this one in the not-too-distant future.

Norman H. Edelman, M.D.
Teodoro V. Santiago, M.D.

Contents

1 Sleep and Breathing in History and Literature

Philip L. Schiffman

> Sleep, next society and true friendship, man's best contentment, doth securely slip his passions and the world's troubles.
>
> —John Donne

Since antiquity man has been fascinated by sleep. He has looked forward to it and has dreaded it, loved it and feared it, theorized about it and baffled over it. Throughout, he has never entirely understood it. This has been reflected over the centuries in folklore, literature, art, music, philosophy, theater, and medicine.

This introductory chapter explores these cultural records of man's theories and perceptions on the essence of sleep throughout the ages. As the breadth of two and a half millenia of ideas makes a comprehensive review impossible, this chapter will concentrate on select works of special interest within the following areas: the relationship of sleep to death, dreams, the nature and function(s) of sleep, and the relationship of sleep to health and disease.

SLEEP AND DEATH

> His life is a watch or a vision
> Between a sleep and a sleep
>
> —Algernon Charles Swinburne
> from *Atlanta in Calydon*

From his earliest writings, we can see that man has perceived a close relationship between sleep and death. At times he has found them difficult to

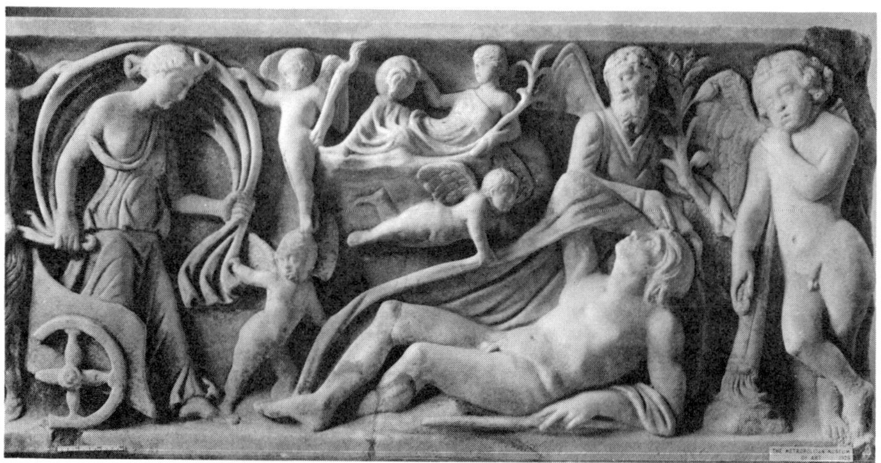

Fig. 1-1 Selene, the moon Goddess saw and fell in love with the handsome but mortal shepherd Endymion who was asleep on Mount Latmus. She visited him often and they had 50 daughters. In one legend, Jupiter offered Endymion a choice of punishments. He could die by any means he chose or he could live in perpetual peaceful sleep. Endymion chose the latter. In another legend, Selene put Endymion into a perpetual sleep so that he would never change. In either legend, Endymion still sleeps today in a state of perpetual youth and is still occasionally visited by Selene. Many second and third century A.D. Roman Sarcophagi have been found adorned by reliefs depicting this story. Above is a picture of part of such a relief from a second century A.D. Sarcophagus. Note Endymion asleep, staff in hand, his head resting on the lap of Somnus, god of sleep. To the right is Eros. To the left is Selene, the moon Goddess (a moon crescent on her forehead). Further to the left on the actual sarcophagus, but out of view of this picture, is a slumbering shepherd and his flock. (The Metropolitan Museum of Art, Fletcher Fund, 1924. [24.97.13])

distinguish as stated in the Bible, "The deepest sleep resembles death" (I Samuel:26:12) and in the Talmud, "sleep and death are similar. They are only different in degree, in that individual organs function more feebly: sleep is one-sixtieth (i.e., one piece) of death . . ." (Berachoth 576). Also, Aristotle[2] wrote, "Persons, too, who have fallen into a deep trance, and have come to be regarded as dead, ..." This instilled in man both a fear of sleep (fear of dying while asleep) and a sense of hope (that death may not be final, but only a prolonged period, similar to sleep).

This perceived linkage between sleep and death can best be seen in mythology[3,4] (Fig. 1-1). Sleep (Hypnos in Greek mythology and Somnus in Roman mythology) and Death (Thanatos) are twin brothers, both sons of Night (Nyx). Hypnos brings mortals solace and fair dreams. The Dreams, whose numbers are infinite are sons of Hypnos. Morpheus, one of the sons of Hypnos (also called the god of dreams), is a molder or shaper of dreams seen by man and of man. Hypnos induces man to sleep by touching him with a magic wand or fanning him with his wings. The cave of the abode of Hypnos lies in stillness and darkness by the River Lethe, whose murmuring waters invite sleep. His dwelling has two gates, one of ivory through which issues false and flattering visions and one of horn through which true dreams pass.

The god of sleep even has power over other gods, some mightier than he. This is seen in the Iliad[5]. Hera despised Paris and his Trojan people, but the mighty Zeus would not permit the Greeks to conquer them and thus their war was stalemated. Hera conspired with Hypnos to put Zeus to sleep so that Poseidon might interfere on behalf of the Greeks while Zeus slumbered.

In contrast to his brother, Thanatos closes the eyes of mortals forever. His abode lies by the River Styx which no mortal may pass and return.

The linkage of sleep and death can be seen over and over again in the works of William Shakespeare.[6] In *Macbeth* he calls sleep "the death of each day's life." Hamlet, in his famous soliloquy repeatedly equates sleep with death:

> to die, to sleep;
> to sleep: perchance to dream: ay, there's the rub,
> For in that sleep of death what dreams may come . . .

In *Henry IV, Part II*, the king refers to the time of his death as when he will be "sleeping with my ancestors."

Like Aristotle, Shakespeare also believed that the very deepest sleep could mimic death and used this as an important device in the plots of two plays, *Cymbelline* and the well-known *Romeo and Juliet*. For example, in *Cymbelline*, Imogen, the king's daughter swallows what she believes to be a soothing potion in order to relieve the anxieties she has developed over the miscommunications with her banished husband. She falls into a deathlike sleep as the medicine is actually an exceedingly strong sleeping potion prepared by the court physician and she is mistaken for dead by her brothers.

Repeatedly, poets have referred to the dead as "the sleeping." This is seen in John McCrae's "In Flanders Field":

> If ye break faith with us who die
> We shall not sleep, though poppies grow
> In Flanders Field.

This interchanging of the terms is also seen in several works that followed in response to "In Flanders Field." John Mitchell wrote in "Reply to In Flanders Field," "Oh! sleep in peace where poppies grow," J. A. Armstrong urged the dead to "sleep peacefully, for all is well," in "Another Reply to the In Flanders Field," and in "America's Answer" R. W. Lilliard wrote,

> and we will keep
> True faith with you who lies asleep

with each a cross to mark his bed,
In Flanders Fields.

Thus it is not surprising that sleep and death have been linked in our thought and language. A dead body is "laid to rest" and bid to "rest in peace" (rest implies a restorative function to sleep).

DREAMS

> When we dream we do not know that we are dreaming. In our dreams we may even interpret our dreams. Only after we are awake do we know we have dreamed. Finally, there comes a great awakening, and then we know life is a great dream.
>
> —Chuang Tzu[7] (Fourth Century B.C.)

Undoubtedly no aspect of sleep has fascinated man more through the ages than dreams. Man has speculated on their causes and their meanings, postulating dreams to be a gift of (the) god(s) or to arise from within; he has considered dreams to be prophetical of the future, nonsense, or derived from the past. He has marvelled at their irrationality (Fig. 1-2). Life itself has even been thought of as a dream (not just figuratively in a song) with death an awakening (Chuang Tzu, above) or attributed to the dream of a superior being, Vishnu.

The Greeks disagreed on the origin of dreams. Herodotus[8] states that pictures arising in the mind while waking in the day may occupy dreams at night, but he also believed that the gods could give man warnings of the future in dreams. Galen believed that the soul created two kinds of dreams:[9]

> The soul does not only form during sleep the sense data of the condition of the body, but also from the customary activities of the day: some of these are our thoughts, and some are disclosed by the soul as prophecies as can be proved by experience.

Aristotle[10] thought dreams to be the misinterpreted perceptions by the sense organs of both internal and external stimuli. Thus an innocuous sound could, during sleep, be perceived as thunder. Moreover, Aristotle thought that different personality types would perceive the same stimulus differently. His example is that a coward, in his dreams, would interpret as a threatening enemy what the amorous person, in his dreams, would interpret as an object of desire. Aristotle[11] however dismisses dreams as not having any prophetic meaning. He attributes those dreams that do come true to coincidence or foresight. He dismisses divine intervention as being the cause of prophetic dreams, as many dreams do not come true and argues that "common people" are just as likely to have their dreams come true, dismissing as absurd that a God would send a prophetic dream to any but the noblest and wisest.

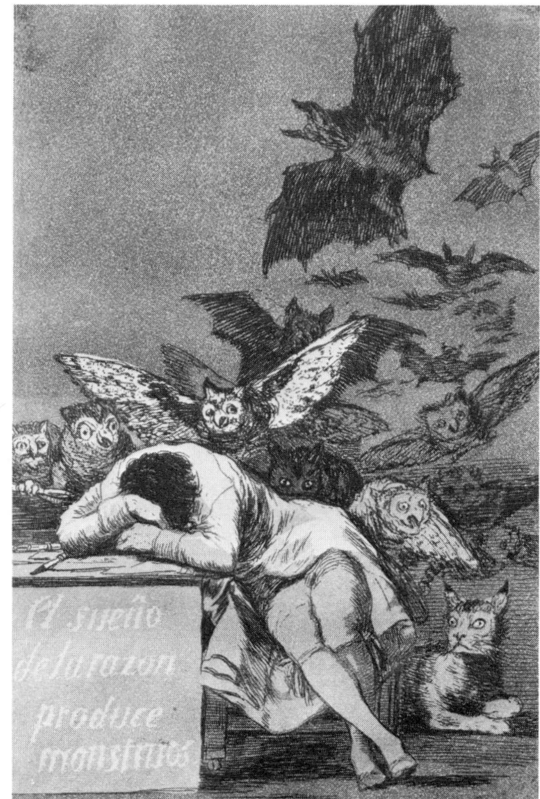

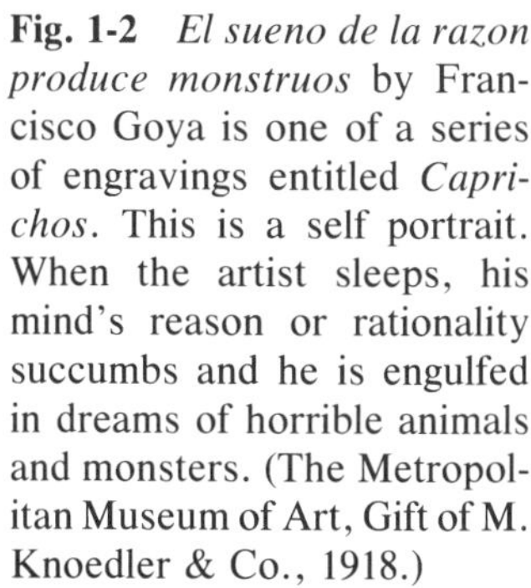

Fig. 1-2 *El sueno de la razon produce monstruos* by Francisco Goya is one of a series of engravings entitled *Caprichos*. This is a self portrait. When the artist sleeps, his mind's reason or rationality succumbs and he is engulfed in dreams of horrible animals and monsters. (The Metropolitan Museum of Art, Gift of M. Knoedler & Co., 1918.)

Through the ages the disagreements continued, varying on one hand, from the Roman, Epicurus, who denied dreams have any relationship to conscious or psychological processes, attributing them to atoms entering the sleeping mind from without[12], to the modern western ideas of Freud who stated, "Every dream will reveal itself as a psychological structure, full of significance and one which may be assigned to a specific place in the psychic activities of the waking state."[13]

Dream interpretation and prophecy was important to the ancients. The Greeks, Aeschylus in particular, credit Prometheus (prometheus is Greek for foresight) as the founder of the "science" of dream interpretation. In "Prometheus Bound" Prometheus states:[14]

> It was I who arranged all the ways of seercraft, and I first adjudged what things come verily true from dreams; and to men I gave meaning to the ominous cries hard to interpret.

In different eras and cultures the prophetic dream took different forms. It could be direct as it often is in the epics of Homer and Virgil, with a vision

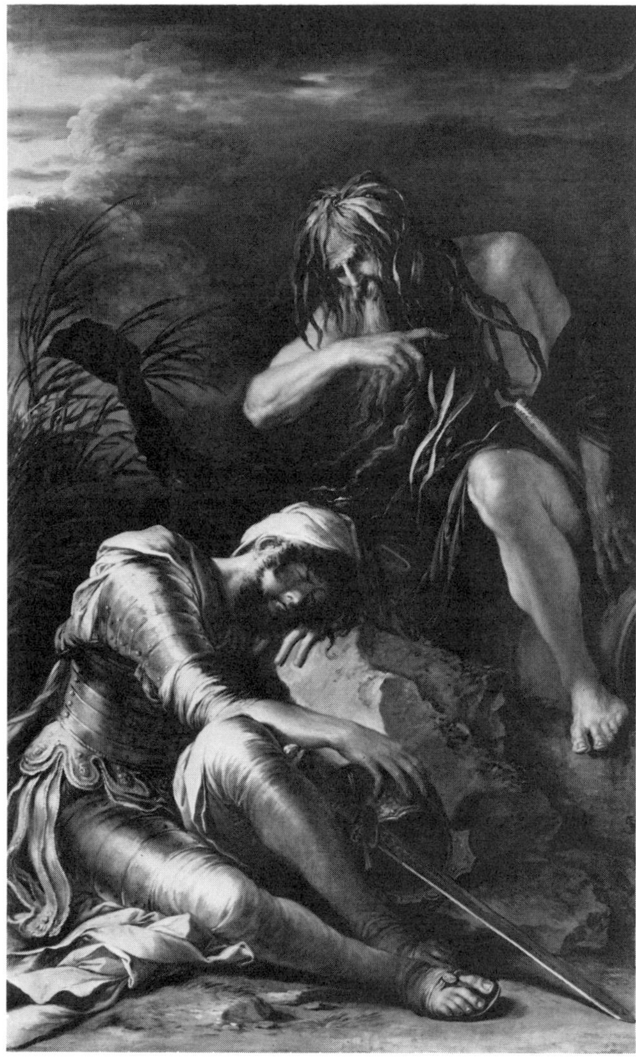

Fig. 1-3 *The Dream of Aeneas* by Salvator Rosa depicts a scene from *The Aeneid* by Virgil. While asleep on the bank of the river Tiber, Aeneas has a dream. Tiberinus, the god of the river, appears amid the mist and the poplars, a wreath of reeds upon his head, and predicts the end of Aeneas' trials and his conquest of Latium. (The Metropolitan Museum of Art, Rogers Fund, 1965. [65.118])

speaking directly to the recipient, given foreknowledge, as was seen by Aeneas when he slept on the banks of the Tiber[15] (Fig. 1-3). (Note however, Epicurus was one of Virgil's mentors.) The prophesy could also be in symbolic form within the dream, requiring interpretation. Prophesies could be forthright or misleading. The Talmud (Berachoth 55a) states that morning dreams have the most significance.[1] However, it is warned in Ecclesiastes:

> Divinations and omens and dreams are folly . . . unless they are sent from the most high as a visitation, do not give your mind to them. For dreams have deceived many . . .

In the bible, Joseph is involved with three sets of pairs of dreams (significant or true dreams often come in pairs. In book VII of Herodotus[8], Xerxes is moved to attack Hellas only after he has had his second prophetic dream); the first pair are Joseph's own; and the last two pairs he interprets for others. In Genesis 37:6–11, Joseph dreams he is binding sheaves in the field when his sheaf arises and his brothers' sheaves surround his, bowing down to it. In his second dream the sun, moon, and eleven stars bow down to him. The symbolism, that Joseph's parents and eleven brothers will one day bow down to him is evident to his brothers who ridicule him, not believing the dreams to be divinely inspired. In Genesis 40:5–19, Joseph interprets the dreams of Pharoah's imprisoned butler and baker and his predictions that in three days the butler will be freed and the baker executed come true. In the last set, in Genesis 41:1–7, Pharoah dreams of seven fat cattle arising from the Nile followed by seven lean cattle that swallow the first. He then dreams of a stalk of corn arising with seven full ears, followed by a second stalk with seven lean ears that swallow the first. The butler remembers Joseph, and Pharoah has him interpret his dreams. Joseph correctly predicts seven years of plenty followed by seven years of famine. Ultimately Joseph's family comes to Egypt and Joseph's dreams are fulfilled.

Dreaming may lead to insights unattainable by the conscious mind. In Genesis 28:12–16, Jacob dreamed of seeing a ladder to heaven with angels ascending on the spot where he slept. A vision of God appears in the dream and tells him it is a holy place. "And Jacob awakened out of his sleep, and he said: 'Surely the Lord is in this place and I knew it not'." Thus Jacob clearly sees in a dream that which is inapparent when awake.

There are other examples of facts revealing themselves in sleep rather than in the wake state. The nineteenth century chemist, August Kekule struggled for years over the structure of benzene. In 1865 Kekule dreamed:

> the atoms gamboled before my eyes . . . My mind's eyes . . . now distinguished larger formations of various shapes. Long rows, in many ways more densely joined; everything in movement, winding and turning like snakes. And look, what was that? One snake grabbed its own tail, and mockingly whirled before my eyes. As if struck by lightening I awoke; . . .

Kekule spent the rest of the night working out the details of a benzene ring composed of six carbon and six hydrogen atoms, opening up a new field within organic chemistry.[16]

Dreams have also served as stimuli for artistic accomplishment. Robert Louis Stevenson is reported to have derived story plots from his vivid and "sometimes horrifying dreams." Two such stories are "Olalla" and "The Strange Case of Dr. Jekyll and Mr. Hyde.[17] Similarly, a dream stimulated Giuseppe Tartini to write his "Il Trillo del Diavalo" ("Devils Trill Sonata"). He describes:[18]

> I dreamed that I had made a compact with the devil . . . I heard him play a solo so singularly beautiful . . . that it surpassed all the music I had ever heard . . . I lost my power of breathing, and the violence of the sensation awoke me . . . The work that this dream suggested and which I wrote at that time is doubtless the best of my compositions. I call it the Devil's Trill Sonata.

Tartini also describes that when he first awoke, try that he might, he could not remember the exact tune the devil played. The dream did however inspire him to compose his best work.

In the late nineteenth century, Sigmund Freud ushered in a new age of dream interpretation, one in which the message is accepted as coming from within rather than from an external source. While many dreams contain content that is complex in nature, and far beyond the intent or scope of this chapter, it is of interest to discuss at least one "typical dream" (A typical dream is one that is almost universal in nature and interpretation). One such dream[13] that most readers of this book are likely to have had is the "examination dream." Freud wrote that "everyone who has received his certificate of matriculation after passing his final examination at school complains of the persistence with which he is plagued by anxiety-dreams in which he has failed, or must go through his course again, etc." Freud notes that the higher the level of accomplishment, the higher the level of the examination the dream is about. But it is always an examination that has already been successfully passed. Freud states that the dream usually occurs when the dreamer is under pressure to complete another task. Freud interprets it as a subconscious message to the dreamer that he need not worry about the present endeavor. After all he knows he really did succeed despite his worry over the past. Freud states he tested this hypothesis by fruitlessly searching for a dreamer who actually had failed the examination.

Many sleepers experience the sensation of falling on the initiation of sleep, which probably is the origin of the common term, "falling asleep" (falling however is another "typical dream"). The longest fall into sleep ever written occurred in the dream story "Alice's Adventures in Wonderland," written by Lewis Carroll.[21] It starts with Alice entering a rabbit's hole and metaphorically falling asleep:

> Alice began to get rather sleepy . . . when suddenly thump! down she came upon a heap of sticks and dry leaves, and the fall was over.

Brevity dictates the exclusion of the five middle paragraphs describing what Alice does during the fall, which undoubtedly is the longest recorded fall to sleep. Freud believed that the fall in a dream is reminiscent of the childhood pleasure of being flung into the air and caught by an adult.[13] However he also states that it is a common dream among young girls and that in females it may have the connotation of "erotic temptation" or the "fallen woman." Thus, the Freudian symbolism of the deep, long hole and other symbolisms within the story produce an obviously erotic dream story written by Carroll for Alice (presumably unintentionally).

NATURE AND FUNCTION OF SLEEP

Sleep is a reconciling,—
 A rest that peace begets;
Doth not the sun rise smiling,
 When fair at even he sets?
Rest you then, rest, sad eyes,—

—John Dowland

The mechanism and function of sleep have always been points of speculation. The Greek physician Alcmaeon of Croton taught that sleep is caused by the retirement of blood into the larger vessels and that waking occurred on its reversal.[20] Aristotle[2] defined the awake condition as one in which the individual is capable of exercising his sense-perception and defined sleep as the opposite of this. He thought sleep to occur when hot vapors rise up in the body and ascend to the head requiring the separation of the pure and impure blood (this occurring in the heart). By far, the simplest explanation of the nature of sleep was expressed by Virgil[21] in the following passage from *The Aeneid* which was also the inspiration for Pierre Chuvis deChavanne to paint *The Sleep* (Fig. 1-4):

> It was just the time when first slumber comes to heal human suffering, stealing on men by heaven's blessing with balmiest influence.

Sleep is a gift of the Gods, its function restorative.

Wilse Webb[22] has grouped the theories on the function(s) of sleep into five categories (Table 1-1). The oldest and most widely held is the *restorative theory*, i.e., that sleep is a time in which the body and/or the mind restores itself (repairs damage and/or removes toxins that have built up during the day). Aristotle[20] thought that the soul was composed of "light atoms" located in the head and circulating through the body, giving it life, but always trying to leave the body. The air contained more "soul atoms" and those lost could be replaced by breathing. Death occurred when pressure outside the body was too great, breathing ceased, and the soul atoms left without replacement. Aristotle

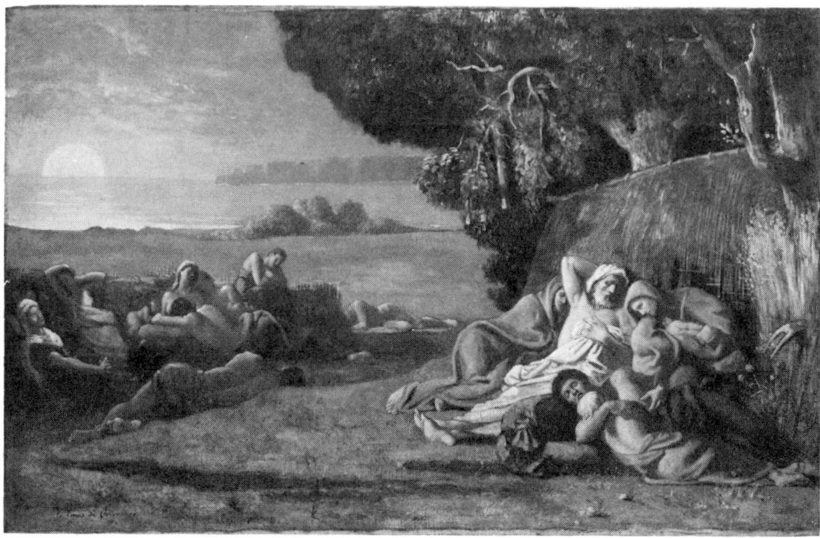

Fig. 1-4 *Sleep* by Pierre Puvis de Chavannes was inspired by *The Aenid* of Virgil Book II, Lines 268–269. (The Metropolitan Museum of Art.) The Theodore M. Davis Collection. Bequest of Theodore M. Davis, 1915. [30.95.253])

thought that sleep was similar to death, but a milder form. Thus, the wear and tear of the day led to a net loss of "soul atoms" and the body slept. Belief in the restorative theory can also be seen in Macbeth:[6]

> Sleep that knits up the ravelled sleeve of care, The death of each day's life, sore labour's bath, Balm of hurt minds, great nature's second course, Chief nourisher in life's feast.

Obviously the harder one works, the greater will be the body's need for restoration and the deeper the sleep. "The sleep of the labouring man is sweet, whether he eat little or much; but the fullness of the rich will not suffer him to sleep" (Ecclesiastes 5:12).

While the restorative theory remains the most widely accepted theory

Table 1-1. Theories on the Function of Sleep.

Restoration theory	A time during which the organism can repair damage and/or remove toxins
Energy conservation theory	Limits the organism's energy requirement
Protective theory	Prevent wear and tear on organism
Ethologic theory	A behavioral adaptation of the organism that is protective in adverse environments
Instinct theory	Inate to the organism

(Webb, WB: Theories of sleep function and some clinical implications In Drucker-Colin R, Shkurovich M, Sterman MB (eds): The Functions of Sleep. Academic Press, New York, 1979.)

today, some objections have been raised. Meddis[23] questions the interindividual variability in humans and interspecies variability in sleep requirements. If sleep restoration is a necessity, why is it that more is necessary for some than for others? If some animal species have evolved that need little or no sleep, why haven't others?

The *energy conservation* theory of the function of sleep postulates that the decreased energy requirements for an organism during sleep conserves energy. Thus by limiting energy expenditure at times of inactivity the animal becomes more energy efficient.[24,25] However, the strategy used in balancing energy requirements and substrate may vary. Comparing two metabolically similar animals it is found that the shrew spends almost no time sleeping and is constantly eating; alternatively the bat is one of the more prodigious sleepers.[23]

The *protective theory* is a modification of the restorative theory, speculating that sleep is instituted by the organism to prevent damage before it would occur. Thus, in the protective theory, sleep prevents that which is repaired in the restorative theory.

The *ethological theory* is especially intriguing, differing radically from the classical conceptions of the function of sleep. To some extent, all of the previously discussed theories have dealt with the organisms somatic well being on a physiologic basis. This theory deals with sleep as an evolutionary behavioral adaptation.[22,23,25] It proposes that there are times when an animal may be so disadvantaged compared to its predators that its best defense is immobility. Since the animal may not be smart enough to understand this (their instinctive urges could cause it to flee from a swifter predator) sleep enforces immobility. One argument in favor of this idea is the instinctive urge of many animals to do their sleeping in a known protective environment such as a nest. Thus it is not surprising that many humans complain of an inability to sleep in a strange environment, such as a hotel, or even outside their own bed (instinctively, insecurity leads to inability to sleep).

In one evolutionary scenario,[25] early mammals developed daytime sleep in an era when reptiles dominated the land. Foraging for food was less dangerous for these "small and insignificant creatures" at night when the cold blooded reptiles slowed down. They could then "scurry back" to the protection of their dens, to remain immobilized by sleep in the day. Eventually carnivorous mammals evolved, adapted to prey on the other mammals and the smaller, less protected reptiles that slowed at night. When reptiles lost their dominance, it then became more advantageous for most mammals to sleep nights and forage days.

Allison and Cicchetti[26] also believe sleep to be a behavioral adaptation that helps a species survive in its environment. They divide species two ways, by the security of their sleep environment and by whether they are predators or prey. They point out that animals with secure sleep environments, such as bats, sleep better than grazing animals, such as sheep or antelopes. This is certainly consistent with the above theory. (One mammal, Dall's porpoise, is reputed not to sleep at all; there is no place to hide in the ocean!) They also point out that predators, such as cats are good sleepers while animals heavily preyed upon, such as rabbits, are poor sleepers. Although this is consistent with a behavioral theory of sleep, it is potentially inconsistent with the ethologic theory as predators should not have to sleep. The only explanation that could consolidate these observations into one theory is that sleep, in the predators, is a hereditary holdover from a time when they were not predators. Because predators are not at risk while asleep, this trait has persisted.

The last theory, the *hereditary theory*, claims that sleep is inate to those animals that do it. This, however, neither explains why the organism evolved to require sleep, nor is it exclusive of any of the above theories. It is actually a requirement for the energy conservation, protective, and ethologic theories.

SLEEP IN HEALTH AND DISEASE

We watched her breathing through the night,
Her breathing soft and low,
As in her breast the wave of life
Kept heaving to and fro
. . . . .
Our very hopes belied our fears,
Our fears our hopes belied,—
We thought her dying when she slept,
And sleeping when she died.
. . . . .
—Thomas Hood

The corrollaries to the restorative theory of sleep function is its necessity for health, its importance to the healing of the sick and the detrimental effect when it is withheld. The importance of a good and regular sleep pattern to health was stated by Benjamin Franklin, "Early to bed, and early to rise, makes a man healthy, wealthy, and wise." and by Hippocrates[27] "Both sleep and insomnolency, when immoderate are bad." Sleep is important in the healing of the ill: "if he sleeps he will get well" (John 11:12) and "Sleep and dreaming are good signs in the sick" (Berachoth 57b).[1] However, the quality of the sleep is important. According to Hippocrates[27]:

> In whatever disease sleep is laborious, it is a deadly symptom: but if sleep does good, it is not deadly.

Along with sleep comes temporary relief of pain. "He that sleeps feels not the toothache."—Cymbelline.[6] For this reason, sleep (anesthesia) is induced prior to surgery. The first such induction was in Genesis 2:21, when Adam was put to sleep to have his rib removed.

In recent years, respiratory physiologists and clinicians have taken delight in finding examples of disorders described in the older nonmedical literature.

Sleep disorders can roughly be divided into two groups:

1. Disorders associated with too little sleep.
2. Disorders associated with too much sleep (hypersomnolence).

The most common sleep complaint among patients by far is insomnia.

> Even thus last night, and two nights more I lay,
> And could not win thee, sleep! by any stealth:
> So do not let me wear the night away:
> Without thee what is all the morning's wealth!
> Come blessed barrier between day and day,
> Dear mother of fresh thoughts and joyous health.
>
> —William Wordsworth

However, a large percent of those who complain of insomnia actually have sleep latencies and total sleep times similar to controls. Joseph Heller[28] probably sensed this when he described Captain Flume in *Catch 22*. Chief White Halfoat had threatened to one night slit the captain's throat from "ear to ear," which kept the captain awake night after night.

> Actually, Captain Flume slept like a log most nights and merely *dreamed* he was awake. So convincing were these dreams of lying awake that he awoke from them each morning in complete exhaustion and fell right back to sleep.[28]

Physical illness may interfere with sleep. When sleep loss is protracted, it may lead to the consequences of sleep deprivation, which may contribute to the patients' further deterioration. Syndromes following cardiac surgery, "post-cardiac surgery delirium,"[29] and in the coronary care unit, "CCU delirium"[30] have been described that abate when the patients finally get an adequate amount of sleep. This is however, probably little different from Hippocrates' description:[27] ". . . when sleep puts an end to delirium, it is a good symptom." Thus, conditions associated with protracted physical and mental pain, and consequent sleep deprivation are not new to the twentieth century, but rather have plagued man since ancient history.

Respiratory-sleep syndromes have mostly been characterized by too much sleep (hypersomnolence is a better term as these patients often suffer from sleep deprivation caused by poor quality sleep). Burwell et al.[31] was probably the first to report a typical description of such a medical condition in the nonmedical literature, coining the term "Pickwickian syndrome" for those individuals with obesity, hypersomnolence, and hypoventilation. Today, we note that most such patients actually have sleep apnea.[32]

The term "Ondine's curse" is often applied to those individuals with idiopathic hypoventilation. It should, however, probably be used to describe hypoventilation secondary to some CNS insult, as the three patients originally described by Severinghaus and Mitchell[33] developed the syndrome following CNS surgery. Additionally, the hypoventilation is not idiopathic in Ritter Hans, the character afflicted with it in the Giraudoux play, but rather a punishment imposed upon the character by the King of the Sea in retribution for his unfaithfulness to the water nymph Ondine. Hans describes his own fate:[19]

> all the things my body once did by itself, it now does by special order . . . I have to supervise five senses, . . . A single moment of inattention, and I forget to breathe. He died, they will say, because it was a nuisance to breathe . . .

Considering his fixation on breathing, one might suspect that Hans actually had hyperventilation syndrome. Since it proved rapidly fatal, we should, however, accept this as true hypoventilation.

As clinicians become more familiar with sleep apnea syndrome, they are apt to diagnose the less severe cases. Similarly, every literary figure that snores, such as Falstaff in *Henry IV, Part I*[34] may now become suspect. However, the person in literature, who by description is most likely to have had sleep apnea syndrome came from much humbler origins (an eight line rhyme) and is the youngest afflicted so far identified. He was a cyanotic lad (''Little Boy Blue'') who developed a justified reputation for sleeping on the job (''He's under the haystack, fast asleep.'') and irrational mood swings (''if you wake him, he's sure to cry''). Of course, it may be argued that shepherds have always been described as sleeping on the job (see Endymion, Fig. 1-1). Perhaps hypersomnolence is an occupational hazard of sheep herders. However, since it is well know that the folk remedy for insomnia, counting sheep, only works for shepherds, it is more likely that hypersomnolent people are drawn to that occupation. Another syndrome to be aware of is pseudo-sleep apnea. On occasion a patient is referred for study who complains of regular episodes of wakening with the sensation of suffocation. At such times they remember dreaming of situations where they cannot breathe or must hold their breath (such as being trapped under water). Although this has not been studied, anecdotally, such patients rarely have sleep apnea syndrome and an alternative diagnosis can usually be found. Joseph Heller described such a case in *Catch-22*.[28] Hungry Joe was described as regularly having nightmares and screaming all night, keeping everyone else awake:

> Late that night Hungry Joe dreamed that Huple's cat was sleeping on his face, suffocating him, and when he woke up, Huple's cat *was* sleeping on his face. His agony was terrifying.

Sleep apnea in infants (near miss episodes of) sudden infant death syndrome (SIDS) was first described by Aristotle who also first warned that alcohol could induce or worsen it:[2]

> The beginning of this malady takes place with many during sleep, and their subsequent habitual seizures occur in sleep, not in waking hours. For when the spirit [evaporation] moves upwards in a volume, on its return downward it distends the veins, and forcibly compresses the passage through which respiration is effected. This explains why wines are not good for infants or for wet nurses (for it makes no difference doubtless, whether the infants themselves, or their nurses, drink them), . . .

Lastly, the first, and one of the most classic presentations of SIDS is described in *I Kings* 3:19–20:

> And this woman's child died in the night, because she overlaid it. And she arose at midnight, and took my son from beside me, while thine handmaid slept, and laid it on her bosom, and laid her dead child in my bosom.

Here is described a city dweller (risk factor), whose mother, a harlot, is of lower socioeconomic class (risk factor) whose previously healthy son (slight male predominance), dies suddenly in his sleep. The cause of death, respiratory, is attributed to the mother's negligence in allowing him to suffocate in the bedding (the first theory on the cause of SIDS). The mother is driven by her anxiety to sociopathic behavior (switching babies) and is ostracized by society, recorded in history forever as an unfit mother.

CONCLUSION

While the importance of sleep has long been recognized (in the twelfth century Moshe Ben Maimon (Maimonides), the court physician to Saladin, listed sleep as one of the six obligations for health[35]), artists, historians, philosophers, poets, and common men have struggled to understand its mysteries. Today, we are not only concerned with sleep as a state by itself, but also how many "well understood" vital body functions are altered during this state in which we spend one third of our lives. These mysteries have become questions to be resolved by physiologists and biochemists rather than by philosophers.

References

1. Preuss J: Biblical and Talmudic Medicine. (Translator and ed Rosner F.) Sanhedrin Press, New York, 1978
2. Aristotle: On sleep and sleeplessness (De somna et viglia). p. 696. In Hutchins RM (ed): Great Books of the Western World. Aristotle I. (Trans Beare JI) William Benton, Chicago, 1952
3. Gayley CM: The Classic Myths. Blaisdell, New York, 1967

4. Grant M, Hazel J: Gods and Mortals in Classical Mythology. G and C Merriam , Springfield, Massachusetts, 1973
5. Homer The Iliad: (Trans Rees E) The Modern Library, New York, 1963
6. Wright WA (ed): The Complete Works of William Shakespeare. Garden City Books, Garden City, New York, 1936
7. Chan W: A Source Book in Chinese Philosophy. Princeton University Press, Princeton, New Jersey, 1973
8. Herodotus: Books I–IX. (Trans Godley AD) Harvard University Press, Cambridge, Massachusetts, 1966
9. Siegel RE: Galen on Psychology, Psychopathology, and Function and Diseases of the Nervous System. S Karger AG, Basel, 1973
10. Aristotle: On dreams (De somniis). p. 702. In Hutchins RM (ed): Great Books of the Western World Aristotle I. (Trans Beare JI) William Benton, Chicago, 1952
11. Aristotle: On prophesying by dreams (De divinatione per Somnum). p. 707. In Hutchins RM (ed): Great Books of the Western World Aristotle I. (Trans Beare JI) William Benton, Chicago, 1952
12. Long AA: Hellinistic Philosophy. Charles Scribner and Sons, New York, 1974
13. Freud S: The Interpretation of Dreams. (Trans Brill AA) Random House, New York, 1950
14. Aeschylus: Prometheus bound. In: Aeschylus II. (Tran Grene D) University of Chicago Press, Chicago, 1952
15. Virgil: The aeneid. In: The Poems of Virgil. William Benton, Chicago, 1952
16. Anschütz R: August Kekulé. In Farber E (ed): Great Chemists. Interscience, New York, 1961
17. Hennessy JP: Robert Louis Stevenson. Simon and Schuster, New York, 1974
18. Ewen D: The Complete Book of Classical Music. Prentice Hall, Englewood Cliffs, New Jersey. 1965
19. Giraudoux J; Ondine A Romantic Fantasy in Three Acts. (Trans Valency M) Samuel French, New York, 1956
20. Phillips ED: Aspects of Greek Medicine. St. Martins Press, New York, 1973
21. Carroll L: The Complete Illustrated Works of Lewis Carroll. Guilliano E (ed), Avenel Books, New York, 1982
22. Webb WB: Theories of sleep function and some clinical implications. In Drucker-Colin R, Shkurovich M. Sterman, MB (eds): The Functions of Sleep. Academic Press, New York, 1979
23. Meddis R: On the function of sleep. Animal Behavior 23:676, 1975
24. Walker JM, Berg RJ: Sleep as an adaptation for energy conservation functionally related to hibernation and shallow torpor. Prog Brain Res 53:255, 1980
25. Snyder F: Toward an evolutionary theory of dreaming. Am J Psychiatry 123:121, 1966
26. Allison T, Cicchetti T: Sleep in mammals: Ecological and constitutional correlates. Science 194:732, 1976
27. Adams FA: Hippocratic Writing. William Benton, Chicago, 1952
28. Heller J: Catch-22, Simon and Schuster, New York, 1955
29. Kornfeld DS, Zimberg S, Malm JR: Psychiatric complications of open-heart surgery. N Engl J Med 273:287, 1965
30. Parker DL, Hodge JR: Delirium in the coronary care unit. JAMA 201:702, 1967
31. Burwell CS, Robin ED, Whaley RD, Bickelmann AG: Extreme obesity associated with alveolar hypoventilation—a Pickwickian syndrome. Am J Med 21:811, 1956

32. Gastaut H, Tassinari CA, Duron B: Polygraphic study of the episodic diurnal and nocturnal (hypnic and respiratory) manifestations of the Pickwick syndrome. Brain Res 2:167, 1966
33. Severinghaus JW and Mitchell RA: Ondine's curse: Failure of the respiratory center automaticity while awake. Clin Res 10:122, 1962
34. Adler JJ: Did Falstaff have the sleep-apnea syndrome? N Engl J Med 308:404, 1983
35. Moshe Ben Maimon: Treatise on Asthma. Muntner S (ed), JB Lippincott, Philadelphia, 1963

2 Respiratory Neuronal Activity in Sleep

John M. Orem

In its discussion of respiratory activity in sleep, this chapter shows, first, that brainstem respiratory activity declines in non-rapid eye movement (NREM) sleep, an effect producing the major characteristics of breathing in that state and, second, that tonic and phasic rapid eye movement (REM) sleep mechanisms influence the respiratory system.

RESPIRATORY ACTIVITY IN NREM SLEEP

Characteristics of Breathing in NREM Sleep

The parameters of breathing in NREM sleep are generally slower or weaker versions of the parameters in wakefulness. For example:

1. The frequency of breathing is slower and more regular in NREM sleep than in wakefulness or REM sleep.[1–4]
2. Peak instantaneous airflow rate[2] and the pressure developed against an occluded airway[5] decrease from wakefulness to NREM sleep.
3. Upper airway resistance increases in sleep. In NREM sleep, the resistance during expiration is greater than in wakefulness, but the resistance during inspiration decreases almost to that in wakefulness. The increase in upper airway resistance is caused by a decrease in upper airway muscle tone.[6–12]
4. Tidal volume increases in NREM sleep as the result of an increased duration of inspiration, but minute ventilation decreases.[2]

5. In NREM sleep, the threshold and/or gain of the response to CO_2 decreases.[1,13–22]

6. The response to hypoxia appears to be diminished in NREM sleep.[13,14,23–25]

7. Ventilatory and muscle responses to airway occlusion are less in NREM sleep than in wakefulness.[26–28]

The number of structures that may participate in the control of breathing in sleep and wakefulness is large. Cortical,[29,30] subcortical telencephalic,[31,32] hypothalamic, and midbrain[10,29,33–35] areas, in addition to the well-known pontine and medullary respiratory areas, participate in the control of breathing. It is likely that each of these areas contributes in some way to the breathing patterns in wakefulness and sleep.

The Activity of Respiratory Neurons in NREM Sleep

In 1974, two groups of investigators reported that medullary respiratory activity decreased in NREM sleep. Studying spinal cats, Puizillout and Ternaux[36] observed a decrease in integrated medullary multiunit respiratory activity during spontaneous sleep and elimination of this activity during the sleeplike behavior induced by vagoaortic stimulation. They noted also an accompanying depression in phrenic nerve activity. The multiunit activity was recorded from the region of the ambiguus nucleus, around the solitary tract, along the medullary midline, and in the hypoglossal nucleus.

Though seldom cited, this finding of a loss of respiratory activity in the hypoglossal nucleus is obviously pertinent to the pathophysiology of sleep apnea.

In the same year as the report by Puizillout and Ternaux,[36] Orem et al.[37] published their study describing single brainstem neurons with activity related to respiration in wakefulness but not in sleep, neurons that they named sleep-sensitive (Fig. 2-1). They studied 28 respiratory neurons in the medulla just caudal to the facial nucleus and found that 79 percent (n = 22) changed their relationship to respiration in sleep. Five of those sensitive to sleep did not lose their respiratory rhythmicity, but only reduced their intraburst discharge frequency. This work was done at Stanford University, where they early recognized sleep apnea as a significant clinical problem, and the authors concluded that the results "show a normal potential for respiratory failure in sleep and suggest the possibility that apneic disorders may be a clinical expression of this potential."

Much is known about the locations and types of respiratory neurons in anesthetized and decerebrate animals but not in unanesthetized, intact animals. There have been studies designed to map the extent of brainstem respiratory activity in unanesthetized animals,[38–41] but the results from these studies were based on statistical procedures the validity of which has been subsequently questioned.[42,43] In a recent study, Orem, Osorio, Brooks and Dick[43a] detected

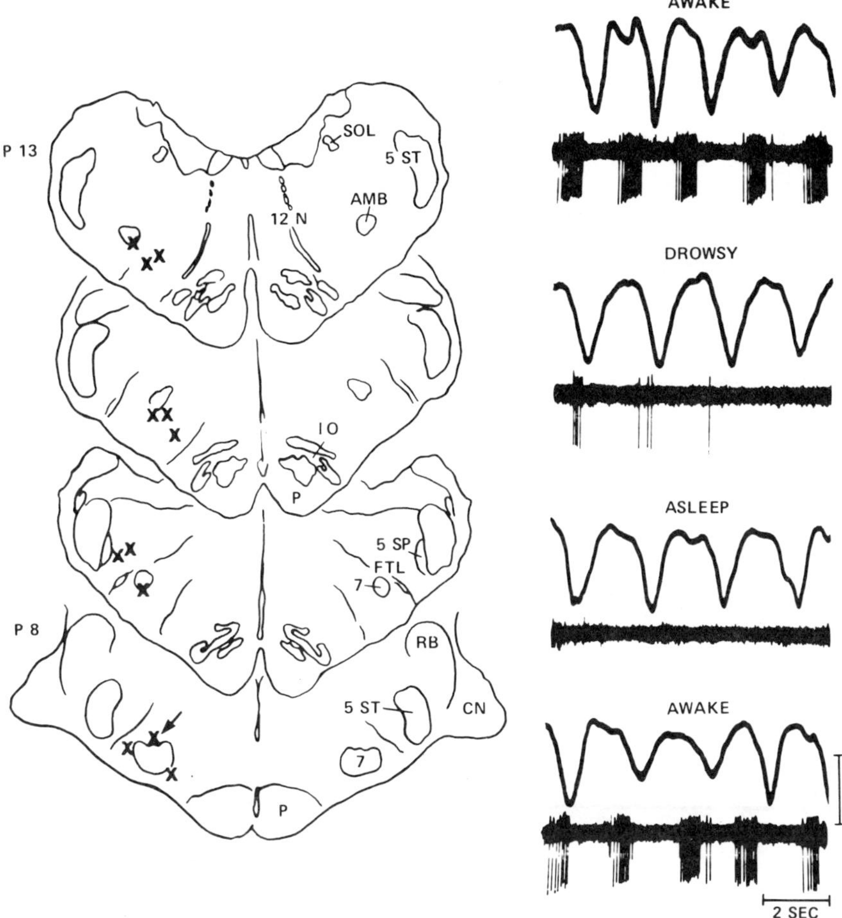

Fig. 2-1 Locations of 12 sleep-sensitive respiratory neurons. Arrow marks the location of the cell whose activity is illustrated on the right. AMB, n. ambiguus; CN, cochlear nucleus; FTL, lateral tegmental field; IO, inferior olive; P, pyramidal tract; RB, restiform body; SOL, solitary tract; 5SP, nucleus of the spinal tract of V; 5ST, spinal tract of V; 7, facial nucleus; 12N, hypoglossal nerve. (Reprinted by permission of the publisher from Changes in the activity of respiratory neurons during sleep by Orem J, Montplaisir J, Dement W: Brain Res 82:309, 1974, by Elsevier Science Publishing Company Inc.)

(using the analysis of variance to discriminate respiratory cells[42]) respiratory activity in the unanesthetized cat in a zone ventral to and within the region of neurons that form the retrofacial and ambiguus nuclei. These authors classified the cells as inspiratory or noninspiratory on the basis of cycle-triggered histograms and as strong or weak on the basis of the η^2 value of their activity (Figs. 2-2, 2-3, and 2-4; Ref. 44). The dichotomous classification of activity as

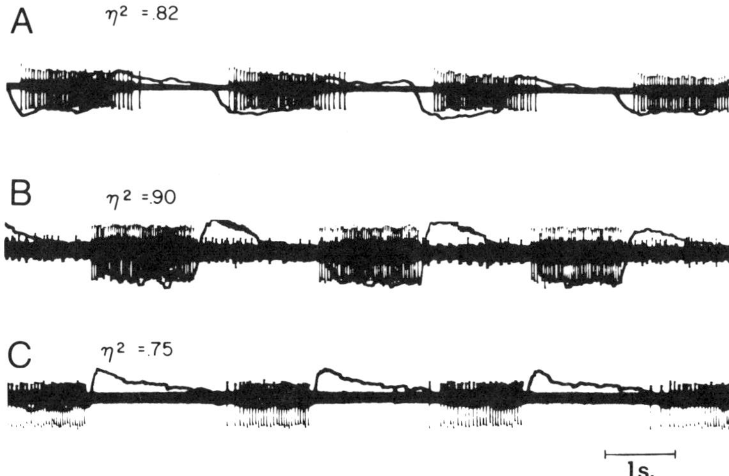

Fig. 2-2 Three Cells (A, B, and C) with high η^2 values. η^2 values in this and the following figures refer to the proportion of the total variability of the activity of the cell that can be attributed to respiratory modulation. Downward deflections of airflow tracings in this figure and in Figs. 2-3 and 2-4 indicate inspiration. (Orem J, Dick T: Consistency and signal strength of the respiratory neuronal activity. J Neurophysiol 50:1098, 1983.)

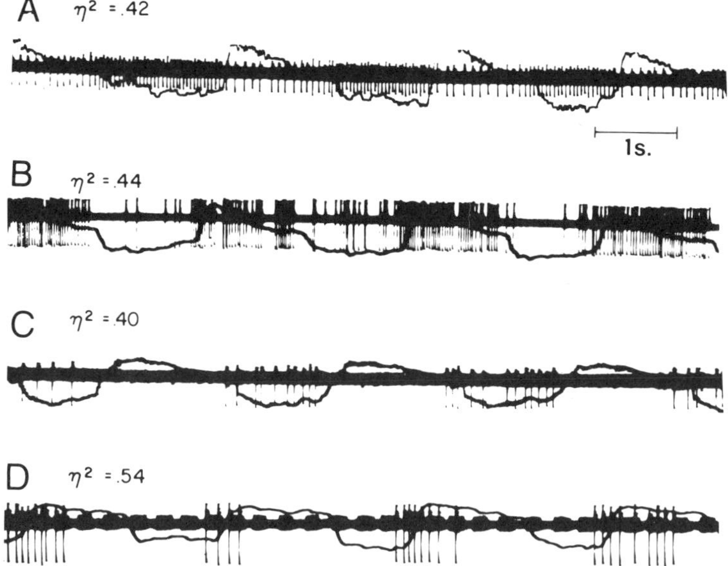

Fig. 2-3 Four Cells (A, B, C, and D) with medium η^2 values. These cells, and those in Fig. 2-2, are members of the group of strong cells. (Orem J, Dick T: Consistency and signal strength of respiratory neuronal activity. J Neurophysiol 50:1098, 1983.)

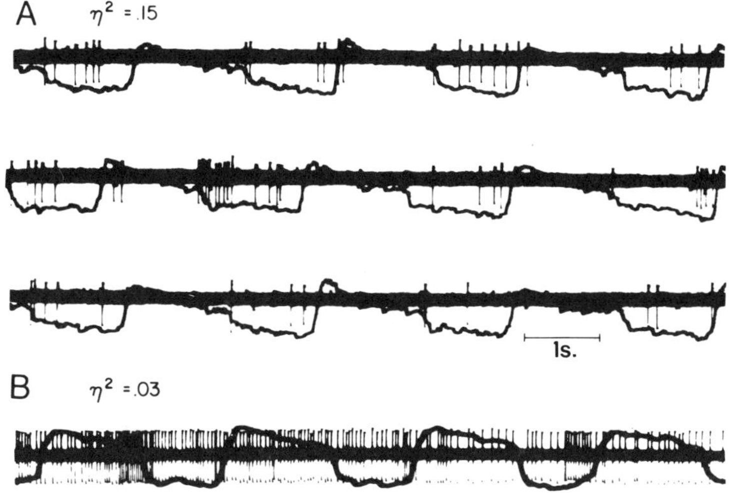

Fig. 2-4 Two Cells (A and B) with low η^2 values (weak cells). (Orem J, Dick T: Consistency and signal strength of respiratory neuronal activity. J Neurophysiol 50:1098, 1983.)

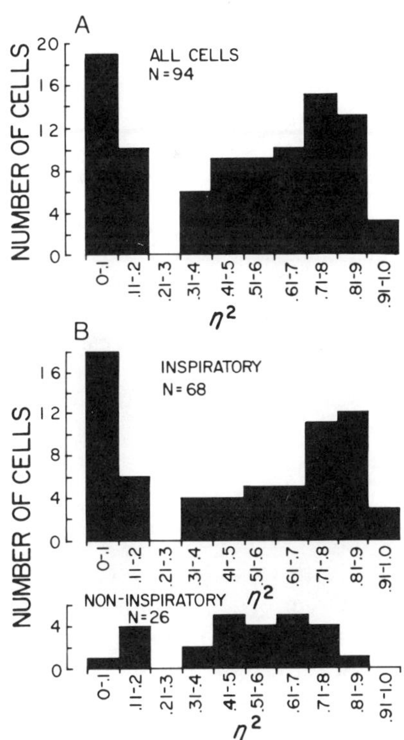

Fig. 2-5 Frequency histograms of cell types. (A) The frequency distribution of all cells, inspiratory and noninspiratory, along the dimension of consistency and signal strength of their respiratory activity. There are two populations: one having high η^2 values (0.31 to >0.90) and the other having low η^2 values (<.021). The cells in the former groups are strong respiratory cells; those in the latter group are weak respiratory cells. (B) The upper histogram shows the distribution of inspiratory cells along the dimension of consistency and signal strength of their respiratory signals. The lower histogram shows the distribution of noninspiratory cells. Both inspiratory and noninspiratory cells show two distinct populations, but the strong inspiratory cells tend to have greater η^2 values than the strong noninspiratory cells. (Orem J, Osorio I, Brooks E, Dick T: Activity of respiratory neurons during NREM sleep. J Neurophysiol 54:1144, 1985.)

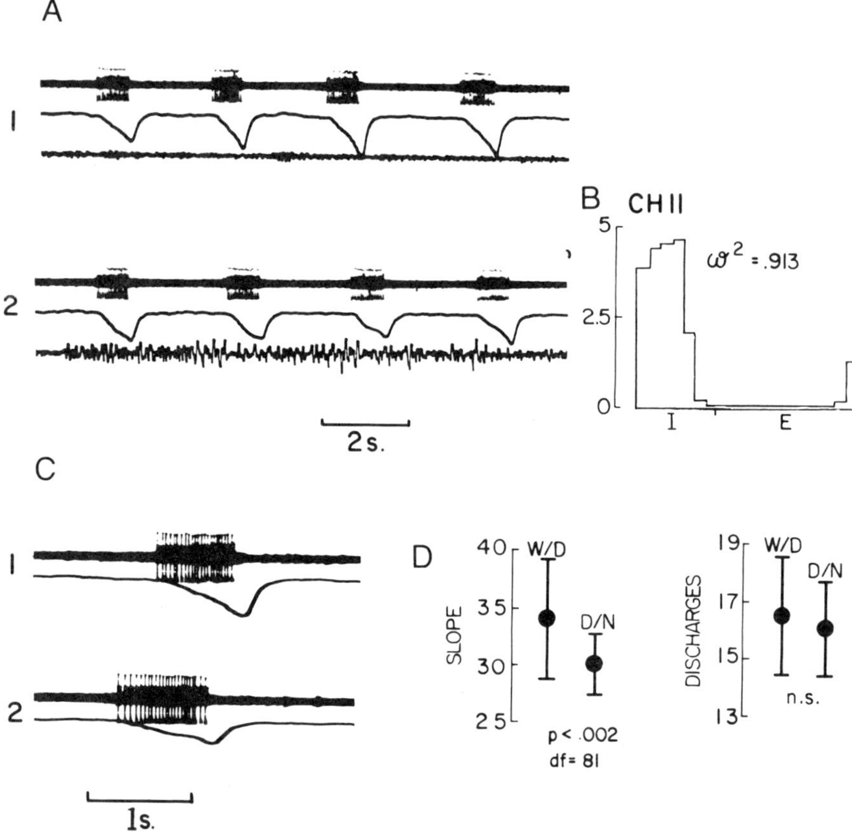

Fig. 2-6 A strong inspiratory cell in wakefulness (A part 1) and NREM sleep (A part 2). (B) The cycle-triggered histogram of the cell shows that it was inspiratory. The η^2 value (indicated as ω^2 in this figure) was 0.913. (C) A breath in wakefulness (part 1) and a breath in NREM sleep (part 2). There seems a slight reduction in discharge rate in NREM sleep—a suggestion confirmed statistically by an analysis of the slope of the cumulative number of discharges. The results of this analysis are shown in D. The average slope in wakefulness/drowsiness (W/D) was significantly greater than that in drowsiness/NREM sleep (D/N). The number of discharges per breath did not differ in the two states (right part of D).

strong or weak was based on the finding that the distribution of the number of cells with various η^2 values was distinctly bimodal (Fig. 2-5).

Orem et al.[43a] found that most ventral medullary respiratory cells were less active in NREM sleep than in wakefulness (Figs. 2-6 and 2-7). These results confirm those of Puizillout and Ternaux[36] and Orem et al.[37] and demonstrate a decrease in excitation in the respiratory centers in sleep. This decreased excitation, hypothesized long ago[45] is possibly the outstanding respiratory fea-

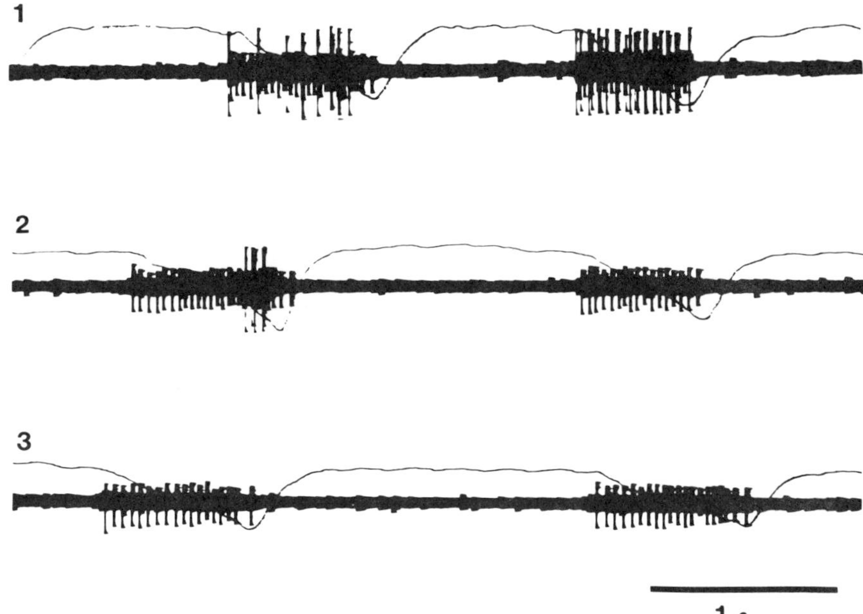

Fig. 2-7 The activity of a weak (large action potentials) and a strong (small action potentials) inspiratory cell during wakefulness (1), drowsiness (2), and NREM sleep (3). The activity of the weak cell varied from breath to breath in wakefulness and drowsiness and was absent in sleep. The activity of the strong cell, although persistent, was reduced quantitatively in sleep. A downward deflection of the instantaneous airflow-rate tracing signals inspiration. (Orem J, Osorio I, Brooks E, Dick T: Activity of respiratory neurons during NREM sleep. J Neurophysiol 54:1144, 1985.)

ture in NREM sleep and accounts for the reduction of many characteristics of breathing in that state.

In the study by Orem et al.[43a] the majority of cells, inspiratory and noninspiratory, strong and weak, were less active in NREM sleep than in wakefulness, but the effect of sleep, expressed as the percentage change in rate, was greater for weak than for strong cells; and, within the class of strong cells, greater for those with lower η^2 values than for those with higher η^2 values (Fig. 2-8). These results are predictable if (1) the η^2 value of activity is related inversely to the amount of nonrespiratory afference causing that activity and (2) the effect of sleep is to reduce primarily the nonrespiratory afference to respiratory neurons.

For most of the strong inspiratory cells recorded by Orem et al.[43a] the reduced firing rate in sleep was a manifestation of a general inverse relationship between their rate and the duration of inspiration. A similar relationship between the frequency of discharge of medullary respiratory neurons and the duration of inspiration has been demonstrated in experiments in which breath-

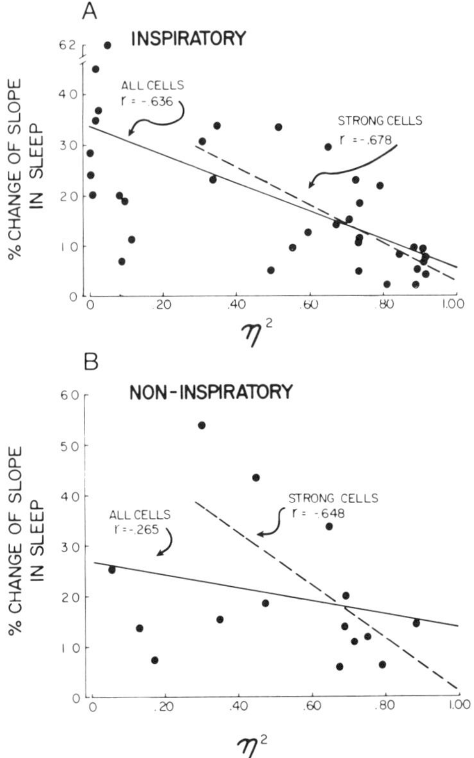

Fig. 2-8 The percent change in slope of the activity of respiratory cells in sleep compared to wakefulness as a function of the η^2 value of the activity. This figure shows the percent change in slope for inspiratory (A) and noninspiratory (B) cells whose activities were less, significantly or not significantly, in sleep. The negative relationship between the percent change in slope and the η^2 value of the activity, depicted here, was strongest within the classes of strong cells. (Orem J, Osorio I, Brooks E, Dick T: Activity of respiratory neurons during NREM sleep. J Neurophysiol 54:1144, 1985.)

ing rates were manipulated by heating the hypothalamus of urethane-anesthetized cats.[46] In the study of Orem et al.,[43a] this relationship was peculiar to strong inspiratory cells: the level of activity of weak inspiratory cells was not related from breath to breath to the duration of inspiration.

Recordings have been made in the pontine pneumotaxic center during sleep and wakefulness. Lydic and Orem[47] recorded single respiratory neurons in the pons of the unanesthetized cat, and 75 percent of these cells were less active in NREM sleep but more active in REM sleep than in wakefulness. Sieck and Harper[48] reported complex state changes in the activity of the pneumotaxic center. These changes included variations in the relationship between the respiratory cycle and the activity of the cells. The authors noted that "respiratory correlations during QS (NREM sleep), in particular, appeared to be absent or attenuated compared with those seen in AW (wakefulness) and REM sleep states" (Ref. 48, p. 89). In addition, this study showed that, in general, activity of nucleus parabrachialis medialis neurons decreased from wakefulness to NREM sleep but increased from NREM sleep to REM sleep, a result they considered consistent with the possible phase-switching role of this region.

These results show that brainstem respiratory neurons with activity phasic with breathing are fewer in number and are less active in NREM sleep than in wakefulness. The generality of this finding mitigates the lack of information on the afferent and efferent relationship of the cells that have been studied. It is unlikely that decreased central respiratory activity in sleep results from a reduced chemical stimulus secondary to a lowered metabolic rate, because (1) there is a relative hypercapnia (greater chemical stimulus) in NREM sleep and (2) breath-to-breath variations in discharge rate as a function of the duration of the breath (itself a function of the state) indicate that the variations in discharge rate occur rapidly with changes in the state of consciousness.

The cause of the changes in NREM sleep is not known. Breathing slows in NREM sleep even after isolation of the respiratory centers from vagal and other proprioceptive activity.[3,4,49,50] Vagal blockade combined with hyperoxia and metabolic alkalosis depresses the rate of breathing during NREM sleep.[51] Evidently, the slowed breathing in NREM sleep is determined centrally and accentuated by removal of afferent respiratory stimuli.

The Wakefulness Stimulus for Breathing

Many workers have proposed that the absence of a wakefulness stimulus[52] explains (1) the reduced respiratory rate and diminished peak airflow rates during NREM sleep,[2] (2) the increased upper airway resistance of NREM sleep,[9,53] (3) upper airway occlusion in the sleep apnea syndrome[54] (4) the discontinuous augmentation pattern of laryngeal muscle activity in response to occlusions during sleep and wakefulness[27] (Fig. 2-9), and (5) the shift to the right and decrease in slope of the ventilatory response to CO_2 during NREM sleep.[55] One might add to this list the reduction of the population of active respiratory neurons and the decreased activity of those remaining active.

Some characteristics of the wakefulness stimulus are known. It does not act exclusively through the metabolic control system. Although the ventilatory response to hypercapnia increases during wakefulness, breathing is stimulated in wakefulness even when chemical stimuli are removed[51,52] or not adequately detected, as in the central hypoventilation syndrome.

The wakefulness stimulus seems to vary with the level of arousal: humans breathe more when doing mental arithmetic than when they are not[56] and more when awake than when asleep. If the respiratory stimulus is an arousal stimulus rather than a wakefulness stimulus, it might also vary with the depth of NREM sleep.

The neural substrate of the wakefulness stimulus may be in the region between the caudal pons and posterior hypothalamus, an area necessary for waking consciousness. Whereas stimulation of parts of this area causes arousal,[57] bilateral lesions produce coma.[29,58] Studies of single neurons[59–61] show that, usually, midbrain reticular neurons have higher discharge rates during wakefulness than during NREM sleep. Moruzzi[62] proposes that this region is essential for waking consciousness and must be inactivated by basal forebrain or medullary sleep centers before sleep can occur.

Trains of high-frequency pulses (30 Hz for 5 to 30 s) applied to the midbrain

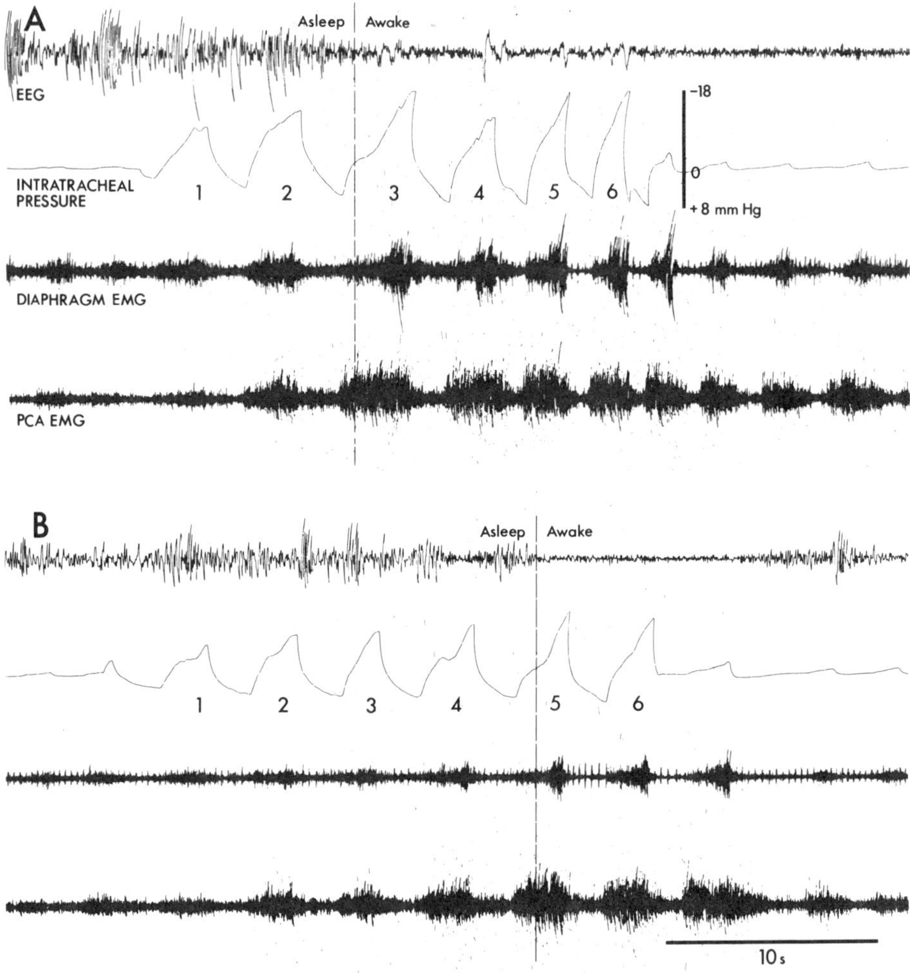

Fig. 2-9 Two polygraphic records showing arousal, laryngeal and diaphragmatic responses to occlusion during NREM sleep. In A, the animal awoke after the second occluded breath, and there was then a large increase in laryngeal activity. Diaphragmatic activity also increased but not as dramatically. In B, the animal awoke on the fifth occluded breath. EEG, electrocorticogram from percruciate cortex; PCA, posterior cricoarytenoid muscle. Occluded breaths are signaled by the large fluctuations in intratracheal pressure. (Reprinted by permission of the publisher from Laryngeal and diaphragmatic responses to airway occlusion in sleep and wakefulness by Orem J, Dick TE, Norris P: Electroencephalogr Clin Neurophysiol 50:151, 1980, by Elsevier Science Publishing Company Inc.)

reticular formation and posterior hypothalamus produce (1) a reduction in the duration of the expiratory phase of the respiratory cycle, (2) an increase in slope of integrated phrenic activity, and (3) an increase in the peak amplitude of integrated phrenic activity.[33] Stimulation of the midbrain reticular formation induces phase-switching of the respiratory cycle also.

The pathways and mechanisms of the reticular influences on respiratory activity are unknown. Phrenic activity is facilitated by midbrain and diencephalic stimulation even in animals that are vagotomized, transected at low cervical levels of the spinal cord, paralyzed, and artificially ventilated.[33] Short latency driving of the posterior cricoarytenoid muscle (PCA) muscles and phase-switching of the respiratory cycle can be obtained even after bilateral dorsolateral pontine (pneumotaxic center) lesions combined with bilateral vagotomy and transection of the spinal cord at C8.[10]

Direct projections from the midbrain reticular formation to the dorsal and ventral medullary respiratory groups have not been reported. Edwards[63] reports connections to the facial nucleus, but his drawings show scattered projections into the region of the retrofacial and ambiguus nuclei. There are no midbrain reticular projections to the dorsal respiratory group, but there are projections to the dorsolateral pons.

The midbrain reticular formation activates the forebrain,[57] and the cortex could mediate reticular influences on pontine and medullary respiratory areas; however, decerebrate rats increase their rate of breathing upon arousal from sleep (Dr. A. Netick, personal communication), and the predominant cortical influence on breathing may be inhibitory. Decorticate cats have abnormally vigorous ventilatory responses to hypoxia,[30] and cortical lesions in humans cause exaggerated ventilatory responses to CO_2, leading to Cheyne-Stokes breathing.[64,65]

Beck et al.[66] studied the relationship between electrocortical arousal and a conditioned respiratory response. Tones were paired with foot-shocks that stimulated breathing. After training, the tones alone elicited a change in breathing, but, in general, the conditioned respiratory response did not occur unless cortical desynchronization occurred also. With overtraining, however, conditioned respiratory responses occurred sometimes without cortical arousal, confirming Popov's earlier observation.[67] A lesioning study confirmed these findings. Conditioned respiratory responses were either absent or equivocal when lesions prevented desynchronization of the electroencephalogram (EEG) to the stimulus[68] (i.e., an arousal-like pattern) but there were exceptions when unquestionable respiratory responses occurred without electroencephalographic arousal.

Midbrain respiratory-related activity exists but it is weak and intermittent (Fig. 2-10, Ref. 43). In two samples of midbrain neurons (the first involving 203, the second 281, unambiguous single neurons), Orem and Netick[43] found that 15 percent and 5.7 percent, respectively, discharged in patterns related to respiration; however, repeated analyses of these midbrain respiratory cells revealed that their respiratory activity was intermittent. The intermittence was

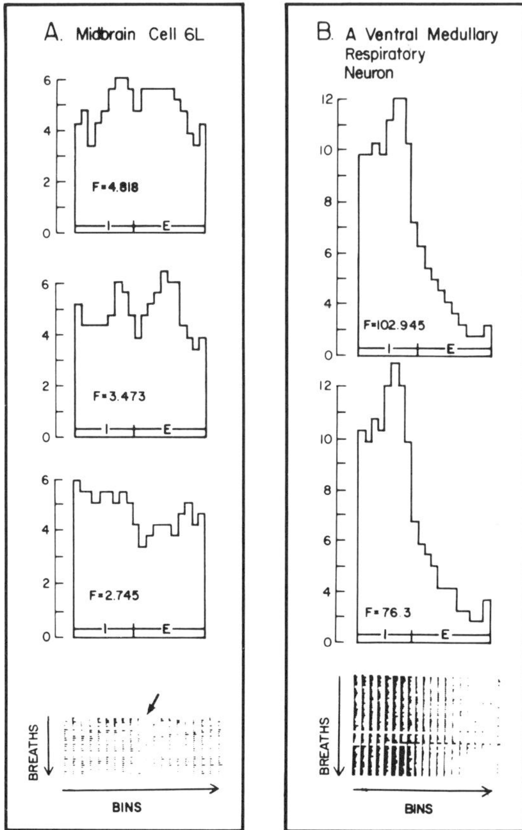

Fig. 2-10 Cycle-triggered histograms of a midbrain and a medullary respiratory neuron. The vertical scale shows average action potential counts/breath determined from 50 breaths. Each bin on the horizontal scale is 5 percent of the respiratory cycle. Note the variable shapes of the cycle-triggered histograms of the midbrain cell. The activity of this cell was significantly related to breathing on 10 of 11 trials of 50 breaths each. The significant feature seemed to be a pause in activity occurring at the I to E transition. This can be seen (arrow) from the raster display at the bottom of the figure. In this display, a row shows the activity during a single breath. Different breaths are shown in each row. The blank rows were the result of false triggering of the oscilloscope and do not indicate breaths during which there was no neuronal activity. The columns represent the 20 bins of each breath, and the number of dots (merging to form horizontal lines of different lengths) indicate the number of discharges occurring during a bin. The columns are aligned so that the equivalent fractions of the respiratory cycle are represented as the same column across breaths. The cycle-triggered histograms and the raster display at the right show the activity of a medullary respiratory neuron recorded in a chronic unanesthetized cat. Note the consistency of the shape of the cycle-triggered histogram and the clear pattern in the raster display. (Reprinted by permission of the publisher from Characteristics of midbrain respiratory neurons in sleep and wakefulness in the cat by Orem J, Netick A: Brain Res 244:231, 1982, by Elsevier Science Publishing Company Inc.)

so great that, except for three cells, it was impossible to exclude the possibility of a false-positive error. This finding differs from the higher percentage of respiratory related cells found in the midbrain by Vibert et al.[41] The difference may lie in the analytic approach.[42,43]

In our study the respiratory-related activity of a midbrain intermittent respiratory neuron tended to be more likely in wakefulness than in NREM sleep, but this tendency was not significant statistically. The projections of the intermittent respiratory cells are unknown, but they behaved similarly to cells that project rostrally. Just like rostrally projecting cells, the intermittent respiratory neurons were more active in wakefulness than in NREM sleep, whereas caudally projecting cells, according to Steriade,[69] are more active in NREM sleep than in wakefulness.

Conclusion

Breathing in NREM sleep is less vigorous than breathing in wakefulness. This effect is the result of a reduction in the population of active respiratory neurons and a decrease in the level of activity of those remaining active. Weak respiratory cells are affected more by sleep than strong respiratory cells—indicating perhaps that the effect of sleep is to reduce primarily the nonrespiratory afference to respiratory neurons. In the case of some strong inspiratory cells, the reduction in rate during sleep is a manifestation of a general, state-independent relationship between discharge rate and the duration of inspiration.

Both medullary and pontine respiratory activity are diminished in NREM sleep. The cause of this reduction in respiratory activity is unknown. Although the metabolic rate may be less in NREM sleep than in wakefulness, the chemical stimulus to breathe is apparently greater (there is a relative hypercapnia in NREM sleep). The reduced breathing in NREM sleep seems determined centrally and is accentuated by removal of afferent respiratory stimuli. There is in wakefulness a stimulus to breathe, which is lost in sleep. The neural basis of this stimulus is not known, but various studies show that brainstem regions that produce electrocortical arousal also excite the respiratory system.

RESPIRATORY ACTIVITY IN REM SLEEP

Characteristics of Breathing in REM Sleep

In REM sleep, th combination of reduced airflow rates[2,4] and shorter inspiratory times[2,3] produces tidal volumes that are less than those in NREM sleep or wakefulness. Atonia of the intercostal muscles reduces or eliminates costal breathing in REM sleep.[70,71] Upper airway respiratory muscles are also atonic or hypotonic.[9,11,72] Apneas and hyperpneas occur as the extremes of very irregular breathing. Ventilatory responses to chemical stimuli and other respiratory reflexes are weakened during phasic REM-sleep activity,[73,74] and laryngeal and diaphragmatic responses to occlusions are inconsistent and variable.[27]

The breathing pattern of REM sleep does not depend upon variations in chemoreceptor,[75] vagal,[4,49,76] or thoracic[49,50] afferent activity. Irregular breathing during REM sleep is seen in the pontine animal[77] and in the neonate.[78]

"Voluntary" Control of Breathing in REM Sleep

For several years after the discovery of REM sleep, researchers believed that dreams explained the physiological irregularities of REM sleep. For example, Dement and Wolpert[79] proposed that the eye movements of REM sleep were the sleeper's response to the dream; that is, the sleeper was scanning or watching his or her dream. Similarly, they believed that dreams caused cardiovascular and respiratory irregularities. These explanations for the physiology of REM sleep were, however, countered by other theories. The relationship of respiratory changes to eye-movement bursts and the large amount of REM sleep (accompanied by respiratory and cardiovascular irregularities) in neonates suggested that the physiological manifestations of REM sleep were an integral part of the brainstem processes producing sleep and not merely responses to dreams. Spreng et al.[80] suggested, "We therefore could have autonomic nervous system changes during stage REM sleep which are related primarily to dream content, those which are associated with neurophysiological triggering of REM-bursts, and in some cases the two could overlap and either augment or suppress the response" (p. 332).

The recent version of this issue involves distinctions between the automatic and voluntary (or behavioral) respiratory systems. The pontomedullary respiratory groups constitute an automatic respiratory system. Damage in these groups or in the ventral cervical cord where their fibers course results in a failure of automatic respiration. Patients with these lesions can breathe on command, but are apneic and require artificial respiration when asleep or when administered anesthetics.[81]

According to Plum,[82] the voluntary respiratory system depends upon forebrain structures. Evidence for this includes the aphasias associated with left hemispheric damage to Broca's area, respiratory apraxia (inability to voluntarily hold the breath) resulting from presumed cortical damage, and pseudobulbar palsy, in which voluntary control of breathing can be interrupted selectively. In addition, electrical stimulation studies show influences on breathing when stimulation is applied to cortical and limbic structures.[31,82,83]

The voluntary and automatic systems may remain separate until converging on the respiratory motoneurons. Plum[82] has hypothesized that whereas the spinal pathway of the automatic system courses in the ventrolateral quadrant, the voluntary system runs with the lateral corticospinal fibers. Lesions of the ventrolateral quadrants eliminate automatic breathing,[84] but there is no clear evidence that the dorsolateral columns have a role in the mediation of voluntary control of breathing. Meyer and Herndon[85] reported that a patient with bilateral infarction of the pyramids and the adjacent ventromedial portion of the medulla breathed spontaneously and regularly but was unable to initiate any voluntary control of his respiration. This patient had a pharyngeal and hypoglossal paralysis also, indicating possible interruption of corticobulbar fibers to medullary respiratory areas. The evidence from this case does not exclude therefore some participation of medullary respiratory neurons in the voluntary control of breathing.

The patient studied by Meyer and Herndon[85] had evidently no detectable decline or irregularity in the breathing pattern while asleep and did not need artificial respiration to sleep.[82] This finding has important implications for the participation of the voluntary system in breathing during REM sleep.

There would appear to be little role for the voluntary system in breathing during NREM sleep; however, the distinction between voluntary and automatic systems may be difficult in many cases. For example, in the cat in the semiprone curled position, intercostal muscle is lateralized with greater activity on the upward-concave side than on the downward-convex side.[86] We may presume that the cat assumes this position voluntarily, but the asymmetrical pattern of intercostal activity persists throughout NREM and REM sleep, when it is difficult to imagine the response as voluntary.

There are no established procedures for neurophysiological investigations of the voluntary system in animals. Consequently, there is little to report on this subject; however, the activity of medullary respiratory neurons, elements of the automatic respiratory system, corresponds exactly to the pattern of breathing in REM sleep[87,88]—a finding difficult to explain if one asserts that the voluntary system is separate from the automatic system and responsible for some of the irregularities of breathing in REM sleep.

Tonic and Phasic REM-Sleep Influences on Respiration

Two REM sleep processes, one tonic, the other phasic, appear to influence breathing. REM sleep has not been divided into stages, but Moruzzi[89] distinguished tonic events (those lasting throughout the period) from phasic events (those occurring only intermittently). The muscle atonia and desynchronized EEG are examples of tonic events; eye movements, pontogeniculooccipital (PGO) waves, and myoclonic twitches are phasic events.

In REM sleep, the activity of medullary respiratory neurons is related positively to the amount of PGO activity[88] (Fig. 2-11). The positive relationship is evident when the number and frequency of neuron discharges are correlated with the number and frequency of PGO waves in the same period (Fig. 2-12). Orem[88] recorded 22 cells and 7 populations from the dorsal and ventral medullary respiratory groups. Six of the cells were expiratory; one was a transitional inspiratory–expiratory neuron, and the others were inspiratory. The value of the correlation between medullary respiratory neuron and PGO activity varied from cell to cell. In general, cells with high activity levels had larger correlations

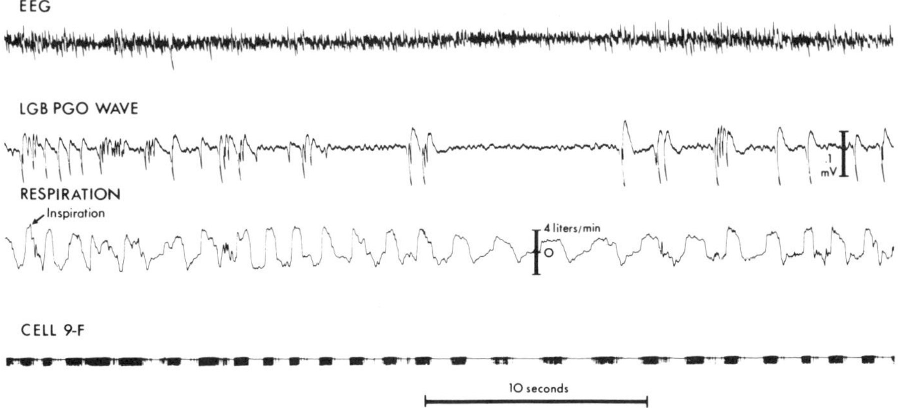

Fig. 2-11 Polygraphic record of REM sleep. EEG, electroencephalogram; LGB PGO wave, pontogeniculooccipital waves recorded from thalamic dorsal lateral geniculate body. Bottom trace shows activity of a respiratory neuron recorded in ventral medullary respiratory group. Note variation in PGO activity and tendency for periods of dense activity to be associated with activation of respiratory neuron and increased breathing rates. (Orem J: Medullary respiratory neuron activity: Relationship to tonic and phasic REM sleep. J Appl Physiol 98:54, 1980.)

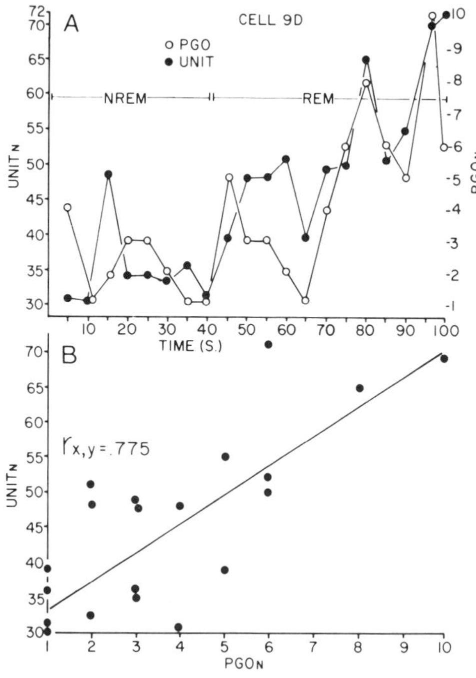

Fig. 2-12 The relationship between number of discharges of a respiratory neuron and density of PGO activity. In A, unit *n* and PGO *n* were summed and plotted every 5 s. In B, the same data are plotted relating unit *n* to PGO *n*. (Orem J: Medullary respiratory neuron activity: Relationship to tonic and phasic REM sleep. J Appl Physiol 48:54, 1980.)

with PGO activity. Because cross-correlation histograms did not show peaks of medullary activity occurring 300 msec before or after PGO waves, it may be that phasic REM processes activate, indirectly or multisynaptically, medullary respiratory neurons.

Either apneas or hyperpneas can occur during intense phasic REM activity.[55,87,90–92] The behavior of medullary respiratory neurons is consistent with the occurrence of hyperpneas but not apneas.

Orem[93] calculated correlations between the number of diaphragmatic motor unit discharges and the number of PGO waves, using the same procedures employed in the study of medullary neurons. The amount of PGO activity did not predict the amount of diaphragmatic activity: sometimes there was a positive relationship between diaphragmatic and PGO activity; at other times the relationship was negative, but most often it was near zero. Polygraphic recordings showed, however, that diaphragmatic activity was suppressed or fractionated during bursts of PGO activity (Fig. 2-13), and sometimes cross-correlation histograms showed a depression in diaphragmatic activity coinciding with PGO waves (Fig. 2-14). These results and the absence of a significant correlation between the amount of PGO activity and the amount of diaphragmatic activity suggest that whereas some phasic REM sleep influences inhibit diaphragmatic activity transiently, other phasic REM sleep influences excite it diffusely. A model of opposing phase REM sleep influences on respiratory motor neurons (one influence being excitatory from upper respiratory motor neurons, the other influence being inhibitory from nonrespiratory REM sleep systems) has been proposed.[93]

Pompeiano et al.[94] have proposed, on the basis of a considerable amount of excellent work, that the atonia of REM sleep is the result of an active inhibitory process rather than the withdrawal of excitatory influences—a theory supported by recent intracellular recordings showing hyperpolarization of trigeminal and spinal motoneurons in REM sleep.[95–101] The intercostal muscles and some of the muscles of the upper airways are atonic or hypotonic in REM sleep, and it is likely that they, as other skeletal muscles, are actively inhibited.

Lesions of the caudal locus coeruleus and subcoeruleus produce REM sleep without the generalized muscle atonia.[102] During REM sleep, animals with this syndrome, responding, we presume, to their dreams, engage in a variety of motor activities, including generalized myoclonic twitching, leaping, exploration, grooming, and biting. They seem to react to imaginary stimuli and may appear to be attacking or experiencing rage or fear.[103] Vocalizations are rare, consisting of weak and plaintive meows. Purring does not occur in these[103] or normal (Orem, unpublished observations) animals during REM sleep.

Anatomical studies show projections from the locus coeruleus and subcoeruleus (regions that when lesioned produced REM sleep without atonia) to the spinal cord and to the nucleus reticularis magnocellularis.[104,105] Stimulation of the latter region produces nonreciprocal inhibition of spinal motoneurons in anesthetized and decerebrate animals[106,107] but reciprocal motor responses in

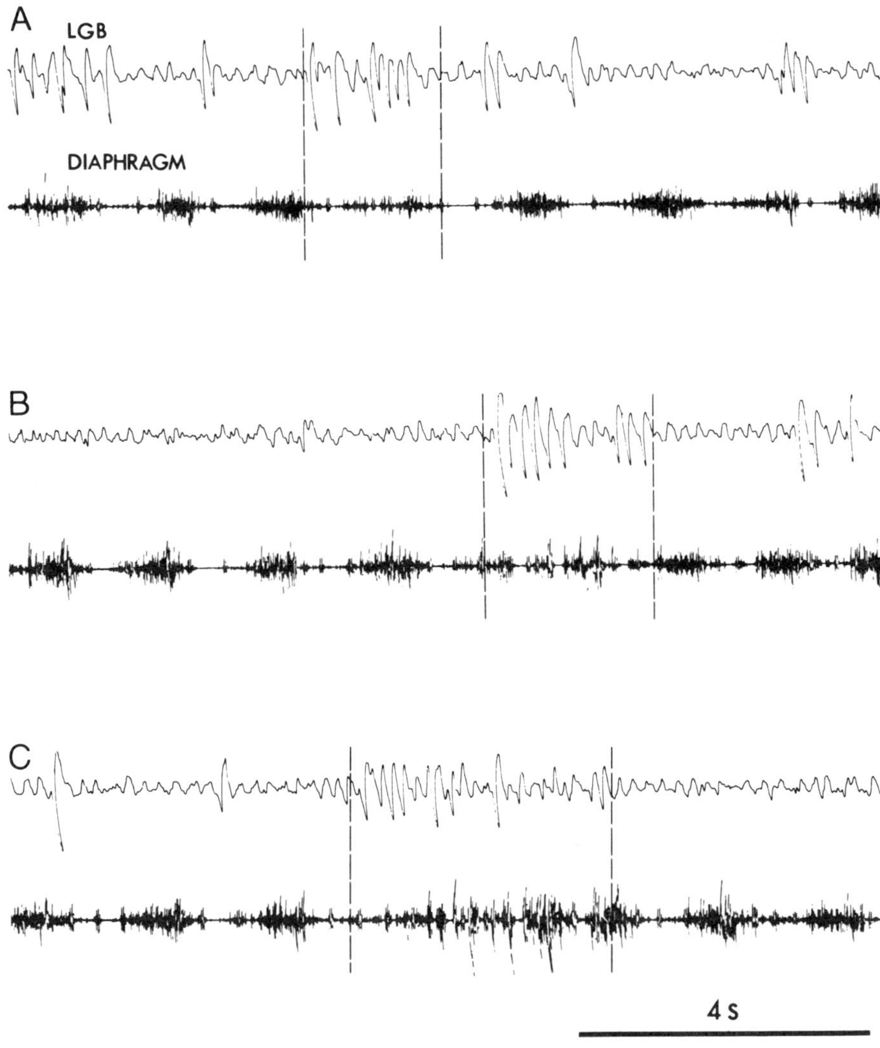

Fig. 2-13 Three episodes of diaphragmatic and PGO activity recorded from the same cat in the same REM sleep period. This figure illustrates the tendency for bursting PGO activity to fractionate diaphragmatic activity. A: The denoted PGO burst (between the vertical dashed lines) almost completely suppresses diaphragmatic activity. B, C: The diaphragmatic activity is fractionated into short bursts. LGB, PGO wave activity recorded from the lateral geniculate body. (Orem J: Neuronal mechanisms of respiratory in REM sleep. Sleep 3:251, 1980. Raven Press, New York.)

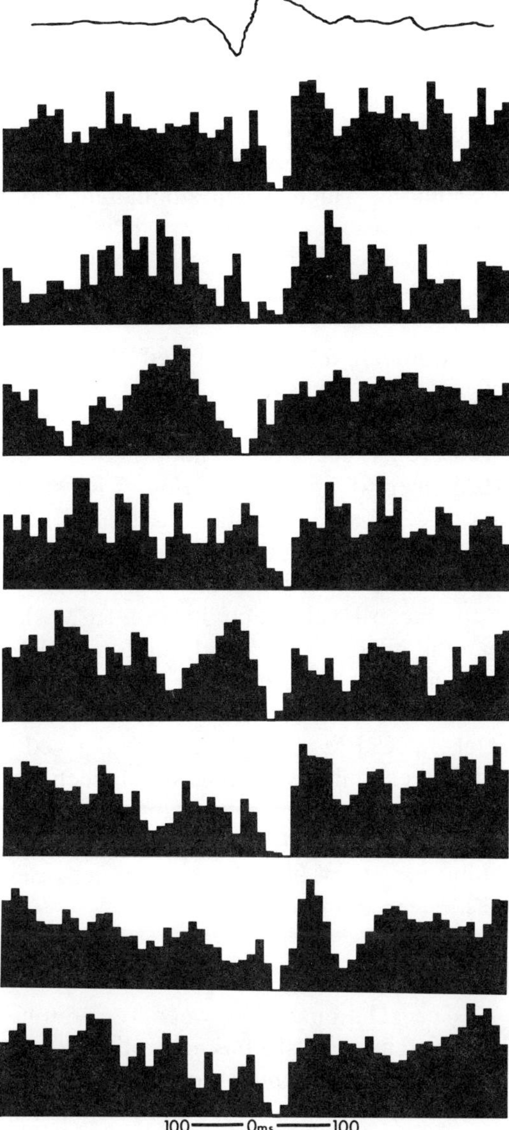

Fig. 2-14 Cumulative discharge histograms of diaphragmatic activity for the period 300 msec before to 300 msec after PGO waves. The waveform at the top is a PGO wave with the initial deflection coinciding with time 0. The histograms are from different diaphragmatic recordings in different animals, but all show a depression in activity coinciding with the PGO wave. The histograms were constructed from the summation of activity occurring around approximately 150 PGO waves. (Orem J: Neuronal mechanisms of respiration in REM sleep. Sleep 3:251, 1980, Raven Press. New York.)

awake animals.[108] Neurons that are purported to act selectively in REM sleep have been found in this region.[109] These cells discharge tonically throughout REM sleep with modulations correlated with phasic REM activity. They are similar, if not identical, to the cells recorded earlier by Netick et al.[110] The latter cells are tonically active during REM sleep, and their discharge frequency is positively related to the rate of breathing. Sakai et al.[109] suggest that these cells may mediate the atonia of REM sleep, but, unable to find such cells in unrestrained cats, Siegel et al.[111] claim that the apparent REM-sleep specificity of the cells depends upon restraint of the animals.

In summary, most evidence suggests an active inhibition of postural muscles during REM sleep. Two suprasegmental regions may participate in producing this inhibition: the region around the caudal locus coeruleus, where lesions produce REM sleep without atonia; and the nucleus reticularis magnocellularis, which, when stimulated, produces inhibition of alpha-motoneurons. The atonia of respiratory as well as nonrespiratory muscles may be mediated by these structures. If this is true, then dorsolateral pontine lesions should eliminate the atonia of the intercostal and upper airway muscles in REM sleep.

Although Moruzzi[89] divided REM sleep events into tonic events and phasic events, Orem[88] has argued that REM sleep does not exist in two pure forms, one tonic and the other phasic. Because PGO waves, which are phasic REM sleep events, occur throughout the REM sleep period, the state of purely tonic REM sleep (defined as a period of REM sleep without phasic activity) is brief and rare. Orem[88] examined the tonic REM sleep state of respiratory neurons by (1) extrapolating the functions relating PGO and respiratory activity to the hypothetical condition of zero PGO activity and (2) comparing the derived level to the mean level of activity in NREM sleep. If the derived level was higher than the NREM sleep level, the tonic REM sleep influence was considered to be excitatory; if it was lower, it was considered inhibitiory.

Cells within the ventral medullary group tended to have higher activity levels in NREM sleep than in the derived tonic REM sleep state (indicating a reduced excitability in tonic REM sleep) whereas the discharge levels of some dorsal respiratory group cells tended to increase in tonic REM sleep. However, phasic excitation of ventral group cells more than compensated for the tonic inhibition: 10 of 14 ventral group cells discharged at higher average rates in REM sleep than in NREM sleep.

Conclusion

The relationship between respiratory and PGO activity indicates that breathing in REM sleep is controlled in part by processes specific to that state. These processes produce complex and even antagonistic effects at different levels of the nervous system, effects that can lead either to apnea or hyperpnea. Although PGO waves are generated in the pons,[112] the relationship of these waves to respiratory changes does not preclude a role for the voluntary respiratory system in the breathing pattern of REM sleep. Indeed the motor behavior in REM sleep of cats with pontine lesions occurs in association with bursts of PGO waves, which may be then the activators of the dream and of the voluntary respiratory system. The distinction between physiological changes related to dream content and those related to neurophysiological triggering of rapid eye movements may therefore be false because rapid eye movements are related to dreaming.

Respiration is also influenced by tonic REM sleep processes. The intercostal and some upper airway muscles become hypotonic in REM sleep. Interpretation of the atonia of these muscles is complicated because of the dual afferents, postural and respiratory, to the motoneurons of some of these muscles (e.g., the intercostal muscles), but there is no evidence that central respiratory drive from medullary respiratory areas decreases sufficiently to account for the hypotonia; therefore, we might reasonably suspect that the atonia results from active inhibition of these motoneurons, just as there is an active inhibition of nonrespiratory motoneurons with postural activity.

ACKNOWLEDGMENT

I acknowledge gratefully Ms. Judith Keeling who edited the manuscript and Ms. Alma Wood who assisted me in its preparation.

REFERENCES

1. Bulow K: Respiration and wakefulness in man. Acta Physiol Scand 59(Supp 209):1, 1963
2. Orem J, Netick A, Dement WC: Breathing during sleep and wakefulness in the cat. Respir Physiol 30:265, 1977
3. Phillipson EA, Murphy E, Kozar LF: Regulation of respiration in sleeping dogs. J Appl Physiol 40:688, 1976
4. Remmers JE, Bartlett D, Putnam MD: Changes in the respiratory cycle associated with sleep. Respir Physiol 28:227, 1976
5. Kawata K, Kotakehara Y, Hosaka K et al: Airway occlusion pressure during sleep in normal adolescents. Abstracts, 4th International Congress on Sleep Research, Bologna, Italy, 1983, p. 41
6. Anch AM, Remmers JE, Sauerland EK, DeGroot WJ: Oropharyngeal patency during waking and sleep in the Pickwickian syndrome: Electromyographic activity of the tensor veli palatini. Electromyogr Clin Neurophysiol 21:317, 1981
7. Berger RJ: Tonus of extrinsic laryngeal muscles during sleep and dreaming. Science 134:840, 1961
8. Megirian D, Sherrey JH: Respiratory functions of the laryngeal muscles during sleep. Sleep 3:289, 1980
9. Orem J, Lydic R: Upper airway function during sleep and wakefulness: experimental studies on normal and anesthetized cat. Sleep 1:49, 1978
10. Orem J, Lydic R, Norris P: Experimental control of the diaphragm and laryngeal abductor muscles by brain stem arousal systems. Respir Physiol 38:302, 1979
11. Sauerland EK, Harper RM: The human tongue during sleep: Electromyographic activity of the genioglossus muscle. Exp Neurol 51:160, 1976
12. Sauerland EK, Orr WC, Hairston LE: EMG patterns of the oropharyngeal muscles during respiration in wakefulness and sleep. Electromyogr Clin Neurophysiol 21:307, 1981

13. Birchfield RI, Sieker HO, Heyman A: Alterations in respiratory function during natural sleep. J Lab Clin Med 54:216, 1959
14. Birchfield RI, Sieker HO, Heyman A: Alterations in blood gases during natural sleep and narcolepsy. Neurology 8:107, 1958
15. Bulow K. Ingvar DH: Respiration and state of wakefulness in normals, studied by spirography, capnography and EEG. Acta Physiol Scand 51:230, 1961
16. Coccagna G, Lugaresi E: Arterial blood gases and pulmonary and systemic arterial pressure during sleep in chronic obstructive pulmonary disease. Sleep 1:117, 1978
17. Magnussen G: Studies on the Respiration During Sleep: A Contribution to the Physiology of Sleep Function. Lewis, London, 1944
18. Phillipson EA, Kozar LF, Rebuck AS, Murphy E: Ventilatory and waking responses to CO_2 in sleeping dogs. Am Rev Respir Dis 115:251, 1977
19. Reed DJ, Kellogg RH: Changes in respiratory response to CO_2 during natural sleep at sea level and at altitude. J Appl Physiol 13:325, 1958
20. Reed DJ, Kellogg RH: Effect of sleep on hypoxic stimulation of breathing at sea level and altitude. J Appl Physiol 15:1130, 1960
21. Straub H: I. Uber schwankungen in der tatigkeit des atemzentrums, speziell im schlaf. Dtsch Arch Klin Med 117:397, 1915
22. Townsend RE, Prinz PN, Obrist WD: Human cerebral blood flow during sleep and waking. J Appl Physiol, 35:620, 1973
23. Douglas N, White D, Weil J, Pickett C et al: Hypoxic ventilatory response decreases during sleep in normal men. Am Rev Respir Dis 125:286, 1982
24. Henderson-Smart DJ, Read DJC: Reduced lung volume during behavioral active sleep in the newborn. J Appl Physiol 46:1081, 1979
25. Jeffery HE, Read DJC: Ventilatory responses of newborn calves to progressive hypoxia in quiet and active sleep. J Appl Physiol 48:892, 1980
26. Iber C, Berssenbrugge A, Skatrud JB, Dempsey JA: Ventilatory adaptation to resistive loading during wakefulness and non-REM sleep. J Appl Physiol 52:607, 1982
27. Orem J, Dick TE, Norris P: Laryngeal and diaphragmatic responses to airway occlusion in sleep and wakefulness. Electroencephalogr Clin Neurophysiol 50:151, 1980
28. Santiago TV, Goldblatt K, Winters K et al: Respiratory consequences of methadone: the response to added resistance to breathing. Am Rev Respir Dis 122:623, 1980
29. Plum F, Posner JB: The Diagnosis of Stupor and Coma. FA Davis, Philadelphia, 1972
30. Tenney SM, Ou LC: Ventilatory response of decorticate and decerebrate cats to hypoxia and CO_2. Respir Physiol 29:81, 1977
31. Reis DJ, McHugh PR: Hypoxia as a cause of bradycardia during amygdala stimulation in monkey. Am J Physiol 214:601, 1968
32. Zhang JX, Harper RM, Frysinger RC: Neuronal discharge patterns in the central nucleus of the amygdala during sleep-waking states. 13th Annual Meeting Society for Neuroscience, Boston Massachusetts, Abstract:1163, 1983
33. Cohen MI, Hugelin A: Suprapontine reticular control of intrinsic respiratory mechanisms. Arch Ital Biol 103:317, 1965
34. Gauthier P, Monteau R, Dussardier M: Inspiratory on-switch evoked by stimulation of mesencephalic structures: A patterned response. Exp Brain Res 51:261, 1983

35. Martin HM, Booker WD: The influence of stimulation of the midbrain upon the respiratory rhythm of the mammal. J Physiol 1:370, 1878
36. Puizillout JJ, Ternaux JP: Variations d'activite toniques, phasiques et respiratoires, au niveau bulbaire pendant l'endormement de la preparation 'encéphale isolé'. Brain Res 66:67, 1974
37. Orem J. Montplaisir J, Dement W: Changes in the activity of respiratory neurons during sleep. Brain Res 82:309, 1974
38. Vibert JF, Bertrand F, Denavit-Saubie M, Hugelin A: Discharge patterns of bulbo-pontine respiratory unit populations in cat. Brain Res 114:211, 1976
39. Vibert JF, Bertrand F, Denavit-Saubie M: Three dimensional representation of bulbo-pontine respiratory networks architecture from unit density maps. Brain Res, 114:227, 1976
40. Bertrand F, Hugelin A, Vibert JF: Quantitative study of anatomical distribution of respiratory related neurons in the pons. Exp Brain Res 16:383, 1973
41. Vibert JF, Caille D, Bertrand F et al: Ascending projection from the respiratory centre to mesencephalon and diencephalon. Neurosci Lett 11:29, 1979
42. Netick A, Orem J: Erroneous classification of neuronal activity by the respiratory modulation index. Neurosci Lett 21:301, 1981
43. Orem J, Netick A: Characteristics of midbrain respiratory neurons in sleep and wakefulness in the cat. Brain Res 244:231, 1982
43a. Orem J, Osorio I, Brooks E, Dick T: Activity of respiratory neurons during NREM sleep. J Neurophysiol 54:1144, 1985
44. Orem J, Dick T: Consistency and signal strength of respiratory neuronal activity. J Neurophysiol 50:1098, 1983
45. Harrison TR, King CE, Calhoun JA, Harrison WG: Congestive heart failure. XX. Cheyne–Stokes respiration as the cause of paroxysmal dyspnea at the onset of sleep. Arch Intern Med 53:891, 1934
46. Pleschka K, Wang SC: The activity of respiratory neurons before and during panting in the cat. Pflugers Arch 353:303, 1975
47. Lydic R, Orem J: Respiratory neurons of the pneumotaxic center during sleep and wakefulness. Neurosci Lett 15:187, 1979
48. Sieck GC, Harper RM: Pneumotaxic area neuronal discharge during sleep-waking states in the cat. Exp Neurol 67:79, 1980
49. Foutz AS, Netick A, Dement WC: Sleep state effects on breathing after spinal cord section and vagotomy in the cat. Respir Physiol 37:89, 1979
50. Netick A, Foutz AS: Respiratory activity and sleep-wakefulness in the deafferented paralyzed cat. Sleep 3:1, 1980
51. Sullivan CE, Kozar LF, Murphy E, Phillipson EA: Primary role of respiratory afferents in sustaining breathing rhythm. J Appl Physiol 45:11, 1978
52. Fink BR: Influence of cerebral activity in wakefulness on regulation of breathing. J Appl Physiol 16:15, 1961
53. Orem J, Netick A, Dement WC: Increased upper airway resistance to breathing during sleep in the cat. Electroencephalogr Clin Neurophysiol 43:14, 1977
54. Krieger J, Kurtz D: EEG changes before and after apnea. In Guilleminault C, Dement WC (eds): Sleep Apnea Syndromes. Alan R Liss, New York, 1978
55. Phillipson EA: Control of breathing during sleep. Am Rev Respir Dis 118:909, 1978
56. Rigg JRA, Inman EM, Saunders NA et al: Interaction of mental factors with hypercapnic ventilatory drive in man. Clin Sci Mol Med 52:269, 1977

57. Moruzzi G, Magoun HW: Brain stem reticular formation and activation of the E.E.G.. Electroencephalogr Clin Neurophysiol 1:455, 1949
58. Lindsley DB, Schreiner LH, Knowles WB, Magoun HW: Behavioral and EEG changes following chronic brain stem lesions in the cat. Electroencephalogr Clin Neurophysiol 2:483, 1950
59. Huttenlocher PR: Evoked and spontaneous activity in single units of medial brain stem during natural sleep and waking. J Neurophysiol 24:451, 1961
60. Kasamatsu T: Maintained and evoked unit activity in the mesencephalic reticular formation of the freely behaving cat. Exp Neurol 28:450, 1970
61. Manohar S, Noda H, Adey WR: Behavior of mesencephalic reticular neurons in sleep and wakefulness. Exp Neurol 34:140, 1972
62. Moruzzi G: The sleep-waking cycle. Ergeb Physiol 64:1, 1972
63. Edwards SB: Autoradiographic studies of the projections of the midbrain reticular formation: Descending projections of nucleus cuneiformis. J Comp Neurol 161:341, 1975
64. Heyman A, Birchfield RI, Sieker HO: Effects of bilateral cerebral infarction on respiratory center sensitivity. Neurology 8:694, 1958
65. Brown HW, Plum F: The neurologic basis of Cheyne–Stokes respiration. Am J Med 30:849, 1961
66. Beck EC, Doty RW, Kooi KA: Electrocortical reactions associated with conditional flexion reflexes. Electroencephalogr (Montreal) 10:279, 1958
67. Popov NA: Etudes electroencephalographiques du probleme des reflexes conditionnes II. Annee Psychol, 47–48:97, 1946–47
68. Doty RW, Beck EC, Kooi KA: Effect of brain stem lesions on conditional responses of cats. Exp Neurol 1:360, 1959
69. Steriade M: Midbrain reticular discharge related to forebrain activation processes. In Szentagothais J, Palkouits M, Hamori J (eds): Advances in physiological Science. Vol. I. Regulation Functions of the CNS. Motion and Organization Principles. Pergamon, Budapest, 1981
70. Tabachnick E, Muller N, Levison H, Bryan AC: The behavior of the respiratory muscles during sleep. Physiologist 23:1, 1980
71. Parmeggiani PL, Sabattini L: Electromyographic aspects of postural, respiratory and thermoregulatory mechanisms in sleeping cats. Electroencephalogr Clin Neurophysiol 33:1, 1972
72. Remmers JE, DeGroot WJ, Sauerland EK, Anch AM: Pathogenesis of upper airway occlusion during sleep. J Appl Physiol 44:931, 1978
73. Sullivan CE, Murphy E, Kozar LF, Phillipson EA: Ventilatory responses to CO_2 and lung inflation in tonic versus phasic REM sleep. J Appl Physiol 47:1304, 1979
74. Sullivan CE: Breathing in sleep. In Orem J. Barnes CD (eds): Physiology in Sleep. Academic Press, New York, 1980
75. Guazzi M, Freis ED: Sino-aortic reflexes and arterial pH, PO_2, and PCO_2 in wakefulness and sleep. Am J Physiol 217:1623, 1969
76. Dawes GS, Fox HE, Leduc BM et al: Respiratory movements and rapid eye movement sleep in the foetal lamb. J Physiol 220:119, 1972
77. Jouvet M: Recherches sur les structures nerveuses et les mecanismes responsables des differentes phases du sommeil physiologique. Arch Ital Biol 100:125, 1962
78. Roffwarg HP, Muzio JN, Dement WC: Ontogenetic development of the human sleep-dream cycle. Science 152:604, 1966

79. Dement W, Wolpert EA: The relation of eye movements, body motility, and external stimuli to dream content. J Exp Psychol 55:543, 1958
80. Spreng LF, Johnson LC, Lubin A: Autonomic correlates of eye movement bursts during stage REM sleep. Psychophysiology 4:311, 1968
81. Severinghaus JW, Mitchell RA: Ondine's curse-failure of respiratory center automaticity while awake. Clin Res 10:122, 1962
82. Plum F: Neurological integration of behavioural and metabolic control of breathing. p. 159. In Porter R (ed): Breathing: Hering–Breuer Centernary Symposium. Churchill, London, 1970
83. Nelson DA, Ray CD: Respiratory arrest from seizure discharges in limbic system. Arch Neurol 19:199, 1968
84. Newsom DJ, Plum F: Separation of descending spinal pathways to respiratory motoneurons. Exp Neurol 34:78, 1972
85. Meyer JS, Herndon RM: Bilateral infarction of the pyramidal tracts in man. Neurology 12:637, 1962
86. Dick TE, Parmeggiani PL, Orem JM: Intercostal muscle activity of the cat in the curled, semiprone sleeping posture. Respir Physiol 56:385, 1984
87. Orem J, Dement WC: Neurophysiological substrates of the changes in respiration during sleep. In Weitzman ED (ed): Advances in Sleep Research. Vol II. Spectrum, New York, 1976
88. Orem J: Medullary respiratory neuron activity: Relationship to tonic and phasic REM sleep. J Appl Physiol 48:54, 1980
89. Moruzzi G: Active processes in the brain stem during sleep. Harvey Lect 58:233, 1963
90. Aserinsky E, Kleitman N: Regularly occurring periods of eye motility and concomitant phenomena, during sleep. Science 118:273, 1953
91. Shapiro A, Goodenough DR, Biederman I, Sleser I: Dream recall and the physiology of sleep. J Appl Physiol 19:778, 1964
92. Hobson JA, Goldfrank F, Snyder F: Respiration and mental activity in sleep. J Psychiatr Res 3:79, 1965
93. Orem J: Neuronal mechanisms of respiration in REM sleep. Sleep 3:251, 1980
94. Pompeiano O: The neurophysiological mechanisms of the postural and motor events during desynchronized sleep. Proc Assoc Res Nerve Ment Dis 45:351, 1967
95. Nakamura Y, Goldberg L, Chandler S, Chase MH: Intracellular analysis of trigeminal motoneuron activity during sleep in the cat. Science 199:204, 1978
96. Chandler SH, Chase MH, Nakamura Y: Intracellular analysis of synaptic mechanisms controlling trigeminal motoneuron activity during sleep and wakefulness. J Neurophysiol 44:359, 1980
97. Chandler SH, Nakamura Y, Chase MH: Intracellular analysis of synaptic potentials induced in trigeminal jaw-closer motoneurons by pontomesencephalic reticular stimulation during sleep and wakefulness. J Neurophysiol 44:372, 1980
98. Chase MH, Chandler SH, Nakamura Y: Intracellular determination of membrane potential of trigeminal motoneurons during sleep and wakefulness. J Neurophysiol 44:349, 1980
99. Morales FR, Chase MH: Intracellular recording of lumbar motoneuron membrane potential during sleep and wakefulness. Exp Neurol, 68:821, 1978
100. Glenn LL, Foutz AS, Dement WC: Membrane potential of spinal motoneurons during natural sleep in cats. Sleep 1:199, 1978

101. Glenn LL: Intracellular analysis of motoneurons during sleep. Ph.D. dissertation, Stanford University, Stanford California, 1979
102. Henley K, Morrison AR: Release of organized behaviour during desynchronized sleep in cats with pontine lesion. Psychophysiology 6:245, 1969
103. Sastre JP, Jouvet M: Le comportement onirique du chat. Physiol Behav 22:979, 1979
104. Sakai K, Sastre JP, Salvert D, et al: Tegmentoreticular projections with special reference to the muscular atonia during paradoxical sleep in the cat: An HRP study. Brain Res 176:233, 1979
105. Tohyama M, Sakai K, Touret M et al: Spinal projections from the lower brain stem in thc cat as demonstrated by the horseradish peroxidase technique. II. Projections from the dorsolateral pontine tegmentum and raphe nuclei. Brain Res 176:215, 1979
106. Magoun HW, Rhines R: An inhibitory mechanism in the bulbar reticular formation. J Neurophysiol 9:165, 1946
107. Jankowska E, Lund S, Lundberg A, Pompeiano O: Inhibitory effects evoked through ventral reticulospinal pathways. Arch Ital Biol 106:124, 1968
108. Sprague JM, Chambers WW: Control of posture by reticular formation and cerebellum in the intact, anesthetized and unanesthetized and in the decerebrate cat. Am J Physiol 176:52, 1954
109. Sakai K, Kanamori N, Jouvet M: Activitiés unitaires specifiques du sommeil paradoxal dans la formation reticulée chez le chat non-restreint. C R Acad Sci (Paris) 289:557, 1979
110. Netick A, Orem J, Dement WC: Neuronal activity specific to REM sleep and its relationship to breathing. Brain Res 120:197, 1977
111. Siegel JM, Wheeler RL, McGinty DJ: Activity of medullary reticular formation neurons in the unrestrained cat during waking and sleep. Brain Res 179:49, 1979
112. Jouvet M: The role of monoamines and acetylcholine-containing neurons in the regulation of the sleep-waking cycle. Ergeb Physiol 64:166, 1972

3 Control of Breathing During Sleep

Richard A. Parisi
Judith A. Neubauer

Characteristic changes in breathing occur between wakefulness and sleep. Rapid eye movement (REM) and non-rapid eye movement (NREM) sleep are fundamentally different states of central neural activity, nearly as different from each other as from the awake state. In this chapter, the relative changes in magnitude and pattern of quiet spontaneous respiration in wakefulness, NREM and REM sleep will be discussed as well as their mechanisms, including what we know about ventilatory and arousal responses to chemical and mechanical stimuli. Although some of these changes may be considered appropriate adjustments to the altered metabolic demands and ventilatory mechanics of each state, the functional basis of some differences in respiratory control is unknown.

SPONTANEOUS BREATHING

Studies of respiration during sleep have been conducted in humans and several other mammalian species.[1–6] These studies provide a large and occasionally conflicting body of information regarding differences in quiet breathing during wakefulness and sleep. Some discrepancies may be species-related, and therefore findings not confirmed in humans will be so identified. However, more significant differences may be methodological. For example, the use of facemasks or mouthpieces to measure ventilation may result in a slower and deeper breathing pattern during wakefulness. Both magnitude and pattern of ventilation, particularly during sleep, could be affected by the reduced airway resistance in tracheostomized animals in which the upper airway was bypassed. Unless stated otherwise, the information presented in this section has been demonstrated to be applicable to breathing through the normal upper airway, and studies employing different methods of measuring ventilation are compared whenever possible.

Minute Ventilation, Pattern, and Gas Exchange

Minute ventilation falls progressively by 5 to 18 percent from wakefulness through the light and deep stages of NREM sleep.[1,2,4,6] The changes in ventilation are accompanied by increasing alveolar and arterial CO_2 tensions of approximately 2 mmHg,[1,2,5–7] indicating that a fall in metabolic CO_2 production does not fully explain the observed hypoventilation during this state. In sleeping humans, the reduction in ventilation is due to small reductions in tidal volume with little or no change in breathing frequency.[2,7] In contrast, a significant decrease in frequency has been noted in several studies of sleeping cats[3,4] and dogs[5] of 23 to 32 percent, at times accompanied by an increase in tidal volume of up to 30 percent. The relative consistency of these findings within species despite use of different methods suggests true species differences in respiratory pattern changes during sleep.

REM sleep is characterized by marked breath-to-breath variability, making averaged respiratory measurements more difficult to interpret. Consistent findings include an increase in breathing frequency primarily due to shortening of expiratory time, and reduction of mean tidal volume to 61 to 73 percent of awake measurements.[2,4,6] Although the bulk of evidence now indicates that ventilation decreases by about 10 perccent from NREM levels, disagreement exists in the literature. In his study of human subjects breathing through a mouthpiece with the nose clipped, Bulow[1] stated that ventilation during REM sleep was approximately equal to that measured during drowsiness (and thus greater than in NREM sleep) and Phillipson et al.[5] reported minute ventilation during REM sleep greater than waking levels in tracheostomized dogs. These discrepancies illustrate the difficulty of interpreting "steady-state" measurements in such a variable state. Carbon dioxide tension during REM sleep increases by 1 to 2 mmHg compared to NREM sleep.[2,5,6] Arterial blood oxygen tension may decrease to a greater degree. The mechanism for the widened alveolar–arterial PO_2 gradient during REM sleep[6] has not yet been agreed upon, but in part must reflect the simple effect of alinearity of the O_2 dissociation curve during non-steady-state hypoventilation.

Mechanics

Changes in pulmonary mechanics during sleep occur primarily for two reasons: (1) change of posture, and (2) changes in drive to the respiratory muscles. Quiet breathing during wakefulness in man is accomplished primarily by diaphragmatic contraction with a lesser contribution by the parasternal intercostal muscles. In the upright posture, this pattern of inspiratory muscle activation results in increased lung volume through outward movement of the chest wall, accounting for about 70 percent of tidal volume, and a smaller displacement of abdominal volume.[8,9] Because of gravitational effects, the same pattern of muscle activity produces greater abdominal than chest wall displacement in the supine posture. This may be explained primarily by increased abdominal compliance due to loss of postural tone of the abdominal muscles.[10] The supine posture is also associated with a decreased functional residual capacity,[11,12] and the reduced lung volume is associated with an increase in intrathoracic airway resistance.[13] Also, lung compliance has been found to decrease in the supine posture, possibly due to increased pulmonary blood volume.[14] Another result of the reduced end-expiratory lung volume in the supine posture is predisposition to small airway closure in the most dependent lung zone at end expiration, a factor that is of greater significance in the elderly or patients with lung disease because of their already increased "closing volumes" and the potential deleterious effect on already impared ventilation-perfusion relationships.[15]

During NREM sleep, the relative motion of the chest wall is greater than that of the abdomen,[7] due to a relative increase in inspiratory intercostal activity compared to wakefulness as well as decreased tone in the expiratory intercostals.[16] Lung compliance does not change, nor does intrathoracic airway resistance.[17]

A different pattern is present during REM sleep. In this state, inspiratory airflow is generated almost entirely through contraction of the diaphragm, as the intercostal muscles are almost totally inhibited by active state-specific central neural mechanisms correlated with the frequency of characteristic dorsal pontine discharges (pontogeniculooccipital, or PGO waves).[18] As a result, thoracic and abdominal movements are both decreased. Paradoxical inward motion of the chest wall may even occur during REM sleep due to intercostal atonia, especially in infancy when the chest wall is less stable.[19]

Substantial changes in upper airway resistance occur during sleep due to different levels of activity of muscles that influence the aperture of the extrathoracic airway.[20–22] Upper airway resistance is quite low during wakefulness, although accounting for the greatest fraction of total airway resistance.[23] Inspiratory resistance is lower than expiratory resistance because of phasic contractions of the upper airway dilator muscles. Both inspiratory and expiratory resistance increase in NREM sleep, and rise further during REM sleep.[20] The inspiratory decrease in resistance may also be lost during REM sleep as both tonic and phasic components of pharyngeal dilator activity are inhibited, particularly during periods of intense PGO activity.[24] These changes in upper airway function during sleep have major significance in the pathophysiology of sleep-disordered breathing due to intermittent upper airway occlusion.[25]

Cerebrovascular Control

Since the overall metabolic rate of the brain does not change appreciably during sleep, the PCO_2 in the local environment of the medullary chemoreceptor may be altered by changes in arterial PCO_2 or in local blood flow.[6] Thus, differences in the relationship between arterial CO_2 tension and brain blood flow may be expected to influence breathing by affecting the fundamental chemical respiratory stimulus at the receptor level. Brain blood flow increases linearly with increasing arterial PCO_2, and the small increase in $PaCO_2$ seen during NREM sleep is reflected in a predictable increase in brain blood flow of no more than 15 percent.[6,26,27] Perfusion of the whole brain, including regional flow to the medulla, has been shown to increase sharply during REM sleep by as much as 80 percent, and tends to fluctuate much more than in NREM sleep. Santiago et al.[6] have shown that the surge of flow during REM sleep was out of proportion to the small rise in $PaCO_2$ observed in goats, and that fluctuations in brain blood flow were temporally correlated with tidal volume in an inverse manner. A similar relationship has been preliminarily reported between brain blood flow and peak integrated diaphragmatic EMG activity,[28] suggesting that a change in cerebrovascular control may contribute to the hypoventilation of REM sleep by causing a wash-out of CO_2 from the environment of the medullary chemoreceptor. However, further study is required before a direct causal relationship can be confirmed.

RESPIRATORY RESPONSES TO CHEMICAL STIMULI

Hypercapnia and hypoxia stimulate breathing during sleep in a manner qualitatively similar to their effects during wakefulness, although their potency is diminished to varying degrees during sleep. Generally these responses maintain the arterial blood gas tensions around a set point with little variation within a given state. Since the ventilatory response to CO_2 is linear while the response to O_2 is hyperbolic, increasing ventilation only when the PO_2 is reduced below 60 mmHg, the level of alveolar ventilation during normal tidal breathing is predominantly a function of the PCO_2. In normal individuals with PO_2 maintained above levels that significantly stimulate breathing, the reduction by sleep of ventilatory response to hypercapnia is adequate to explain the small increases in PCO_2 and reduction in PO_2. In hypercapnic and hypoxemic patients, in whom hypoxic drive may also play an important role in setting the level of respiration, sleep state-related reductions of both hypercapnic and hypoxic responses may further impair the already abnormal awake blood-gas tensions. Further, in addition to their ability to elicit a respiratory response, hypoxia and hypercapnia of sufficient magnitude also produce arousal from both NREM and REM sleep. Since frequent arousals can alter the quality of sleep, the hypoxic and hypercapnic patient may exhibit complications associated with partial sleep deprivation.

Hypercapnia

Hypercapnic ventilatory response has been extensively studied during sleep in humans and animals.[1,7,29–32] Progressive hypercapnia results in a linear increase in minute ventilation regardless of state. Thus, the slope of the ventilation/PCO_2 response is a useful index of CO_2 responsiveness, steep slopes signifying greater responses. The position of the curve and the extrapolated intercept to zero ventilation yield some measure of the PCO_2 threshold for stimulation of ventilation. Thus, in addition to a reduction in slope, a shift of the curve toward increased PCO_2 levels is often interpreted as a diminished CO_2 sensitivity.

Several investigators have found a decrease in the slope of the response line as well as a rightward shift (toward lower minute ventilation for a higher PCO_2) during NREM sleep compared to the awake response. Generally, the slope of the response during wakefulness in humans ranges from 1 to 5 L/min/mmHg with a PCO_2 intercept of about 33 mmHg.[33] During NREM sleep this slope is reduced up to 53 percent.[7,29,31,32] During REM sleep, the CO_2 response decreases further although difficulty in interpretation arises from the intrinsic respiratory variability in this state and thus the weaker correlation between the stimulus (PCO_2) and response (ventilation). In general, the REM CO_2 response slope is reported to be from 28 to 75 percent of the awake response. Measurement of the ventilatory response to CO_2 during REM sleep is further complicated by the effect of the density of phasic REM activity superimposed on the tonic effects of this state. In a study of sleeping dogs, Sullivan et al.[34] found that the hypercapnic ventilatory response in tonic REM sleep was similar to the response in NREM sleep, while it was markedly diminished and possibly absent during phasic REM sleep. Although these findings have not been substantiated in subsequent human and animal studies, they are provocative as they may be explained by the inhibition of respiratory output by phasic REM activity.[35] Further evidence in support of the ability of phasic REM activity to depress respiratory responses has been shown for the genioglossus muscle, an oropharyngeal dilator activated in inspiration during stimulated breathing. The inspiratory activity of the genioglossus as measured by the integrated electromyogram in sleeping goats is totally abolished during phasic REM at both low and high PCO_2.[36] Thus, there may be a distinction between the influences of tonic and phasic REM activity on respiratory responses, but the substantiation of these differences may be limited by the brevity and variability of phasic REM episodes.

Progressive hypercapnia produces arousal from both NREM and REM sleep. Chemoreceptor stimulation through neural connections with the brainstem reticular activating system or greater stimulation of mechanoreceptors by the increase in ventilation may contribute to the arousal response. Arousal by progressive hypercapnia has been found to occur at a higher PCO_2 in REM (60 mmHg) than NREM (54 mmHg) sleep in dogs,[30] but no consistent state-related differences were found in humans.[29]

Hypoxia

Ventilatory response to hypoxia is fundamentally different from CO_2 response in that (1) it is mediated primarily by the peripheral chemoreceptors, which play only a minor role in CO_2 sensitivity, and (2) the relationship between PO_2 and ventilation is hyperbolic, so that little change in ventilation occurs above an arterial PO_2 of 60 mmHg. Arterial oxygen saturation, on the other hand, is linearly related to minute ventilation. Hypoxic ventilatory response may therefore be expressed as the negative slope of V_E/SaO_2 or in terms of the hyperbolic equation describing the V_E/Po_2 relationship.[37] These two methods have been found to describe hypoxic responses comparably, and are assumed to be interchangeable for the purpose of this discussion.

Early studies of hypoxic ventilatory response during sleep reported that no significant decrease occured from wakefulness to either NREM or REM sleep.[38–40] However, arterial PCO_2 was not controlled in most of these studies, and was allowed to decrease as ventilation was stimulated by progressive hypoxia. In sleeping humans studied during progressive isocapnic hypoxia,[41] the ventilatory response was shown to decrease by approximately 41 percent during NREM sleep and 69 percent during REM sleep compared to wakefulness, suggesting a methodologic difference between this and previous studies. A recent comparative study by Santiago et al.[42] demonstrated that failure to maintain isocapnia can mask the decrease in hypoxic response in sleeping goats.

It is well known that hypoxia disturbs normal sleep. One of the most common complaints of sojourners to high altitude is insomnia with frequent awakenings and lack of refreshing sleep.[43] It appears from animal studies[44] that hypoxemia produces a shift toward lighter stages of sleep with less time spent in deeper sleep (Stages III–IV NREM and REM). Therefore, daytime somnolence of hypoxic patients or sojourners to altitude may be a side effect of insufficient deep sleep secondary to frequent awakenings.

Several studies have attempted to quantify the amount of hypoxemia necessary to cause arousal. A greater degree of hypoxia has been found to be required to produce arousal from REM than NREM sleep in dogs,[39] with arousal occuring from NREM at an SaO_2 of 87 percent and from REM at 70 percent. However, arousal responses to hypoxia in cats was shown by Neubauer et al.[45] to occur at a much lower SaO_2 of approximately 47 percent during NREM or 43 percent during REM sleep when care was taken to minimize contamination of results with spontaneous arousals.

The mechanism of frequent arousals during hypoxia is not clearly understood. Possible explanations have included a hypoxia-induced increase in the activity of the reticular activating system secondary to stimulation of peripheral chemoreceptors. Although studies in sleeping dogs[39] found that arousal with hypoxia was abolished after carotid sinus denervation, the study by Neubauer et al.[45] found the arousal response to hypoxia unaffected by this procedure in sleeping cats. Since sleep is not a passive neural process but involves the activation of specific neural circuitry, and neurons with higher metabolism will be most affected by lowered oxygen supply, then arousal may merely represent a switching from one group of active neurons to another.

RESPIRATORY RESPONSES TO NEUROMECHANICAL STIMULI

Various mechanical stimuli can influence magnitude and pattern of breathing. Arousal from sleep can also be produced by these same stimuli. Those neuromechanical reflexes that have been studied during sleep as well as wakefulness and which are felt to be most relevant to respiratory control under physiologic conditions will be discussed.

Lung Volume-Related Feedback

As lung volume increases during inspiration, pulmonary stretch receptor stimulation feeds back to the respiratory controller via the vagus nerve to terminate inspiratory activity. The influence of this reflex loop may be assessed by examining the inverse correlation of tidal volume and inspiratory time, or by measuring the duration of apnea induced by an involuntary airway occlusion at end-inspiration, the classic Hering-Breuer reflex. Although it has been shown that this reflex exerts a greater influence on breathing pattern in many other mammals than in humans,[46] vagal feedback has been demonstrated to affect inspiratory volume-time relationships in anesthetized humans during tidal breathing,[47] and may therefore play a role in the generation of respiratory pattern during sleep. Respiratory pattern has been studied in awake and sleeping animals before and after chronic bilateral vagotomy.[3,5] Tidal volume and inspiratory time are both increased following vagotomy in awake animals, while mean inspiratory flow rate (V_T/T_I) does not change. The same effects on the respiratory cycle found in wakefulness were produced by vagotomy during NREM and REM sleep. Neither the slower breathing frequency of NREM sleep nor the rapid, shallow and irregular pattern of REM sleep were different in comparison to wakefulness after vagotomy. The duration of apnea produced by lung inflation in dogs was found to be greater during NREM sleep than wakefulness, and reduced during REM sleep, particularly during periods of intense phasic REM activity.[34] It may be that this finding is also species related, since no depression of the lung inflation reflex by phasic REM activity was observed in the opossum.[48] It may be concluded that the influence of vagally mediated volume-related feedback on respiratory pattern does not account for a significant portion of the changes in respiratory pattern during sleep.

Mechanical Load Compensation

When the ventilatory apparatus is mechanically loaded during inspiration by increasing resistance to airflow (flow-resistive load) or by decreasing total thoracic compliance (elastic load), an unconscious effort is made to maintain tidal volume at the unloaded level. Mechanical loads may be internal, such as the flow-resistive load imposed by obstructive lung disease or the elastic load of pulmonary fibrosis, or may be applied externally in the laboratory. This load compensation is accomplished by increasing output to the inspiratory muscles, and can be observed on the first breath after a load is imposed. The strength of the load-compensating reflex can be assessed by measuring respiratory output independent of mechanics as reflected by diaphragmatic EMG activity or mouth occlusion pressure with and without an externally-applied load under comparable conditions of chemical respiratory drive. Studies in animals and man have shown that the flow-resistive and elastic load-compensating reflexes are diminished during both NREM and REM sleep.[49–51] Since inspiratory airflow resistance increases due to reduced tone in the upper airway dilator muscles during sleep, especially REM sleep, it may be advantageous for diaphragmatic activity not to increase in response to this challenge, for such an increase might generate a force sufficient to overcome the pharyngeal dilators and cause complete airway occlusion.[52]

Airway Occlusion

Complete occlusion of the airway, which may be thought of as an infinite mechanical load, causes arousal from NREM and REM sleep. In tracheostomized animals airway occlusion during NREM sleep results in a progressive increase in inspiratory effort followed by an arousal within a few breaths.[53,54] Occlusion during REM sleep also produces arousal, but after a more prolonged and variable period of time. With the exception of patients with obstructive sleep apnea, airway occlusion in humans has only been systematically studied by obstructing airflow through a mask or mouthpiece externally. This contrasts with the animal studies that utilized tracheostomies in that inspiratory efforts against the external occlusion would generate negative pressure within the upper airway, where pressure-sensitive receptors are known to be present.[55] External airway occlusion in humans[56] results in considerably earlier arousal from REM than NREM sleep (mean= 6.2 sec vs. 20.4 sec), a finding that contrasts with the more prolonged occlusive events seen in patients with obstructive sleep apnea, suggesting that pressure receptors in the upper airway may play a role in the arousal response to airway occlusion during REM sleep. Apparently the arousal response to occlusion involves an interaction between the mechanoreceptor stimulation, particularly in the upper airway, and the progressive chemoreceptor stimulation by the accompanying hypercapnia and hypoxia. The latter is supported by the delay in occlusion-induced arousal in dogs produced by carotid body denervation.[54]

Airway Irritation

One would expect that superficial airway receptors sensitive to noxious stimuli, which initiate cough during wakefulness, may also protect against airway occlusion by causing arousal from sleep. Sullivan et al.[57,58] have demonstrated that stimulation of irritant receptors in either the larynx or large intrathoracic airways by intraluminal injection of water can produce arousal in sleeping dogs, although greater volumes were required during REM than NREM sleep.

SUMMARY

Respiratory phenomena associated with sleep include decreased minute ventilation during NREM and REM sleep, and changes in pattern of breathing. Breathing frequency is reduced during NREM sleep, but REM sleep is characterized by irregular, rapid and shallow breathing. These characteristic breathing patterns persist following vagotomy in animals, and therefore are not due to changes in vagally-mediated feedback from lung afferents. Respiratory irregularities during REM sleep have been found to correlate with phasic pontine discharges (PGO waves) and also with fluctuations in brain blood flow during this state. Ventilatory responses to hypercapnia and hypoxia are depressed to a greater degree in REM than NREM sleep. Arousal caused by progressive hypercapnia occurs at a lower CO_2 tension during NREM sleep, and the threshold for hypoxic arousal is at a higher SaO_2 during NREM than REM sleep. Ventilatory compensation for mechanical inspiratory loads is absent or markedly depressed during all sleep stages. Arousal may also be produced by airway occlusion or irritation. The time to arousal may differ between sleep states and across species depending on the method of study, although generally more intense stimuli are required to induce arousal from REM and NREM sleep.

REFERENCES

1. Bulow K: Respiration and wakefulness in man. Acta Physiol Scand 59 (Suppl.):1, 1963
2. Douglas NJ, White DP, Pickett CK et al : Respiration during sleep in normal man. Thorax 37:840, 1982
3. Remmers JE, Bartlett Jr D, Putnam MD: Changes in the respiratory cycle associated with sleep. Respir Physiol 28:227, 1977
4. Orem J, Netick A, Dement WC: Breathing during sleep and wakefulness in the cat. Respir Physiol 30:265, 1977
5. Phillipson EA, Murphy E, Kozar LF: Regulation of respiration in sleeping dogs. J Appl Physiol 40:688, 1976
6. Santiago TV, Guerra E, Neubauer JA, Edelman NH: Correlation between ventilation and brain blood flow during sleep. J Clin Invest 73:497, 1984
7. Gothe B, Altose MD, Goldman MD, Cherniack NS: Effects of quiet sleep on resting and CO_2-stimulated breathing. J Appl Physiol 50:724, 1981
8. Konno K, Mead J: Measurement of the separate volume changes of rib cage and abdomen during breathing. J Appl Physiol 22:407, 1967

9. Sharp JT, Goldberg NB, Druz WS, Danon J: Relative contributions of rib cage and abdomen to breathing in normal subjects. J Appl Physiol 39:608, 1975
10. Campbell EJM: An electromyographic study of the role of the abdominal muscles in breathing. J Physiol 117:222, 1952
11. Behrakis PK, Baydur A, Jaeger MJ, Milic-Emili, J: Lung mechanics in sitting and horizontal body positions. Chest 83:643, 1983
12. Linderholm H: Lung mechanics in sitting and horizontal postures studied by body plethysmographic methods. Am J Physiol 204:85, 1963
13. Vincent MJ, Knudson R, Leith DE et al : Factors influencing pulmonary resistance. J Appl Physiol 29:236, 1970
14. Agostini E, Mead J: Statics of the respiratory system. p. 103. In Fenn WO, Rahn H (eds): Handbook of Physiology (Sect. 3 Respiration). American Physiologic Society, Washington, D.C., 1965
15. Leblanc P, Ruff F, Milic-Emili J: Effect of age and body position on "airway closure" in man. J Appl Physiol 28:448, 1970
16. Lopes JM, Tabachnik E, Muller NL et al : Total airway resistance and respiratory muscle activity during sleep. J Appl Physiol 54:773, 1983
17. Hudgel DW, Martin RJ, Johnson B, Hill P: Mechanics of the respiratory system and breathing pattern during sleep in normal humans. J Appl Physiol 56:133, 1984
18. Netick A, Orem J, Dement W: Neuronal activity specific to REM sleep and its relationship to breathing. Brain Res 120:197, 1977
19. Tusiewicz K, Moldofsky H, Bryan AC, Bryan MH: Mechanics of the rib cage and diaphragm during sleep. J Appl Physiol 43:600, 1977
20. Orem J, Netick A, Dement WC: Increased upper airway resistance to breathing during sleep in the cat. Electroencephalogr Clin Neurophysiol 43:14, 1977
21. Sauerland EK, Orr WC, Hairston LE: EMG patterns of oropharyngeal muscles during respiration in wakefulness and sleep. Electromyogr Clin Neurophysiol 21:307, 1981
22. Guilleminault C, Hill MW, Simmons FB, Dement WC: Obstructive sleep apnea: Electromyographic and fiberoptic studies. Exp Neurol 62:48, 1978
23. Ferris BG, Mead J, Opie LH: Partitioning of respiratory resistance in man. J Appl Physiol 19:653, 1964
24. Orem J, Lydic R: Upper airway function during sleep and wakefulness: Experimental studies on normal and anesthetized cats. Sleep 1:49, 1978
25. Remmers JE, deGroot WJ, Sauerland SK, Anch AM: Pathogenesis of upper airway occlusion during sleep. J Appl Physiol 44:931, 1978
26. Reivich M, Isaacs G, Evarts E, Kety SS: The effect of slow-wave sleep and REM sleep on regional cerebral blood flow in cats. J Neurochem 15:301, 1968
27. Townsend RE, Prinz PN, Obrist WD: Human cerebral blood flow during sleep and waking. J Appl Physiol 35:620, 1973
28. Parisi RA, Santiago TV, Neubauer JA et al : Linkage between brain blood flow and respiratory drive during REM sleep. Clin Res 33:470A, 1985
29. Douglas NJ: White DP, Weil JV et al : Hypercapnic ventilatory response in sleeping adults. Am Rev Respir Dis 127:758, 1982
30. Phillipson EA, Kozar LF, Rebuck AS et al : Ventilatory and waking responses to CO_2 in sleeping dogs. Am Rev Respir Dis 115:251, 1977
31. Netick A, Dugger WJ, Symmons RA: Ventilatory response to hypercapnia during sleep and wakefulness in cats. J Appl Physiol 56:1347, 1984

32. Berthon-Jones M, Sullivan CE: Ventilation and arousal responses to hypercapnia in normal sleeping humans. J Appl Physiol 57:59, 1984
33. Hirshman CA, McCullough RE, Weil JV: Normal values for hypoxic and hypercapnic ventilatory drives in man. J Appl Physiol 38:1095, 1975
34. Sullivan CE, Murphy E, Kozar LF, Phillipson EA: Ventilatory responses to CO_2 and lung inflation in tonic versus phasic REM sleep. J Appl Physiol 47:1304, 1979
35. Orem J: Medullary respiratory neuron activity: Relationship to tonic and phasic REM sleep. J Appl Physiol 48:54, 1980
36. Parisi RA, Neubauer JA, Frank M et al : Correlation between genioglossal and diaphragmatic responses to hypercapnia in sleeping goats. Am Rev Respir Dis 131:A295, 1985
37. Weil JV, Byrne-Quinn E, Sodal IE et al : Hypoxic ventilatory drive in normal man. J Clin Invest 49:1061, 1970
38. Reed DJ, Kellogg RH: Effect of sleep on hypoxic stimulation of breathing at sea level and altitude. J Appl Physiol 15:1130, 1960
39. Phillipson EA, Sullivan CE, Read DJC et al : Ventilatory and waking response to hypoxia in sleeping dogs. J Appl Physiol 44:512, 1978
40. Gothe B, Goldman MD, Cherniack NS, Mantey P: Effect of progressive hypoxia on breathing during sleep. Am Rev Respir Dis 126:97, 1982
41. Douglas NJ: White DP, Weil JV et al : Hypoxic ventilatory response decreases during sleep in normal men. Am Rev Respir Dis 125:286, 1982
42. Santiago TV, Scardella AT, Edelman NH: Determinants of the ventilatory responses to hypoxia during sleep. Am Rev Respir Dis 130:179, 1984
43. Weil JV, Kryger MH, Scoggin CH: Sleep and breathing at high altitude. p. 119. In Guilleminault C, Dement WC (eds): Sleep Apnea Syndromes. Allan R. Liss, New York, 1978
44. Pappenheimer JR: Sleep and respiration of rats during hypoxia. J Physiol London 266:191, 1977
45. Neubauer JA, Santiago TV, Edelman NH: Hypoxic arousal in intact and carotid chemodenervated cats. J Appl Physiol 51:1294, 1981
46. Widdicombe JG: Respiratory reflexes in man and other mammalian species. Clin Sci 21:163, 1961
47. Polacheck J, Strong R, Arens J et al : Phasic vagal influences on inspiratory motor output in anesthetized human subjects. J Appl Physiol 49:609, 1980
48. Farber JP, Marlow TA: Pulmonary reflexes and breathing pattern during sleep in the opossum. Respir Physiol 27:73, 1976
49. Santiago TV, Sinha AK, Edelman NH: Respiratory flow-resistive load compensation during sleep. Am Rev Respir Dis 123:382, 1981
50. Iber C, Berssenbrugge A, Skatrud JB, Dempsey JA: Ventilatory adaptations to resistive loading during wakefulness and non-REM sleep. J Appl Physiol 52:607, 1982
51. Wilson PA, Skatrud JB, Dempsey JA: Effects of slow wave sleep on ventilatory compensation to inspiratory elastic loading. Respir Physiol 55:103, 1984
52. Brouillette RT, Thach BT: A neuromuscular mechanism maintaining extrathoracic airway patency. J Appl Physiol 46:772, 1979
53. Orem J, Dick T, Norris P: Laryngeal and diaphragmatic responses to airway occlusion in sleep and wakefulness. Electroencephalogr and Clin Neurophysiol 50:151, 1980
54. Bowes G, Townsend ER, Bromely SM et al : Role of the carotid body and of afferent

vagal stimulation in the arousal response to airway occlusion in sleeping dogs. Am Rev Respir Dis 123:644, 1981
55. Matthew OP, Abu-Osba YK, Thach BT: Influence of upper airway pressure changes on genioglossus muscle respiratory activity. J Appl Physiol 52:438, 1982
56. Issa FG, Sullivan CE: Arousal and breathing responses to airway occlusion in healthy sleeping adults. J Appl Physiol 55:1113, 1983
57. Sullivan CE, Murphy E, Kozar LF, Phillipson EA: Waking and ventilatory responses to laryngeal stimulation in sleeping dogs. J Appl Physiol 45:681, 1978
58. Sullivan CE, Kozar LF, Murphy E, Phillipson EA: Arousal, ventilatory and airway responses to bronchopulmonary stimulation in sleeping dogs. J Appl Physiol 47:17, 1979

4 Control of Breathing in Children

Gabriel G. Haddad

Though the "purpose" of sleep is not yet clear, considerable knowledge has been accumulated regarding the influence of sleep and state of consciousness on respiratory function. Previous investigations, especially those of the past decade, have shown that sleep may constitute a challenge to cardiorespiratory function[1–4] since potentially life-threatening episodes can occur during sleep. For example, O_2 desaturation occurs in sleep [especially in rapid eye movement (REM) sleep] even in the normal healthy adult subject.[2] PaO_2 also falls in the infant during sleep as compared to wakefulness.[5] This fall in PaO_2 and in O_2 saturation is markedly exaggerated in subjects with already existing cardiorespiratory disease.[3]

The physiologic alterations induced by sleep may have added significance in the young for at least three reasons: (1) infants in early life spend most of their time in sleep (and most of that time is spent in REM sleep); (2) the immaturity of certain systems (e.g., respiratory mechanical system) renders the sleep-induced changes more prominent and clinically more serious (one example is the very compliant chest wall of the newly born); and (3) during early postnatal life, rapid and considerable changes take place in a variety of systems. Engineering control theory predicts that periods of instability can occur during such developmental stages.

The purpose of this chapter is to review some of the important observations made in the past decade on the control of breathing during sleep in the perinatal period. Much of what will be described suggests that the respiratory control system participates, like other control systems, in the overall expression of the complex neurophysiologic nature of each sleep state or state of consciousness. The factors that determine blood gas tensions during sleep and, in this regard, the importance of respiratory muscle activity and metabolic rate will also be discussed. The problem of periodic breathing, apnea and chemosensitivity to respiratory stimuli during sleep in the young will also be reviewed. Finally, the chapter will briefly examine some of the important clinical conditions in infants and children that occur mostly during sleep.

THE FETUS

The study of fetal breathing has been subject to numerous investigations in the past 1 to 2 decades.[6–10] Because respiration in the fetus is exquisitely sensitive to anesthesia and surgical manipulation, the results of many of the older studies that used acutely instrumented, anesthetized animals are difficult to interpret. For this reason, the development of chronically instrumented unanesthetized animal preparations[11,12] and noninvasive ultrasonic technology in the human[13,14] represent major contributions in our ability to study respiratory control in utero.

Although mechanisms underlying respiratory behavior in the fetus have been obscure to a large extent, important observations regarding the nature of fetal breathing movements have been made. Most notable is the finding that the fetus makes episodic breathing movements.[7,15] Since fetal breathing movements follow medullary, phrenic or diaphragmatic neural activity[8], they probably represent the "predecessors" of postnatal breaths and may constitute an in utero "training" program. These breathing episodes are usually associated with a high frequency, low amplitude electroencephalogram (EEG) while long respiratory pauses and respiratory silence are associated with low frequency, high amplitude EEG.[15] Whether the high frequency, low amplitude EEG in the fetus is indicative of REM sleep or wakefulness is not known. The recently developed double window preparation[16], a technique that allows constant visualization of the fetal lamb in utero, may provide additional information about the state of consciousness of the fetus in utero and its relationship to breathing.

By analogy to heart rate and heart-rate variability, investigators have tried to determine whether the pattern and nature of breathing movements could predict the state of the fetus, that is, predict whether the fetus is under stress or not. To date, these efforts have not been successful. This is due in part to the episodic nature of breathing in the fetus: it can normally be in complete respiratory silence for hours with no conventionally accepted evidence of distress.

The reasons for the episodic nature of breathing movements in utero are unclear. Recent studies on decorticate fetal lambs have suggested that the cortex does not, as has previously been assumed, play a role in inhibiting breathing during slow-wave high-amplitude EEG.[17] Other mechanisms therefore should be invoked. It is possible that the general decrease in neuronal afferent activity during fetal life may play a role in the respiratory restraint.[18] At birth, a wide variety of different afferent stimuli such as lung stretch, temperature change, hormonal fluctuation, auditory and visual stimuli may contribute to this increase in afferent neuronal traffic. It is possible that this activates respiratory neuronal circuitry and leads to the continuous pattern of breathing seen in the newly born infant seconds after delivery. These afferent sensory stimuli must play a more important role in modulating breathing than the state of consciousness since, in the presence of these stimuli (postnatal life), the state of consciousness does not have such a dramatic effect on breathing as in their absence (prenatal life).

VENTILATION AND VENTILATORY PATTERN IN EARLY POSTNATAL LIFE

Ever since the discovery of the existence of definable sleep states and states of consciousness in infants and adults,[19,20] studies performed on newborn infants and animals have indicated that sleep state modulates ventilation and the ventilatory pattern postnatally.[21–26] Although there are some contradictory results regarding the effect of sleep state on tidal volume (V_T) and respiratory timing, there is a consensus that ventilation is sleep state-dependent.[21,22,24,25,27] Finer et al.[28], Bolton et al.[21], and Hathorn[25] showed that, at 1 week of age, the respiratory frequency is higher in REM than in quiet sleep, thereby resulting in a higher minute ventilation in the former than in the latter state. Our studies on infants in the first 4 months of life did not show a difference in minute ventilation until the age of 3 months (Fig. 4-1).[22] Before that age, the higher respiratory frequency that characterized REM sleep was associated with a smaller tidal volume. Since we did not use invasive techniques (pneumotachography, neck seals, and esophageal balloons) to measure ventilation as others did,[21,25] the question must be raised as to whether the differences in findings are due to differences in measuring techniques. Such techniques have been shown to alter the ventilatory pattern, especially when facial areas (i.e., trigeminal area) are stimulated.[29,30]

Fewer studies have examined the inspiratory and expiratory components of the respiratory cycle time (T_{TOT}) (inverse of respiratory frequency) in infants as a function of sleep state.[22,25] Both inspiration and expiration are longer during quiet than during REM sleep in human infants in the first few months of life (Fig. 4-2).[22] Interestingly, this difference in the pattern of respiratory timing between REM and quiet sleep exists across ages in humans and some animals.[31,32] However, it is not shared by all mammals. For example, whereas piglets and kittens are similar to humans and show a lower respiratory frequency and longer inspiratory and expiratory durations during quiet than during REM sleep[33] (unpublished observations from our laboratory), puppies show the opposite pattern: they have a shallower and faster breathing pattern in quiet than in REM sleep.[34]

Although respiratory frequency generally follows changes in expiratory time (T_E), inspiratory time (T_I) is an important timing parameter that determines

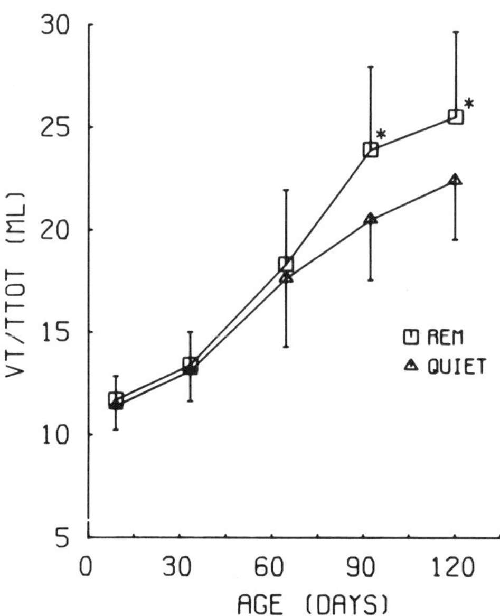

Fig. 4-1 Instantaneous minute ventilation plotted as a function of age at 2 weeks, and 1, 2, 3 and 4 months of life in normal infants in REM and quiet sleep. Note that V_T/T_{TOT} is larger in REM than in quiet sleep after the first 2 months of life. (Haddad GG, Epstein RA, Epstein MAF et al : Maturation of ventilation and ventilatory pattern in normal sleeping infants. J Appl Physiol 46:998, 1979.)

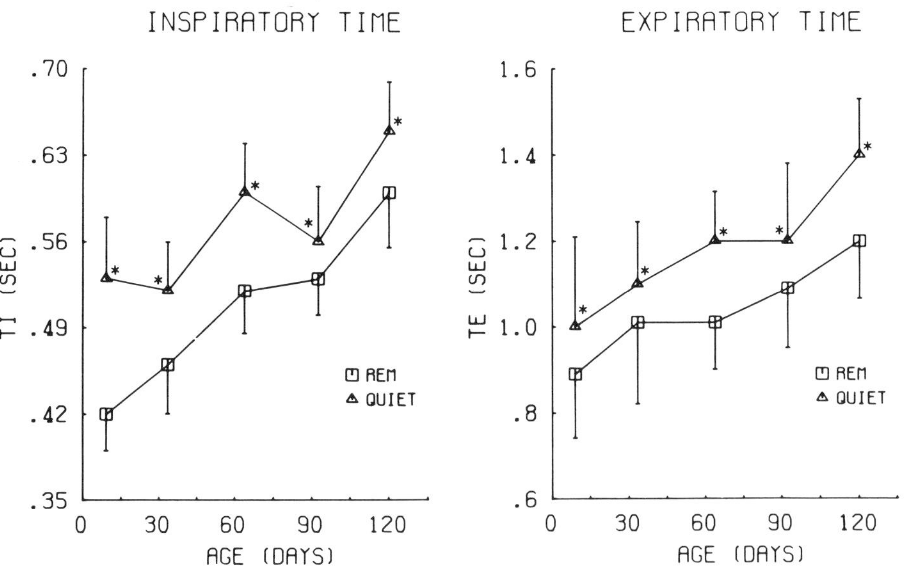

Fig. 4-2 Inspiratory and expiratory time plotted as a function age in normal infants in REM and quiet sleep. Both variables are longer in quiet than in REM sleep. (Haddad GG, Epstein RA, Epstein MAF et al : Maturation of ventilation and ventilatory pattern in normal sleeping infants. J Appl Physiol 46:998, 1979.)

in part tidal volume and minute ventilation. Since T_I and T_E, measured from an airflow trace, correlate closely with neural timing of respiratory events,[35] the shorter T_I and T_E during REM sleep in infants suggests that the termination of neural inspiratory and expiratory activities occurs earlier in REM sleep. The control of respiratory timing is complex but it is believed that the difference in respiratory timing between REM and quiet sleep is central in origin. This is based on the observations that (1) the difference in timing persists after vagotomy[36,31] and total spinal cord transection[37] and (2) increased airway impedance, which occurs more readily in REM than in quiet sleep,[38,39] would tend to increase T_I rather than shorten it. The opposite, however, occurs (shorter T_I in REM sleep) indicating that, if mechanical loading is a phenomenon of REM sleep, it is not an important factor in determining inspiratory duration.

Additional evidence provided by recent studies in our laboratory suggests that the overall ventilatory pattern and not just inspiratory duration is determined by central mechanisms,[40] especially in REM sleep. Our studies, for instance, show that in normal sleeping infants both V_T and T_{TOT} decrease with increasing frequency of rapid eye movements.[40] Because the presence of eye movements depends on the occurrence of the centrally generated pontogeniculooccipital (PGO) waves[41–43], our data suggest that alterations in the CNS modulate the ventilatory pattern in REM sleep. This observation is made even more significant by results of previous studies showing that the breathing pattern in REM sleep is independent of a variety of peripheral inputs to the CNS including vagal,[44] chemosensitive,[45] intercostal muscle,[37] and spinal cord afferent[44] systems.

Since minute ventilation can be written as

$$V = \frac{V_T}{T_I} \times \frac{T_I}{T_{TOT}} \times 60$$

there has been an interest in distinguishing between changes in V that are due to alterations in mean inspiratory flow (V_T/T_I), or "respiratory drive," from those due to respiratory duty cycle (T_I/T_{TOT}).[46,47] In both sleep states, we have shown that, as expected, V increases with age in the first several months and that this increase is solely due to an increase in V_T/T_I, T_I/T_{TOT} being unaltered by age.[24,48] Whether the change in V_T/T_I is the result of an increase in respiratory drive or decrease in respiratory impedance (such as an increase in conductance) is not clear, although there is some evidence to suggest the latter.[49]

Analysis of ventilation is not complete without the examination of its variability since mean levels alone do not provide information about changes in ventilation from breath to breath or over periods of time. These changes in ventilation can be critical in newborn and young infants since their gaseous stores are smaller (relative to their metabolic rate) than those in adults and can therefore manifest alterations in blood gas tensions more readily, especially during sleep.[5,50] Studies performed to date have shown that the variability in

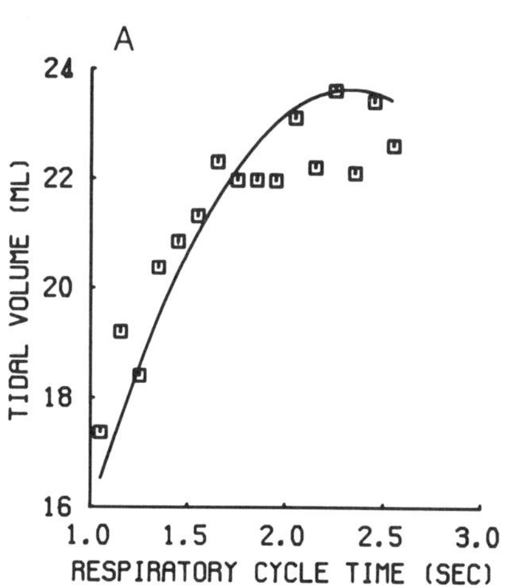

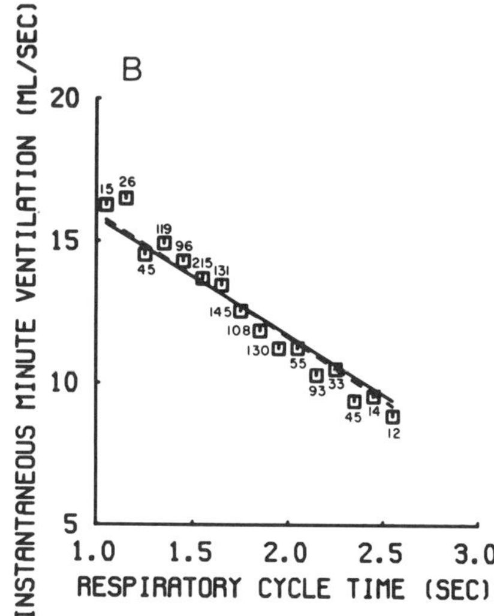

Fig. 4-3 (A) Tidal volume plotted against respiratory cycle time (T_{TOT}) in one infant during sleep. The relation is alinear and at longer T_{TOT} (or lower respiratory frequencies); (B) minute ventilation is decreased. (Haddad GG, Lai TL, Epstein MAF et al : Breath-to-breath variations in rate and depth of ventilation in sleeping infants. Am J Physiol 243: R164, 1982.)

V_T, T_{TOT} and V is 2- to 4-fold greater in REM than in quiet sleep.[24,25] However, the variability of T_I in REM sleep does not seem to be different from that in quiet sleep.[24] Hence the variability of T_{TOT} is primarily due to variability in T_E. This entails that, unlike the off-switching of inspiratory activity, inspiratory on-switching is highly irregular in REM sleep and accounts for a major part of the breathing irregularity found in that state.

Several investigators have previously examined the interrelations between the various parameters of a breath and, in addition to changes in timing, V_T has been shown to vary considerably on a breath to breath basis.[21,24–26,48] Although we agree with Hathorn on some aspects of his analysis,[25,26] we believe that some of our findings are contrary to his because of differences in techniques of data handling. Hathorn showed that V_T and T_{TOT} are positively and linearly related. Our data, on the other hand, show that the regression function of V on T_{TOT} decreases linearly,[24] implying that minute ventilation decreases when respiratory frequency decreases during eupnea (Fig. 4-3). The regression function of V_T on T_{TOT} is therefore of quadratic nature and the amplitude of a breath (V_T) and its duration (T_{TOT}) may not be regulated by the same control mechanisms. There is experimental evidence indeed to suggest that anatomically discrete respiratory nuclei and pathways are primarily responsible for the regulation of either tidal volume or respiratory cycle time.[51–53] How sleep modulates the nature of this relationship is not known. However, the positive relation between V_T and T_{TOT} was lost when one of Dejours' subjects went from wakefulness to sleep.[54] This dissociation between V_T and T_{TOT} can become even more pronounced in certain pathologic states such as in central hypoventilation syndromes of infancy.[55,56]

PERIODIC BREATHING AND APNEA

Although Cheyne-Stokes breathing is only one form of periodic breathing, investigators have tended to group all forms of periodic breathing under the term of Cheyne-Stokes. From a theoretical point of view, this may be attractive. On the other hand, there is no reason to believe that all forms have the same pathogenesis since the pattern of breathing differs from one form to another. For example, the pattern of Biot's breathing is different from that of Cheyne-Stokes.

Because patients with Cheyne-Stokes breathing are clinically unstable, most investigations have been performed in experimental animal and mathematical models.[57–62] These studies[57–59] have shown that there are at least 3 possible explanations for the unstable ventilatory pattern observed in Cheyne-Stokes: (1) an enhanced gain of the respiratory controller, or operation on an alinear portion of the stimulus response curve of the controller; (2) a delay in the transfer of feedback information between the end organ and the controller and sensor; and (3) a decrease in system damping. The gain of the controller can be reflected in the $PaCO_2$ or PaO_2 ventilatory response curve. The transfer of information is probably performed, at least in part, by the circulation. The system buffering capacity depends on the amount of CO_2 and O_2 in the tissues and lungs and the effect of ventilation on these stores.

Premature infants and newcomers to high altitude breathe periodically in a similar manner to Cheyne-Stokes breathing during sleep.[61] Although sleep modifies cardiorespiratory function in a major way, we do not know how sleep induces this type of periodic breathing. However, both premature infants and newcomers to high altitude are relieved of this periodic breathing when the fractional inspired O_2 concentration is increased. This implies that the portion of controller gain due to PaO_2 is enhanced and that the drive to breathing is therefore mainly dependent on the alinear O_2 system, possibly because the sensitivity to CO_2 is decreased.[57–59] Whether sleep changes the circulation time and the size of the gaseous stores is not clear. Since sleep (1) alters cardiac output and systemic vascular reactivity[63,64] and (2) decreases CO_2 production,[65] it might be argued that the gas stores (buffering capacity) and the circulation time (information transfer) may be altered during sleep as well. Full term infants show this periodic breathing almost exclusively in REM sleep and rarely in quiet sleep[66] (unpublished observations from our laboratory) (Fig. 4-4). This contrasts with Bulow's observations and predictions that periodic breathing would occur in quiet sleep in adult humans who have a shift in the CO_2 response curve to the right.[60,61,67] In addition, most infants who show periodic breathing

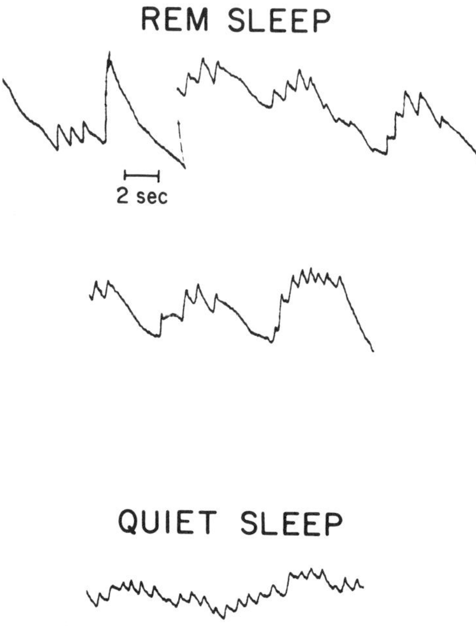

Fig. 4-4 Respiratory waveform (barometric plethysmography) in one normal full-term infant during REM sleep (two upper panels) and during quiet sleep (lower panel) at 17 days of age studied in our laboratory. Note the periodic nature of breathing in REM sleep. (Haddad GG, Mellins RB: Cardiorespiratory aspects of SIDS: An overview. p. 357. In Tildon T, Roeder L, Steinschneider A (eds): Sudden Infant Death Syndrome. Academic Press, New York, 1983.)

are premature, although some are full term.[66] We have rarely seen periodic breathing after the age of 3 to 4 months in normal full-term infants and almost all infants who show periodic breathing have no cardiovascular or neurologic diseases similar to those in the adult with Cheyne-Stokes. Hence, if the pathogenesis and significance of Cheyne-Stokes breathing are not fully understood at the bedside in the adult, they are even less clear in the infant.

The term apnea has been used loosely. The length of the respiratory pause that constitutes an apnea has been ill defined and investigators have considered pauses of >2 to 3 seconds, >6 seconds, >10 seconds, >15 seconds or >20 seconds as apneas.[68–76] Since long respiratory pauses are more likely to be associated with life-threatening alterations of cardiovascular function, it may be more appropriate to categorize respiratory pauses by the presence or absence of simultaneously occurring cardiovascular changes. However, this association has not been studied and, at the moment, respiratory pauses cannot be categorized in this way.

Although there is a great deal of controversy regarding the pathogenesis of respiratory pauses, there is a consensus about certain observations. For instance, normal full-term infants, children and adult humans exhibit respiratory pauses during sleep. Paradoxical as it may seem, we believe that the presence of respiratory pauses and breathing irregularity is a "healthy" sign and that the complete absence of such pauses during sleep may be indicative of abnormalities in the respiratory control system. Actually, extreme regularity of breathing with no pauses occurs in patients with an abnormal behavioral component of the control system.

Independent of age group, respiratory pauses are more prevalent during sleep than during wakefulness. Also, our data and those of others indicate that the frequency and duration of respiratory pauses depend on sleep state in human infants.[68,71,72] Respiratory pauses are more frequent and shorter in REM than in quiet sleep and more frequent in the younger than older infants.[68] Comparisons between children and adults (especially older adults) are not available.

Since the infant has (1) a higher O_2 consumption per unit body weight than the adult and (2) a relatively smaller lung volume and O_2 store, it is possible that short respiratory pauses (on the order of a few seconds each) that may not be clinically important in the adult can present serious consequences in the newborn infant. To date, however, the actual significance of these short pauses, is not known. One reason for this is the technical inadequacy of equipment currently available to measure very fast (seconds) change in blood gas tensions.

Prolonged apneas, on the other hand, can be life-threatening and demand some form of therapy. Comprehensive discussion on the etiology and treatment of prolonged sleep apnea has been given previously.[77–80] Clues to the pathogenesis and possible treatment of prolonged, life-threatening apneas may generally be obtained from answers to questions such as: (1) What are the clinical circumstances of the patient at the time of the generation of these apneas? (2) Are apneic spells associated with cardiovascular (systemic or pulmonary) changes? (3) How chronic has the clinical condition been? (4) In the case of an infant or child, how eventful was the perinatal period? (5) Is the prolonged apnea a result of an increased inhibitory influence or a lack of facilitatory input? (6) Is the etiology central or peripheral?

RESPIRATORY MUSCLES AND SLEEP

The activity of various groups of skeletal muscles, especially postural muscles, has been shown to vary with state of consciousness and sleep state.[43] The activity of respiratory muscles that are crucial to the translation of the central respiratory neural output into airflow, also depends on the neurophysiologic state of the CNS.[39,80–83] It is not surprising therefore that the state of consciousness has a major influence on ventilation through its action on the respiratory musculature. Two examples deserve special note in this regard. First, there is an age-independent, supra-spinal inhibition of alpha-motoneurous in REM sleep.[43,80] As a consequence, the external intercostal muscles (inspiratory muscles) are inhibited. Because (1) external intercostal muscles generally stabilize the chest wall and help the diaphragm during inspiratory efforts and (2)

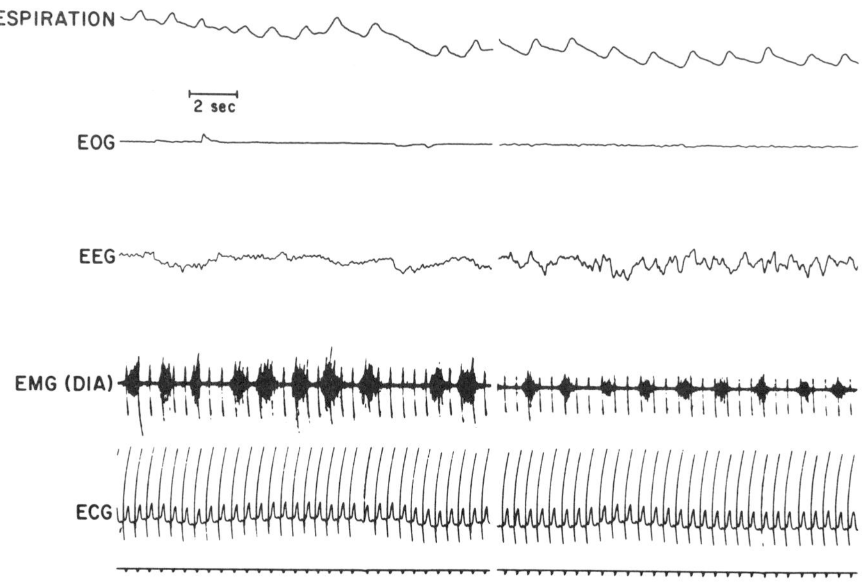

Fig. 4-5 Cardiorespiratory and neurophysiologic signals plotted in time in one infant in REM sleep (left panel) and quiet sleep (right panel) studied in our laboratory. Note the larger electrical activity of the diaphragm [EMG(DIA)] in REM than in quiet sleep.

infants have a very compliant chest wall,[84] the loss of intercostal muscle activity during REM sleep renders the respiratory mechanical system unstable. Young infants, for example, have paradoxical breathing during REM sleep: during inspiration, the chest moves inward at the time when the abdomen moves outward.[38,80,84,85] This type of breathing is inefficient since energy is spent on moving the chest wall inward rather than air into the lungs. Hence, to move a given volume of air into the lungs, young infants generate more pressure and perform more work than do older children and adults. Since the intercostals are inhibited during REM sleep, the extra work of breathing needed is performed by the diaphragm. In support of this notion, Bryan *et al.* have shown on several occasions that the electrical activity of the diaphragm during REM sleep is larger than that during quiet sleep. We have also demonstrated this phenomenon in young infants and an example is represented in Figure 4-5. As a result of this increased load on the diaphragm during REM sleep, diaphragmatic fatigue may occur in newborn infants and may be an important cause of apnea, hypoventilation, and hypercapnia during REM sleep, especially in those premature infants with major respiratory loads such as respiratory distress syndrome, pneumonias, and upper airway obstruction.[81,86,87]

Another example of the influence of the state of consciousness on respiratory function is the effect of sleep state on upper airway muscles and upper airway patency. Several studies have suggested that the motoneurons of the muscles of the upper airways, especially the genioglossal, the palatal and laryngeal, lose their activity during REM sleep.[39,88,89] Since airway patency depends on the activity of these muscles, it becomes evident that REM sleep may provide a neurophysiologic environment that is deleterious to airflow and gas exchange. The biological value of such phenomenon during REM sleep is not apparent. REM sleep, however, is a complex state in which the respiratory muscular system participates in this state's activities. As long as the overall purpose of REM sleep is not clear, it will be difficult to evaluate the benefits and costs to respiratory function during REM sleep.

METABOLIC RATE AND STATE OF CONSCIOUSNESS

With sleep, a decrease in total body metabolic rate occurs.[65] It has also been demonstrated that the metabolic rate is higher in REM than in quiet sleep in both infants and adult humans.[65,90] Since the difference in metabolic rate between quiet and REM sleep is not large, it is possible that the increase is related to the increase in muscular activity that exists during REM sleep. However, we believe that this issue is complicated since studies on adult cats have suggested that profound changes in organ blood flow distribution occur in REM sleep.[64] For instance, brain blood flow increases considerably,[91] iliac artery flow is reduced and mesenteric and renal vascular conductance is augmented.[64] The relation between organ blood flow, O_2 extraction and O_2 consumption has not been well studied during sleep.

Respiratory control in the very young depends critically on metabolism and thermoregulation. We have shown that under certain stresses (such as hypoxia), young puppies decrease rather than increase minute ventilation in order to match it to metabolism which is itself reduced under these circumstances.[34,92] This decrease in ventilation in young subjects contrasts with what has been assumed,[29,93] and does not lead to accumulation of CO_2. There is also evidence suggesting that some apneas occur at a time when metabolism is at its lowest activity, especially during sleep (Dr. Karl Schultz, personal communication).

Another important factor that determines metabolic rate is environmental temperature. During wakefulness, experimental animals increase their O_2 consumption with a reduction in environmental temperature.[94–96] In REM sleep, the sensitivity to changes in environmental temperature is blunted and metabolic rate does not change even after substantial reduction in temperature.[97] In quiet sleep, the response of the same animals is between that of REM sleep and that of wakefulness.[97] An important conclusion from these observations is that studies on respiratory control, especially in the young, should take into consideration not only the state of consciousness but also the metabolic status of the subjects as well as the environmental temperature.

ARTERIAL BLOOD GAS TENSIONS AND STATE OF CONSCIOUSNESS

It has been well documented, especially in the adult, that oxygen saturation may fluctuate and reach low levels during sleep.[2,3,5,89] The lowest levels in O_2 saturation occur in REM sleep and even healthy adult subjects can experience substantial reductions in O_2 saturation in this sleep state.[2] Because there are no means for continuous accurate and precise CO_2 tension measurements, it is not clear whether $PaCO_2$ changes, and if it does, what the magnitude of the change is during these episodes.

Similar fluctuations and reductions in PaO_2 and O_2 saturations are seen in premature infants during REM sleep[5,98] (Dr. C. Bryan, personal communication). The reasons for these reductions are not well understood. However, there are clear differences between REM and quiet sleep and between REM sleep and wakefulness regarding ventilation and cardiovascular functions. Unlike quiet sleep, which produces only mild alterations in the ventilatory output when compared to wakefulness, REM sleep brings about profound changes in ventilation and ventilatory pattern in infants.[21,22,24–26,47] As has been discussed in this chapter, these changes are related in part to the fact that nondiaphragmatic respiratory motoneuron activity is reduced.[40,41,81,85] Other factors that may play a role in influencing blood gas tensions during sleep states are variations in O_2 consumption and changes in lung volume (O_2 stores). Measurable differences in heart rate, cardiac output, mean arterial blood pressure, and regional blood flow to various organs exist between REM and quiet sleep and between REM sleep and wakefulness.[63,64,99–101] How these cardiovascular alterations in REM sleep influence arterial blood gas tensions is not known. It is conceivable, however, that pulmonary blood flow and ventilation/perfusion ratios change with state of consciousness as a consequence. Arterial blood gas tensions in each state may also depend on species. For example, relative to wakefulness and quiet sleep, the dog but not the adult human hyperventilates in REM sleep and reduces its $PaCO_2$ below that of wakefulness.[102]

CHEMOSENSITIVITY TO RESPIRATORY STIMULI

Recent evidence suggests that the ventilatory response to respiratory stimuli matures with age from fetal to adult life.[6,103–105] The response to progressive hypoxia is a good illustration of this developmental process. While the fetus stops initiating respiratory movements when arterial PO_2 is lowered,[6,105] the adult human has a brisk increase in ventilation that levels off after several minutes.[106] The newborn infant's response to a reduction in inspired O_2 concentration, however, is different from those of the fetus and adult.[93,107] All infants, preterm or full term, exhibit a biphasic response when challenged with hypoxia, which is characterized by an initial increase in ventilation followed by a return to baseline or below baseline levels.[93,103,107]

Whether sleep state influences this biphasic response to hypoxia in newborn infants is not known. In addition, the mechanisms responsible for the decrease in ventilation (latter part of the biphasic response) are not well understood. However, recent human and animal studies suggest several possibilities. First, the fall in ventilation may be related to a change in pulmonary mechanics induced by hypoxia.[108] Second, hypoxia may lead to a depression of central respiratory output as measured by phrenic neurogram.[109] The cause of this central respiratory depression is not known. Third, hypoxia leads to a decrease in O_2 consumption and a secondary drop in minute ventilation with no increase in CO_2.[34,92] It might also be noted that although chemoreceptors are active in the fetus and at birth, the "synaptic contacts"[110] of the carotid sinus nerve with the CNS may not be fully mature and the hypoxic depression of the CNS may overwhelm excitatory carotid afferent impulses.

Henderson-Smart and Read,[111] and Jeffrey and Read[112] examined the ventilatory response to progressive hypoxia during sleep in puppies and calves in early life. These studies showed that similar to the response in adults,[113] the response in young animals to progressive hypoxia in REM sleep was not different from that in quiet sleep. These studies cannot be easily compared to those in which the effect of steady levels of hypoxia was examined since the changes in the inhaled gas concentrations in the former are very rapid and only a few breaths generally characterize a given hypoxic level.

Studies examining the steady state ventilatory response to hypoxia which have controlled for state of consciousness or sleep state have been scarce.[33,34] Recent experiments from our laboratory have shown that young and older puppies increased their ventilation in REM sleep in response to hypoxia.[34] In contrast, there was a decrease in ventilation in the younger puppies in quiet sleep (Fig. 4-6). In older puppies, however, ventilation increased with hypoxia in quiet sleep. Therefore, as puppies matured, there was a progressively greater increase in ventilation with hypoxia in quiet sleep. No such maturational changes occurred in REM sleep. Baker and McGinty showed similar results by measuring respiratory frequency in maturing kittens exposed to 10 percent O_2.[33] Their studies showed that hypoxia induced episodes of decreased breathing in quiet sleep but the onset of REM sleep always stimulated breathing. These results in kittens and puppies suggest that REM sleep may provide a more stable environment than quiet sleep in the young when stimulated with hypoxia.

Arousal to a hypoxic stimulus has recently been studied in adult animals and man.[1,12,114] Not surprising is the fact that the level of hypoxia at which arousal occurs varies with species and between subjects within a species.[1,12,114] These studies suggest that although the mechanisms for hypoxic arousal from sleep are complex, the carotid bodies may play a role in some animal species.[12] Of major clinical importance, however, is the observation that most adult human subjects do not arouse to hypoxia even when O_2 saturation falls to low levels such as 70 to 75 percent,[1] saturation levels that can compromise cerebral function. Thus hypoxia may not be an effective arousal stimulus. Similar studies in early life are lacking.

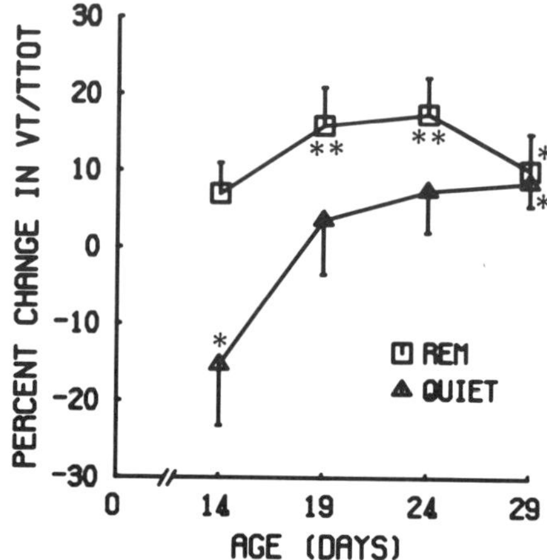

Fig. 4-6 The effect of age and sleep state on ventilatory response to hypoxia. The mean percent change in V_T/T_{TOT} ($FIO_2 = 0.15$) is plotted against age in puppies studied in both REM and quiet sleep. Note that there is an increase in V_T/T_{TOT} in response to hypoxia in REM sleep at all ages but an increase in V_T/T_{TOT} in quiet sleep only at 29 days of age. (Haddad GG, Gandi MR, Mellins RB: Maturation of ventilatory response to hypoxia in puppies during sleep. J Appl Physiol 52:309, 1982.)

CO_2 has been used as a respiratory stimulant in early life in both REM and quiet sleep and studies of responses to both transient progressive increase in CO_2 and steady level CO_2 have been performed.[115–117,23] Our studies on normal infants have shown that the percent increase in ventilation in response to a steady level of CO_2 is virtually the same in both sleep states.[23] Other studies examining the effect of progressively administered CO_2 have demonstrated that the response to CO_2 is depressed in REM sleep, especially during periods characterized by phasic events.[102,112] The mechanisms for this depression in CO_2 responsiveness are not clear. However, in premature infants, uncoupling of thoracoabdominal movements during CO_2 challenge may be at the basis of this depressed ventilatory response.

CLINICAL IMPLICATIONS

Sleep, when compared to wakefulness, seems to represent a form of stress. While there is little doubt that the normal human adult and infant cope well with this form of stress, the subject with lung, chest wall or muscle disease and the very young or premature infant may not be able to sustain such a challenge. The following section describes some clinical conditions that are encountered in infants and children and are probably related to mechanisms that determine cardiorespiratory function during sleep.

Upper Airway Obstruction

Upper airway obstruction (UAO) during sleep is being recognized with increasing frequency in children, from early infancy on to adolescence. In contrast to adults with UAO in whom the etiology of obstruction often remains obscure, many children have anatomic abnormalities that often prove to be the cause of their UAO. A common cause of upper airway obstruction in children is tonsillar and adenoidal hypertrophy due to repeated upper respiratory infections.[118] Other abnormalities include craniofacial malformations (Crouzon's disease), micrognathia (Pierre Robin syndrome) and muscular hypotonia.[118]

The usual site of obstruction in UAO in both infants and adults seems to be the oropharynx, between the posterior pharyngeal wall, the soft palate and the genioglossus.[89,119–122] During sleep (especially REM sleep) upper airway muscles, including those of the oropharynx, lose tone and provide the "medium" to trigger an episode of UAO. It is possible, as has been shown in some animal preparations, that some of these UAO episodes start as central apneas and revert to obstructive episodes. The basis for this change in the nature of the apneic episode is likely to be a difference in PaO_2 or $PaCO_2$ chemosensitivity between the diaphragm and upper airway muscles including the genioglossus.[123–129] Because the sensitivity threshold may be lower for the diaphragm, suction forces by the contracting diaphragm can induce an episode of UAO.[125,129] This is especially the case when the stimulus is not potent enough to induce activity in the upper airway muscles or arousal.

Snoring with recurrent periods of respiratory pauses are commonly present during sleep in children.[124,130] These episodes are more frequent or exaggerated in the presence of upper respiratory infection. Parents will frequently describe periods of increasing chest wall movement without airflow and with cyanosis. These pauses are usually terminated by a loud snort and arousal. Associated with UAO are disturbed sleeping habits including restlessness and arousals from sleep during the night. In older children the syndrome complex may include enuresis, failure to thrive, developmental delays, and poor school performance.[130] Obesity and daytime hypersomnolence are less common in children than in adults with UAO.

Although children with UAO may present to the pediatrician in the early stages of the disease with the chief complaint (expressed by parents) of loud snoring, they may also present with long-standing signs and symptoms of UAO during sleep, right ventricular failure, and cor pulmonale.[118,130] The treatment therefore will vary but should be targeted primarily at the underlying cause of obstruction. Some of these infants will benefit simply by tonsillectomy and adenoidectomy.[118] Others will not be relieved by this operation. In some of these refractory children, successful treatment in our institution has included the chronic insertion of a soft nasopharyngeal tube to ensure a patent oropharyngeal space. This is similar in principle to the reversal of obstructive sleep apnea successfully achieved in adults by continuous positive airway pressure applied through the nose.[131] In some infants in which other means have

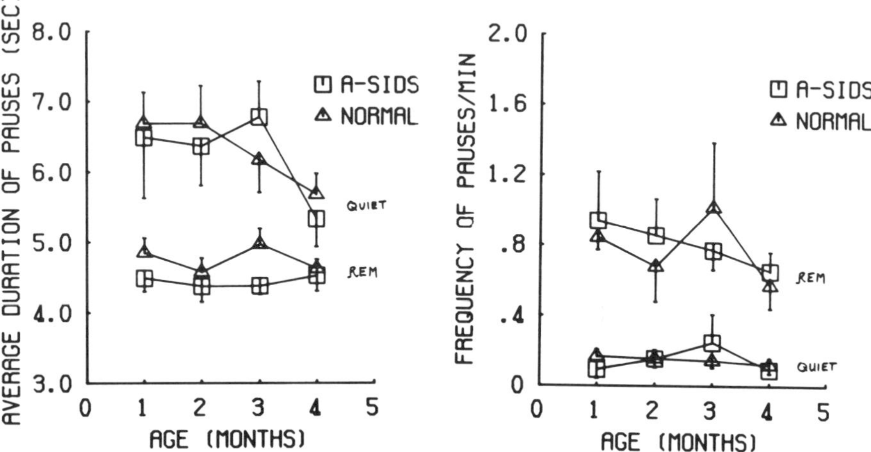

Fig. 4-7 Average duration and frequency of respiratory pauses plotted against age in the first 4 months of life in both REM and quiet sleep in normal full-term infants and age-matched aborted SIDS infants (A-SIDS). Note that differences for both variables exist between sleep states but not between the two infant populations. (Bazzy AR, Haddad GG, Chang SL, Mellins RB: Respiratory pauses during sleep in near-miss sudden infant death syndrome. Am Rev Respir Dis 128:973, 1983.)

failed, it is worthwhile to intervene pharmacologically (respiratory stimulants) before resorting to surgery and chronic tracheostomy.

Sudden Infant Death Syndrome

Sudden infant death syndrome (SIDS) is not an uncommon disorder, occurring between the ages of 1 month and 1 year, with a peak incidence at 2 to 3 months of age. Death occurs in an infant whose clinical history, physical examination, and thorough postmortem study are unremarkable and do not disclose the cause of demise. The terminal episode is presumed to occur during sleep. By definition therefore, normal defense mechanisms have failed in SIDS victims. Many investigators have been led to suspect that these infants have abnormal control systems. In this regard, the cardiorespiratory control system has been probed and cardiorespiratory function examined in various infant populations believed to be at high risk for SIDS. Conflicting data and views, however, have emerged in almost every aspect studied.[66,132] For example, some investigators have shown that high risk infants exhibit prolonged and more frequent respiratory pauses and more numerous episodes of periodic breathing,[73,133–135] whereas others have not (Fig. 4-7).[68,136,137] Similarly, investigators have not agreed on the presence or absence of airway obstruction, decreased responsiveness to CO_2, cardiac arrhythmias, etc.[67,138,139]

Several review articles have appeared on SIDS in the past 2 years in which the results of relevant studies have been summarized and discussed.[67,140–142] Today, SIDS is still an unclassified syndrome the pathophysiology of which seems to involve the cardiorespiratory control system. Abnormalities in the autonomic nervous system and in arousal from sleep have been proposed.[66,133,142] Much remains to be learned of the normal development of cardiorespiratory control.[23,143–145]

Alveolar Hypoventilation Syndromes

There are several forms of alveolar hypoventilation syndrome; the common denominator among them is severe hypoventilation during sleep.[48,146] Riley-Day syndrome and Leigh's subacute necrotizing encephalomyelopathy should constitute part of the differential diagnosis of alveolar hypoventilation syndrome in infants and children.[48]

The etiology of these syndromes is believed to be a defect in the central neural regulation of breathing during sleep. The site of the pathology is not known. Although hypoventilation can develop in patients after CNS infections such as bulbar poliomyelitis,[146] many of these patients are symptomless before hypoventilation develops.[55,146] Mellins et al. described an infant with a severe form of Ondine's curse or failure of automatic control of breathing.[146] We subsequently described a variant of this congenital form in three cases who, in addition to severe alveolar hypoventilation, had Hirschsprung's disease (abnormal control of gastrointestinal motility) and a fixed and rapid heart rate.[55] Since the initial report we have learned of a dozen such cases from the literature or from personal communications. Although heart rate and heart rate variability are abnormal in these patients in all states of consciousness, they hypoventilate primarily in quiet sleep. In fact they can have a normal $PaCO_2$ in wakefulness and a near normal one in REM sleep,[55] and it is during these two states that they can be weaned off the ventilator. $PaCO_2$, however, can rise to considerable levels (over 70 to 80 mmHg) in quiet sleep. By analogy to the circulation, this may be called "persistent fetal ventilation" since it is only during quiet sleep that these infants hypoventilate, a state during which the fetus is normally in near complete respiratory silence.[7,10,15]

In summary, there is increased clinical awareness that life-threatening apnea and upper airway obstruction do occur in infants and children during sleep and that these episodes can result in clinically serious cardiovascular complications as early as in infancy.

REFERENCES

1. Berthon-Jones M, Sullivan CE: Ventilatory and arousal responses to hypoxia in sleeping humans. Am Rev Respir Dis 126:632, 1982
2. Block AJ, Boysen PG, Wynne JW et al : Sleep apnea, hypopnea and oxygen desaturation in normal subjects. N Engl J Med 300:513, 1979

3. Douglas NJ, Calverly PMA, Leggett RGE: Transient hypoxemia during sleep in chronic bronchitis and emphysema. Lancet 1:1, 1979
4. Chipps BE, Mak H, Schuberth KC et al : Nocturnal oxygen saturation in normal and asthmatic children. Pediatrics 65:1157, 1980
5. Hanson N, Okken A: Transcutaneous oxygen tension of newborn infants in different behavioral states. Pediatr Res 14:911, 1980
6. Boddy K, Dawes GS, Fisher R: Foetal respiratory movements, electrocortical and cardiovascular responses to hypoxia and hypercapnia in sheep. J Physiol (London) 243:599, 1974
7. Bowes G, Adamson TM, Ritchie BC et al : Development of patterns of respiratory activity in unanesthetized fetal sheep in utero. J Appl Physiol 50:693, 1981
8. Bystrzycka E, Nail BS, Purves MJ: Central and peripheral neural respiratory activity in the mature sheep foetus and newborn lamb. Respir Physiol 25:199, 1975
9. Chapman RLK, Dawes GS, Rurak DW, Wilds PL: Breathing movements in fetal lambs and the effect of hypercapnia. J Physiol (London) 302:19, 1980
10. Maloney JE, Adamson TM, Brodecky V et al : Modification of respiratory center output in the unanesthetized foetal sheep in utero. J Appl Physiol 39:552, 1975
11. Boddy K, Robinson JS: External method for detection of fetal breathing in utero. Lancet 2:1231, 1971
12. Bowes G, Townsend ER, Kozar LF et al : Effect of carotid body denervation on arousal response to hypoxia in sleeping dogs. J Appl Physiol 51:40, 1981b
13. Patrick J, Natale R, Richardson B: Patterns of human fetal breathing activity at 34–35 weeks gestational age. Am J Obstet Gynecol 132:507, 1978
14. Trudinger BJ, Lewis PJ, Magez J, O'Connor E: Fetal breathing movements in high risk pregnancy. Br J Obstet Gynaecol 85:662, 1978
15. Dawes GS, Fox HE, Leduc BM et al : Respiratory movements and rapid eye movement sleep in the foetal sheep. J Physiol (London) 220:119, 1972
16. Rigatto H, Moore M, Horvath L et al.: Direct observation of the fetus in the chronic sheep preparation using a double wall plexiglass window. Fed Proc 42:1251, 1983
17. Ioffe S, Jansen AH, Chernick V: EcoG and breathing activity in fetal lambs after undercut of the cerebral cortex. J Appl Physiol (In press)
18. Mellins RB, Haddad GG: Respiratory control in early life: An overview. p. 3. In Sutton J, Houston C, Jones, N (eds): Hypoxia, Exercise and Altitude. Alan R. Liss, New York, 1983
19. Dement WC, Kleitman N: Cyclic variations in EEG during sleep and their relation to eye movements, body motility, and dreaming. Electroenceph Clin Neurophysiol 9:673, 1957
20. Kleitman N, Engelmann TG: Sleep characteristics of infants. J Appl Physiol 6:269, 1953
21. Bolton DPG, Herman S: Ventilation and sleep state in the newborn. J Physiol 240:67, 1974
22. Haddad GG, Epstein RA, Epstein MAF et al : Maturation of ventilation and ventilatory pattern in normal sleeping infants. J Appl Physiol 46:998, 1979
23. Haddad GG, Leistner HL, Epstein RA et al : CO_2-induced changes in ventilation and ventilatory pattern in normal sleeping infants. J Appl Physiol 48:684, 1980
24. Haddad GG, Lai TL, Epstein MAF et al : Breath-to-breath variations in rate and depth of ventilation in sleeping infants. Am J Physiol 243:R164, 1982

25. Hathorn MKS: The rate and depth of breathing in new-born infants in different sleep states. J Physiol (London) 243:101, 1974
26. Hathorn MKS: Analysis of the rhythm of infantile breathing. Br Med Bull 31:8, 1975
27. Aserinsky E: Periodic respiratory pattern occurring in conjunction with eye movements during sleep. Science 150:764, 1965
28. Finer NN, Abroms IF, Taeusch HW: Ventilation and sleep states in newborn infants. J Pediatr 89:100, 1976
29. Askanazi J, Silverberg PA, Foster RJ, Hyman AI, Milic-Emili J, Kinney JM: Effects of respiratory apparatus on breathing pattern. J Appl Physiol 48:557, 1980
30. Gilbert R, Auchincloss JH, Brodsky J, Boden W: Changes in tidal volume, frequency and ventilation induced by their measurement. J Appl Physiol 33:252, 1974
31. Remmers JE, Bartlett D Jr, Putnam MD: Changes in the respiratory cycle associated with sleep. Respir Physiol 28:227, 1976
32. Tabachnik E, Muller NL, Bryan AC, Levison H: Changes in ventilation and chest wall mechanics during sleep in normal adolescents. J Appl Physiol 51:557, 1981
33. Baker TL, McGinty DJ: Reversal of cardiopulmonary failure during active sleep in hypoxic kittens: Implications for sudden infant death. Science 199:419, 1977
34. Haddad GG, Gandhi MR, Mellins RB: Maturation of ventilatory response to hypoxia in puppies during sleep. J Appl Physiol 52:309, 1982
35. Miserocchi G, Milic-Emili J: Effect of mechanical factors on the relation between rate and depth of breathing in cats. J Appl Physiol 41:277, 1976
36. Phillipson EA: Regulation of breathing during sleep. Am Rev Resp Dis 115(Suppl.):217, 1977
37. Thach BT, Abroms IF, Frantz ID et al : Intercostal muscle reflexes and sleep breathing patterns in the human infant. J Appl Physiol 48:139, 1980
38. Knill R, Bryan AC: An intercostal-phrenic inhibitory reflex in human newborn infants. J Appl Physiol 40:352, 1976
39. Orem J, Netick A, Dement WC: Increased upper-airway resistance to breathing during sleep in the cat. Electroencephalog Clin Neurophysiol 43:14, 1977
40. Haddad GG, Lai TL, Mellins RB: Determination of ventilatory pattern in REM sleep in normal infants. J Appl Physiol 53:52, 1982
41. McGinty DJ, Harper RM, Fairbanks MK: Neuronal unit activity and the control of sleep states. Adv Sleep Res 1:173, 1974
42. Orem J: Medullary respiratory neuron activity: Relationship to tonic and phasic REM sleep. J Appl Physiol 48:54, 1980
43. Pompaeino O: The neurophysiological mechanisms of the postural and motor events during desynchronized sleep. p. 351. In Kety S, Evarts E, Williams H (eds): Sleep and Altered States of Consciousness. Williams and Wilkins, Baltimore, 1967
44. Foutz AS, Netick A, Dement WC: Sleep state effects on breathing after spinal cord transection and vagotomy in the cat. Respir Physiol 37:89, 1979
45. Guazzi M, Freis ED: Sinoaortic reflexes and arterial pH, PO_2, and PCO_2 in wakefulness and sleep. Am J Physiol 217:1623, 1969
46. Grunstein MM, Milic-Emili J: Analysis of interactions between central and vagal respiratory control mechanisms in cats. IEEE Trans Biomed Eng 25:225, 1978
47. Milic-Emili J, Grunstein MM: Drive and timing components of ventilation. Chest 70:1341, 1976
48. Haddad GG, Epstein RA, Epstein MAF et al : Breath-to-breath control of ventilation in normal infants during sleep. p. 85. In Fitzgerald R, Gautier H, Lahiri

S (eds): The Regulation of Respiration during Sleep and Anesthesia. Plenum, New York, 1978

49. Stocks J, Godfrey S: Specific airway conductance in relation to postconceptional age during infancy. J Appl Physiol 43:144, 1977
50. Haddad GG, Mellins RB: Hypoxia and respiratory control in early life. Ann Rev Physiol 46:629, 1984
51. von Euler C, Herrero F, Wexler I: Control mechanisms determining rate and depth of respiratory movements. Respir Physiol 10:93, 1970
52. Guz A, Nobel MIM, Widdicombe JG et al : The effect of bilateral block of vagus and glossopharyngeal nerves on the ventilatory responses to CO_2 of conscious man. Resp Physiol 1:206, 1966
53. Kreiger AJ, Christensen HD, Sapru HN, Wang SC: Changes in ventilatory patterns after ablation of various respiratory feedback mechanisms. J Appl Physiol 33:431, 1972
54. Dejours P, Puccinelli R, Armand J, Dicharry M: Breath-to-breath variations of pulmonary gas exchange in resting man. Resp Physiol 1:265, 1966
55. Haddad GG, Mazza NM, Defendini R et al : Congenital failure of automatic control of ventilation, gastrointestinal motility and heart rate. Medicine 57:517, 1978
56. Shannon DC, Marsland DW, Gould JB et al : Central hypoventilation during quiet sleep in two infants. Pediatrics 57:342, 1976
57. Cherniack NS, Longobardo GS: Cheyne–Stokes breathing. N Engl J Med 288:952, 1973
58. Cherniack NS, Von Euler C, Hamma I, Kao FF: Experimentally induced Cheyne–Stokes breathing. Respir Physiol 37:185, 1979
59. Cherniack NS, von Euler C, Hamma I, Kao F: Animal models of Cheyne–Stokes breathing. p. 417. In von Euler C, Lagercrantz H (eds): Central Nervous Control Mechanisms in Breathing. Pergamon, Oxford, 1979
60. Cherniack NS, Longobardo GS: Cheyne–Stokes Breathing. N Engl J Med 305:325, 1981
61. Cherniack NS: Respiratory dysrhythmias during sleep. N Engl J Med 305:325, 1981
62. Waggener TB, Frantz III ID, Stark AR, Kronauer RC: Oscillatory breathing patterns leading to apneic spells in infants. J Appl Physiol 52:1288, 1982
63. Khatri IM, Freis ED: Hemodynamic changes during sleep. J Appl Physiol 22:867, 1967
64. Mancia G, Baccelli G, Adams DB, Zanchetti A: Vasomotor regulation during sleep in the cat. Am J Physiol 220:1086, 1970
65. Brebbia DR, Altshuler KZ: Oxygen consumption rate and electroencephalographic stage of sleep. Science 150:1621, 1965
66. Haddad GG, Mellins RB: Cardiorespiratory aspects of SIDS: An overview. p. 357. In Tildon T, Roeder L, Steinschneider A (eds): Sudden Infant Death Syndrome. Academic Press, New York 1983
67. Bulow K: Respiration and wakefulness in man. Acta Physiol Scand 59(Suppl. 209):77, 1963
68. Bazzy AR, Haddad GG, Chang SL, Mellins RB: Respiratory pauses during sleep in near-miss sudden infant death syndrome. Am Rev Respir Dis 128:973, 1983
69. Carse EA, Wilkinson AR, Whyte PL et al : Oxygen and carbon dioxide tensions, breathing and heart rate in normal infants during the first six months of life. J Dev Physiol 3:85, 1981

70. Daily WJR, Klaus M, Meyer HBP: Apnea in premature infants: Monitoring, incidence, heart rate changes, and an effect of environmental temperature. Pediatrics 43:510, 1969
71. Gabriel M, Albani M, Schulte EJ: Apneic spells and sleep states in preterm infants. Pediatrics 57:142, 1976
72. Guilleminault C, Peraita R, Souquet M, Dement WC: Apneas during sleep in infants: Possible relationship with sudden infant death syndrome. Science 190:677, 1975
73. Guilleminault C, Eldridge FL, Simmons FB, Dement WC: Sleep apnea in eight children. Pediatrics 58;23, 1976
74. Henderson-Smart DJ: The effect of gestational age on the incidence and duration of recurrent apnoea in newborn babies. Aust Paediatr J 17:273, 1981
75. Hoppenbrouwers T, Harper RM, Hodgman JE et al : Polygraphic studies of norman infants during the first six months of life. II. Respiratory rate and variability as a function of state. Pediat Res 12:120, 1978
76. Stein IM, White A, Kennedy JL Jr et al.: Apnea Recordings of healthy infants at 40, 44 and 52 weeks postconception. Pediatrics 63:724, 1979
77. Aranda JV, Turmen T: Methylxanthines in apnea of prematurity. Clin Perinatol 6:87, 1979
78. Kattwinkel J: Neonatal apnea: Pathogenesis and therapy. J Pediat 90:342, 1977
79. Rigatto H: Respiratory control and apnea in the newborn infant. Crit Care Med 5:2, 1977
80. Schulte FJ, Busse C, Eichhorn W: Rapid eye movement sleep, motoneurone inhibition and apneic spells in preterm infants. Pediatr Res 111:709, 1977
81. Muller N, Gulston G, Cade D et al : Diaphragmatic muscle fatigue in the newborn. J Appl Physiol 46:688, 1979
82. Sauerland EK, Mitchell SP: Electromyographic activity of intrinsic and extrinsic muscles of the human tongue. Tex Rep Biol Med 33:445, 1975
83. Sauerland EK, Harper RM: The human tongue during sleep: Electromyographic activity of the genioglossus muscle. Exp Neurol 51:160, 1976
84. Bryan MH, Mansell AL, Levison H: Development of the mechanical properties of the respiratory system. p. 445. In Hodson WA (ed): Development of the Lung. Dekker, New York, 1977
85. Bryan MH, Bryan AC: Respiration during sleep in infants. p. 457. In von Euler C, Lagercrantz H (eds): Central Nervous Control Mechanisms in Breathing. Pergamon, Oxford, 1979
86. Lopes JM, Muller NL, Bryan MH, Bryan AC: Synergistic behavior of inspiratory muscles after diaphragmatic fatigue in the newborn. J Appl Physiol 51:547, 1981
87. Muller N, Volgyesi G, Eng P et al : The consequences of diaphragmatic muscle fatigue in the newborn infant. J Pediatr 95:793, 1979
88. Remmers JE, deGroot WJ, Sauerland EK, Anch AM: Pathogenesis of upper-airway occlusion during sleep. J Appl Physiol 44:931, 1978
89. Remmers JE, Anch AM, deGroot WJ: Respiratory disturbances during sleep. Clin Chest Med 1:57, 1980
90. Stothers JK, Warner RM: Oxygen consumption and neonatal sleep states. J Physiol (London) 278:435, 1978
91. Reivich M, Isaacs G, Evarts E, Kety S: The effect of slow wave sleep and REM sleep on regional cerebral blood flow in cats. J Neurochem 15:301, 1968

92. Haddad GG, Gandhi MR, Mellins RB: O_2 consumption during hypoxia in sleeping puppies. Am Rev Respir Dis 123:183, 1981
93. Rigatto H, Brady JP, Verduzco RT: Chemoreceptor reflexes in preterm infants: I. The effect of gestational and postnatal age on the ventilatory response to inhalation of 100% and 15% oxygen. Pediatrics 55:604, 1975
94. Hey EN: The relation between environmental temperature and oxygen consumption in the new-born baby. J Physiol (London) 200:589, 1969
95. Hill JR: The oxygen consumption of newborn and adult mammals. Its dependence on the oxygen tension in the inspired air and on the environmental temperature. J Physiol (London) 149:346, 1959
96. Hill JR, Rahimtulla KA: Heat balance and the metabolic rate of newborn babies in relation to environmental temperature; and the effect of age and of weight on basal metabolic rate. J Physiol (London) 180:239, 1965
97. Glotzbach SF, Heller HC: Central nervous regulation of body temperature during sleep. Science 194:537, 1976
98. Martin RJ, Okkew A, Rubin D: Arterial oxygen tension during active and quiet sleep in the normal neonate. J Pediatr 94:271, 1979
99. Baust W, Bohnert B: The regulation of heart rate during sleep. Exp Brain Res 7:169, 1969
100. Guazzi M, Zanchetti A: Blood pressure and heart rate during natural sleep of the cat and their regulation by carotid sinus and aortic reflexes. Arch Ital Biol 103:789, 1965
101. Snyder F, Hobson JA, Morrison DF, Goldfrank F: Changes in respiration, heart rate, and systolic blood pressure in human sleep. J Appl Physiol 19:417, 1964
102. Phillipson EA, Kozar LF, Rebuck AS, Murphy E: Ventilatory and waking responses to CO_2 in sleeping dogs. Am Rev Respir Dis 115:251, 1977
103. Rigatto H: A critical analysis of the development of peripheral and central respiratory chemosensitivity during the neonatal period. p. 137. In von Euler C, Langercrantz H (eds): Central Nervous Control Mechanisms in Breathing. Pergamon, Oxford, 1979
104. Sankaran K, Wiebe H, Seshia MMK et al : Immediate and late ventilatory response to high and low O_2 in preterm infants and adults subjects. Pediatr Res 13:875, 1979
105. Towell ME, Salvador HS: Intrauterine asphyxia and respiratory movements in the fetal goat. Am J Obstet Gynecol 118:1124, 1974
106. Kagawa S, Stafford MJ, Waggener TB, Severinghaus JW: No effect of naloxone on hypoxia-induced ventilatory depression in adults. J Appl Physiol 52:1030, 1982
107. Cross KS, Oppe TW: The effect of inhalation of high and low concentrations of oxygen on the respiration of the premature infant. J Physiol (London) 117:38, 1952
108. Woodrum DE, Sandaert TA, Mayock DE, Guthrie RD: Hypoxic ventilatory response in the newborn monkey. Pediatr Res 15:367, 1981
109. Lawson EE, Long WA: Central origin of biphasic breathing pattern during hypoxia in newborns. J Appl Physiol 55:483, 1983
110. Lahiri S, Brody JS, Motoyama EK, Velasquez TM: Regulation of breathing in newborns at high altitude. J Appl Physiol 44:673, 1978
111. Henderson-Smart DJ, Read DJC: Ventilatory response to hypoxaemia during sleep in the newborn. J Dev Physiol 1:195, 1979
112. Jeffrey HE, Read DJC: Ventilatory responses of newborn calves to progressive hypoxia in quiet and active sleep. J Appl Physiol 48:892, 1980

113. Phillipson EA, Sullivan CE, Read DJC et al : Ventilation and waking responses to hypoxia in sleeping dogs. J Appl Physiol 44:512, 1978
114. Neubauer JA, Santiago TV, Edelman NM: Hypoxic arousal in intact and carotid chemodenervated sleeping cats. J Appl Physiol 51:1294, 1981
115. Anderson JV, Martin RJ, Abboud EF et al : Transient ventilatory response to CO_2 as a function of sleep state in full term infants. J Appl Physiol 54:1482, 1983
116. Frantz ID, Adler SM, Thach BT, Taeush HW: Maturational effects on respiratory responses to carbon dioxide in premature infants. J Appl Physiol 41:41, 1976
117. Guthrie RD, Standaert TA, Hodson WA, Woodrum DE: Development of CO_2 sensitivity: Effect of gestational age, postnatal age and sleep state. Pediatr Res 13:535, 1979
118. Brouillette RT, Fernbach SK, Hunt CE: Obstructive sleep apnea in infants and children. J Pediatr 100:31, 1982
119. Stark AR, Thach BT: Mechanisms of airway obstruction leading to apnea in newborn infants. J Pediatr 89:982, 1976
120. Stark AR, Thach BT: Recovery of airway patency after obstruction in normal infants. Am Rev Respir Dis 123:691, 1981
121. Thach BT, Brouillette RT: The respiratory function of pharyngeal musculature: Relevance to clinical obstructive apnea. p. 483. In von Euler C, Langercrantz H (eds): Central Nervous Control Mechanisms in Breathing, Pergamon, Oxford, 1979
122. Thach BT, Stark AR: Spontaneous neck flexion and airway obstruction during apneic spells in preterm infants. J Pediatr 94:275, 1979
123. Bartlett Jr D: Effects of hypercapnia and hypoxia on laryngeal resistance to airflow. Respir Physiol 37:293, 1979
124. Brouillette RT, Thach BT: Control of genioglossus muscle inspiratory activity. J Appl Physiol 49:801, 1980
125. Cherniack NS, Longobardo GS, Gothe B, Weiner D. Interactive effects of central and obstructive apnea. p. 553. In Kutas I, Debreczeni LA (eds): Advances in Physiological Sciences, Respiration in CO_2 Storage in Tissues. Pergamon, New York, 1981
126. Longobardo GS, Gothe B, Goldman MD, Cherniack NS: Sleep apnea considered as a control system instability. Respir Physiol 50:311, 1982
127. Strohl KP, Hensley MJ, Hallett M et al.: Activation of upper airway muscles before onset of inspiration in normal humans. J Appl Physiol 49:638, 1980
128. Weiner DJ, Salamone MJ, Nochomovitz M, Cherniack NS: The effect of chemical drive on the electrical activity and force of contraction of the tongue and chest wall muscles. Am Rev Respir Dis 121S:418, 1980
129. Weiner DJ, Salamone MJ, Cherniack NS: Effect of chemical stimuli on nerves supplying upper airway muscles. J Appl Physiol 52:530, 1982
130. Guilleminault C, Korobkin R, Winkle R: A review of 50 children with obstructive sleep apnea syndrome. Lung 159:275, 1981
131. Sullivan CE, Berthon-Jones M, Issa FG, Eves L: Reversal of obstructive sleep apnoea by continuous positive airway pressure applied through the nares. Lancet 1:862, 1981
132. Haddad GG, Leistner HL, Lai TL, Mellins RB: Ventilation and ventilatory pattern during sleep in aborted sudden infant death syndrome. Pediatr Res 15:879, 1981
133. Curzi-Dascalova L, Flores-Guevara R, Guidasci S et al.: Respiratory frequency during sleep in siblings of sudden infant death syndrome victims. Early Hum Dev 8:235, 1983

134. Kelly DH: Incidence of severe apnea and death in infants identified at high risk for sudden infant death syndrome. p. 607. In Tildon T, Roeder L, Steinschneider H (eds): Sudden Infant Death Syndrome. Academic Press, New York, 1983
135. Shannon DC: A quantitative approach to defects in control of the respiratory and cardiovascular systems in SIDS. p. 341. In Tildon T, Roeder L, Steinschneider A (eds): Sudden Infant Death Syndrome, Academic Press, New York, 1983
136. Hodgman JE, Hoppenbrouwers T: Cardio-respiratory behavior in infants at increased, epidemiological risk for SIDS. p. 669. In Tildon T, Roeder L, Steinschneider A (eds): Sudden Infant Death Syndrome, Academic Press, New York, 1983
137. Southall DP, Richards JM, Shinebourne EA: Prospective population-based studies into heart rate and breathing patterns in newborn infants: Prediction of infants at risk of SIDS? p. 621. In Tildon T, Roeder L, Steinschneider A (eds): Sudden Infant Death Syndrome, Academic Press, New York, 1983
138. Schwartz PJ: Autonomic nervous system, ventricular fibrillation, and SIDS. p. 319. In Tildon T, Roeder L, Steinschneider A (eds): Sudden Infant Death Syndrome, Academic Press, New York, 1983
139. Thach BT: The role of pharyngeal airway obstruction in prolonging infantile apneic spells. p. 279. In Tildon T, Roeder L, Steinschneider A (eds): Sudden Infant Death Syndrome, Academic Press, New York, 1983
140. Mellins RB, Haddad GG: Sudden Infant Death Syndrome. p. 1770. In Behrman RE, Vaughn III CVC (eds): Nelson Textbook of Pediatrics, 12th Edition. W.B. Saunders, Philadelphia, 1983
141. Mellins RB, Haddad GG: Cardiorespiratory control in sudden infant death syndrome. p. 51. In Sutton J, Houston C, Jones N (eds): Hypoxia, Exercise and Altitude. Alan R. Liss, New York, 1983
142. Shannon DC, Kelly DH: SIDS and near-SIDS. N Engl J Med 306:959, 1982
143. Guilleminault C, Ariagno RL: Why should we study the infant "near miss for sudden infant death." Early Hum Dev 213:207, 1978
144. Haddad GG, Epstein RA, Epstein MAF et al : The R-R interval and R-R variability in normal infants during sleep. Pediatr Res 14:809, 1980
145. Hoppenbrouwers T, Hodgman JE, Arakawa K et al : Respiration during the first six months of life in normal infants. III. Computer identification of breathng pauses. Pediatr Res 14:1230, 1980
146. Mellins RB, Balfour HH, Turino GM, Winters RW: Failure of automatic control of ventilation (Ondine's curse). Medicine 49:487, 1970

5 Sleep and Breathing During Hypoxia

Jerome Dempsey
Anne Berssenbrugge
James Skatrud

The combination of sleep and arterial hypoxemia presents many varied and interactive effects on the ventilatory control system (Table 5-1). On one hand, sleep state or loss of wakefulnesss exerts significant, inhibitory effects on several critical determinants of ventilatory regulation. These include suppressed influences from the higher central nervous system (CNS) on the neuronal output of inspiratory neurons in the brain stem and a reduced level of activity to both major inspiratory skeletal muscles in the chest wall and to those muscles that control upper airway resistance. These effects may be manifested, as will be shown, in truly fundamental changes in ventilatory responses to specific perturbations imposed during sleep. Hypoxemia, on the other hand, exerts a host of both excitatory and inhibitory effects on ventilatory control (Table 5-1). The net effect of acute hypoxemia is, of course, an excitatory one (in normal adults) as carotid sinus nerve input and ventilation increase in a curvilinear fashion with increasing hypoxemia. This dominant excitatory action is opposed by inhibitory feedback actions of respiratory alkalosis as peripheral chemoreceptor PCO_2 ($PaCO_2$) falls because of alveolar hyperventilation and medullary chemoreceptor PCO_2 ($P_{cereb.ECF}CO_2$) is reduced even further because of hypoxic-induced cerebral vasodilation and increased blood flow. An additional so-called direct central depressant effect of cerebral hypoxia on respiratory center neurons may also exert some additional inhibitory effects attributable to cerebral respiratory alkalosis. The inhibitory cerebral respiratory alkalosis may be counteracted to some extent by augmented cerebral tissue

Table 5-1. Potential Influences of Sleep State and Hypoxemia on the Regulation of Breathing

Sleep State
Inhibition of suprapontine influences on the output and gain of brain stem inspiratory neurons.
Reduced innervation of diaphragm and intercostals.
Reduced innervation of upper airway skeletal muscles.
Hypoxemia
Acute Hypoxemia
Excitatory
Increased carotid sinus nerve activity with curvilinear response and progressively increasing gain.
Increased CNS metabolic acid production and brain ECF [H+] (hypocapnia and severe hypoxia).
Inhibitory
CNS and systemic alkalosis ($\downarrow$ $PaCO_2$ and $\uparrow$ cerebral blood flow).
CNS hypoxia ("direct" effect?).
Carotid sinus nerve efferent activity.
Interactions
Of hypoxemia and alkalosis at peripheral and central chemoreceptors (positive and negative).
Short-term Hypoxemia (days and weeks)
ventilatory "acclimatization"—increased carotid chemoreceptor responsiveness and cerebral fluid acid–base partial compensation.
Long-term (years–generations)
"Blunted" hypoxic response (rest and exercise).

metabolic acid production, which occurs over a wide range of hypocapnia and in the presence of very severe arterial hypoxemia (i.e., PaO_2 = 30 to 35 mmHg).[1] The interactive effects of changes in these two powerful chemical influences—hypoxemia and hydrogen ion—are not completely understood, but in general, coexistence of systemic or whole-body acidity and hypoxemia such as may occur during apnea, show strong, positive interactive effects on both carotid sinus nerve output and on ventilatory output. Curiously, in unanesthetized animals, carotid body responsiveness to stimulation appears to interact in a hypoadditive manner with cerebral fluid acid–base changes, i.e., the more acid the cerebral extracellular fluid (ECF) the less the ventilatory response to carotid chemoreceptor stimulation.[2]

The duration of hypoxemia changes the relative contributions to ventilatory drive as carotid chemoreceptor "responsiveness" may increase during days and weeks of hypoxemia and the carotid bodies are essential to ventilatory acclimatization.[3] On the other hand, with years of long-term hypoxemia, hypoxic ventilatory responsiveness is clearly "blunted," as in the native of high altitude.

Both sleep and hypoxia exert strong, independent effects on ventilatory control. Not unexpectedly, this combination produces highly complex and even unique effects of a fundamental nature on ventilatory output. We shall examine the nature and mechanism of ventilatory control produced by this combination, with our primary frame of reference being that of healthy humans exposed to environmental hypoxia for various durations. The hypoxemia that accompanies sleep in the chronic obstructive lung disease patient or, in the occlusive apnea patient, is of course much more complex because the dimension of increased mechanical impedence to ventilatory drive is added to this already multifaceted regulatory schema. These important clinical entities are covered in detail in other sections of this volume and we will deal with them only as potential applications of principles learned from the specific effects of hypoxia–sleep combinations on breathing patterns.

BREATHING INSTABILITY DURING SLEEP IN HYPOXIA: DESCRIPTION

Hyperventilation is an essential adaptive response to hypoxemia, employing carotid chemoreceptors as critical feedback modulators for homeostatic regulation. This response is initiated within seconds of hypoxic exposure, and increases with time over the first hours, days, and weeks in hypoxia. The importance of this response to homeostasis may best be exemplified during exercise in the sojourner to high altitude who relies solely (in the absence of changes in alveolar-capillary diffusion or ventilation/perfusion distribution) on a marked hyperventilatory response to maintain arterial PO_2 near resting levels even at moderately high altitudes.[4] Another extreme example is the remarkable progressive level of alveolar hyperventilation achieved in acclimatized humans sojourning between 6500 m altitude ($\approx$20 mmHg P_ACO_2) and the 8800 m summit of Mt. Everest ($\approx$7.5 mmHg P_ACO_2). This response was claimed to be sufficient to defend alveolar PO_2 at a constant level of 35 mmHg despite a substantial drop in inspired PO_2.[5] (The stimulus that drove ventilation so much higher between these altitudes, as estimated pH was becoming more alkaline, remains to be found.)

This essential compensatory hyperventilation at high altitudes is not achieved without significant physiological cost. These consequences include, on one hand, the excessive mechanical work done by the chest wall in meeting the high flow rates and volumes required by the tachypneic hyperventilation of exercise in hypoxia.[4] On the other hand, the same homeostatic chemoreceptor feedback system responsible for stability in gas exchange during the waking state is also primarily responsible for causing the instability of ventilatory control and breathing pattern, and wide fluctuations in arterial oxygenation and acid–base status during sleep in hypoxia.

The development of periodic breathing typical of that produced when hypoxemia is induced during non-REM sleep is demonstrated in Figure 5-1 for a normal, healthy adult subject abruptly exposed to a simulated altitude of about 4300 m. The sequence of changes over the initial 10 minutes of hypoxic exposure include the following events. As $P_{ET}O_2$ falls below 60 mmHg, tidal volume is increased and mild hypocapnia of -1 to 2 mmHg occurs. Tidal volume stays elevated and fairly stable and P_ACO_2 drops slightly to about 38 mmHg over the next 2 minutes. For about the next 1.5 minutes, V_T loses some of its breath-to-breath stability and varies in an apparently random fashion.

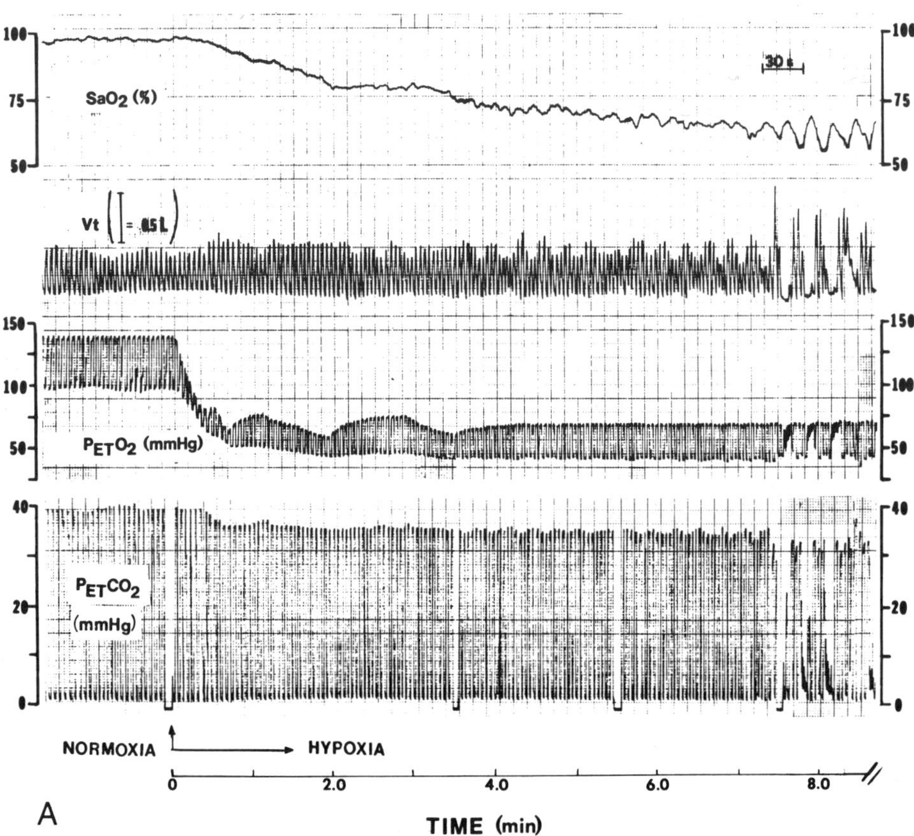

Fig. 5-1 (A) Development of breathing pattern instability and periodicity within the initial few minutes of hypoxic exposure ($F_{I}O_2$ ≈0.12) during non-REM sleep. The subject slept with his head and neck in a flow-through plastic hood into which the inspired gas mixtures were introduced at high flow rates. Arterial 0_2 saturation (SaO_2) was estimated by ear oximetry, and end-tidal PO_2 and PCO_2 were determined by rapid fuel cell and infrared analyzers sampling via a nasal catheter. Tidal volume was estimated body surface measurements over the rib cage and abdomen via inductance plethysmography. (Berssenbrugge A, Dempsey JA, Iber C et al: J Physiol (London) 343:507, 1983.) (Figure continues).

Then from about the 4th to between the 7th and 8th minutes in hypoxia, periodicity of breathing pattern becomes clear in alternating cycles of large and small tidal volumes in clusters of two to four breaths each. The waxing and waning characteristic of breath amplitude within each cluster is particularly obvious during this period. The larger tidal volumes markedly exceed smaller ones by three to fourfold; thus arterial HbO_2 saturation (SaO_2) and alveolar gases also show periodic breath-to-breath fluctuations during this time. Note that $P_{ET}CO_2$ has fallen to ≈36 mmHg by this time. Then, at the 7.5 minute mark, and following a few especially small tidal volumes, a very large inspi-

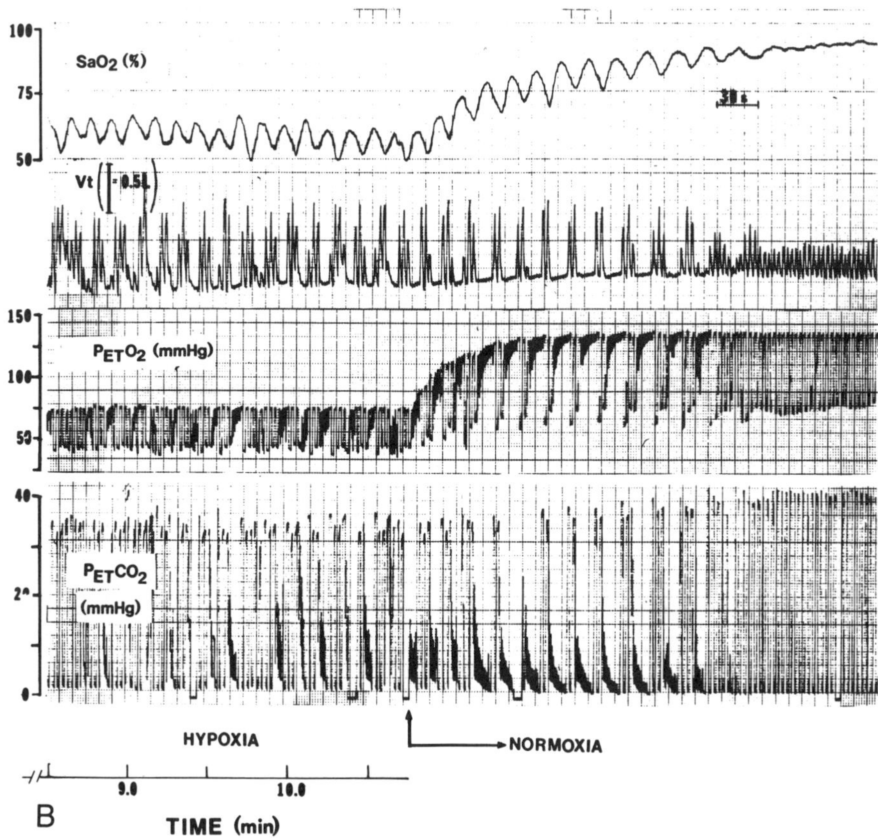

Fig. 5-1 (Continued). **(B)** Continuation of Fig. 5-1A, showing effects of restoration of normoxia.

ration occurred that is about three times the normal control V_T and approximately five times the low V_T in the preceding periodic cluster. This is followed by a drop in P_ACO_2 to 35 mmHg and thereafter the periodic pattern now becomes one of regularly spaced apneic periods with 2 to 3 large V_T's in each breath cluster. P_ACO_2 now fluctuates ± 4 to 6 mmHg and SaO_2 ± 8 to 15 percent within a three-breath cluster; with the highest $P_{ET}CO_2$ and the lowest SaO_2 occurring at end apnea. These cycles will repeat themselves with amazing regularity so long as the hypoxemia and the non-REM sleep state are present. Upon reoxygenation, (see Fig. 5-1B) the gradual return to normocapnia and to a stable breathing pattern are mirror images of the development of instability with hypoxia onset. Note that as SaO_2 rose, the apneic periods lengthened initially and then shortened as the periodic pattern was gradually lost and rhythmicity returned.

Thus, the predominant ventilatory response to sleep in hypoxia is clearly one of breathing "periodicity," a term which has been used to describe a wide variety of unstable, disordered breathing patterns that are other than the rhythmic, reproducible more "orderly" pattern thought to be present in the healthy subject during wakefulness. The classical periodic pattern is, of course, Cheyne-Stokes respiration, in which there is a waxing and waning of tidal volume excursion with apneic pauses.[6] This type of periodic pattern has been described during wakefulness or sleep in a wide variety of cardiovascular and CNS diseases[7,8] and is commonly observed to occur, although only transiently, in normal sleeping subjects during changes in sleep state or in the transition from sleep to arousal.[9,10] In hypoxic sleep, this undulating pattern is most clearly seen in those periods just prior to the development of apneic episodes. (See for example the 5 to 7 minute period of hypoxia onset in Fig. 5-1.) Periodicity with apnea during hypoxic sleep doesn't always clearly show a characteristic crescendo during the three or four breath clusters and occasionally even resembles the abrupt start and stop apneustic or gasping pattern of so-called Biot's breathing produced experimentally by brain stem lesioning.[11] It seems most reasonable for both descriptive and mechanistic considerations, to categorize the self-perpetuating periodicity of hypoxic sleep as Cheyne-Stokes respiration, although we emphasize that mechanisms underlying this phenomena in normal subjects are certainly distinctly different than those described in many of the clinical entities of Cheyne-Stokes respiration.

There are several key characteristics of the periodic breathing pattern of hypoxic sleep that have been noted for some time beginning with the work of Mosso in 1885 and Douglas et al. in 1913.[12] Berssenbrugge et al. have recently analyzed all breaths during all sleep stages taken over one to four nights of hypoxic sleep in normal subjects at 4300 m altitude and compared these data with appropriate sea level controls.[13,14] We use examples from these quantitative data to describe the essential features of the periodic pattern of hypoxic sleep (Figs. 5-2 to 5-4).

First, it is important to note that sleep effects on overall ventilatory volumes and arterial blood acid–base status are similar at sea level and at high altitude. Thus $PaCO_2$ rises 3 to 6 mmHg from wakefulness to non-REM and REM sleep and pH shifts in a mildly acid direction. Average SaO_2 falls during sleep, although this desaturation is, of course, much greater in hypoxia because the awake PaO_2 ($\approx$35 to 40 mmHg) is already on the steep portion of the HbO_2 disassociation curve during wakefulness. As in the waking state, a relative respiratory alkalosis also prevails throughout non-REM sleep in hypoxia.

Cycle length is quite reproducible within and among normal subjects and is probably dependent upon the severity of hypoxemia.[15,16] Thus in these data, at 4300 m, periodic breathing clusters appeared about every 20 seconds and these oscillations were reported to be slightly longer ($\approx$25 sec) at 2500 m to 3200 m and probably slightly shorter at 5400 m.[17] In normoxia, spontaneous temporal variations of several parameters of a breath do occur[18] and at an average cycle time of about 30 seconds in normal adults.[16]

The characteristics of the two to five breaths occurring within each periodic

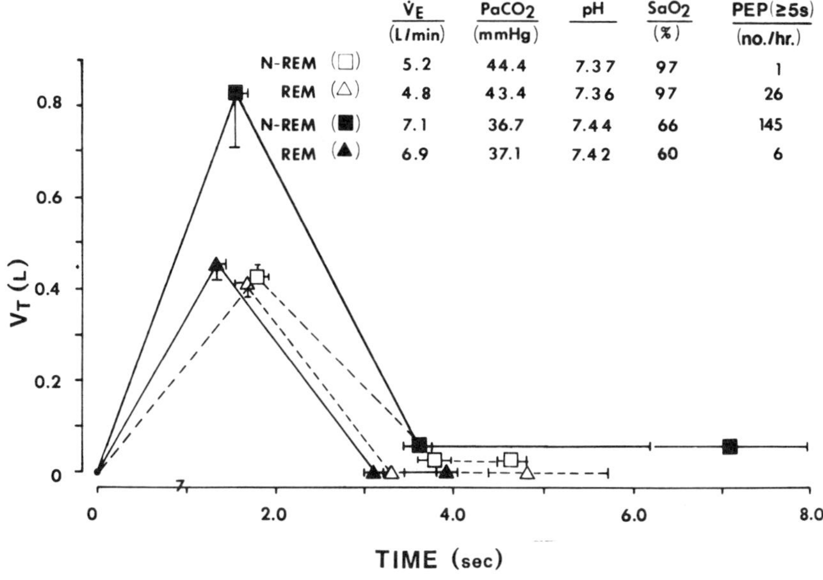

Fig. 5-2 Average spirogram and mean ventilatory measurements from six subjects during non-REM sleep and REM sleep during control conditions in normoxia (□ and △) and during the initial 7 to 9 hours at 4300 m altitude (■, ▲). Expiratory time (T_E) has been subdivided into T_E "short" (that portion of T_E during which expiratory flow is present); and the expiratory pause (EP, or apnea). Non-REM sleep in hypoxia showed marked increases in V_T, V_T/T_I, and $\dot{V}_E$ as well as multiple apneas. Timing of the breathing pattern in REM sleep in hypoxia was like that at sea level. Note that mean values during *wakefulness* included at *sea level*: $PaCO_2 = 40.7 \pm 1.2$ mmHg, pHa = 7.40 ± .01, and $SaO_2 = 98 \pm 0.3$ per cent; and at 4300 m, $PaCO_2 = 33.4 \pm 1.0$, pHa = 7.46 ± .01 and $SaO_2 = 78 \pm 1.2$ percent.

cluster were also quite consistent within and among subjects. Relative to a nonperiodic breathing pattern in normoxic non-REM, in hypoxia these breaths showed increased V_T secondary to augmented mean inspiratory flow (V_T/T_I) (Fig. 5-2). Within a cluster, these augmented inspiratory efforts were commonly confined to the initial breaths with the last breath in the cluster, usually (but not always) equal to or often less than control V_T. Large variability in V_T (and in V_T/T_I and $\dot{V}_E$) is another consistent characteristic of breaths within the periodic clusters in non-REM sleep (Fig. 5-3). Note that a significant fraction of all breaths occur at less than 0.3 L V_T (close to dead-space volume) on the one hand, and also a significant fraction above 1.0 L, on the other. Corresponding ranges for breath-to-breath $\dot{V}_E$ were from less than 3.0 L per minute to greater than 15 L/minute. Surprisingly, alveolar ventilation seemed to be well regulated (for purposes of acid–base homeostasis) during these highly variable periods, as no significant differences in "average" $PaCO_2$ were noted

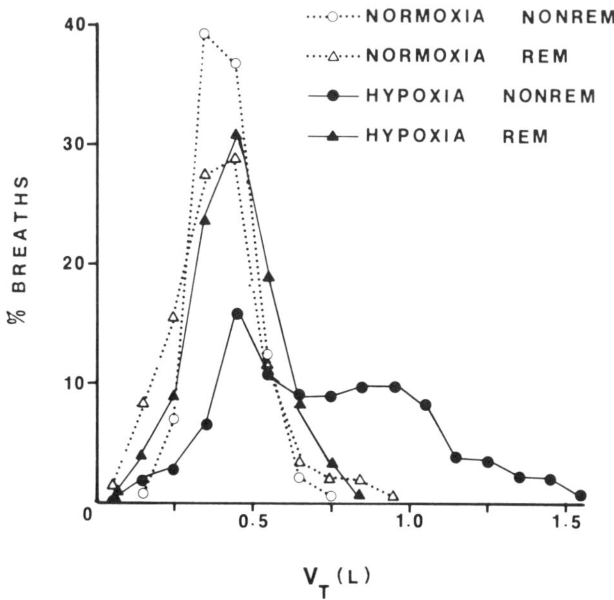

Fig. 5-3 Frequency distribution of tidal volume in six subjects during sleep in normoxia and hypoxia.

between the many samples obtained during the periodic episode and the (many fewer) samples obtained during nonperiodic episodes.

Timing changes in breathing pattern occurred consistently only in the final breath of each cluster. Inspiratory and expiratory times were normal and the expiratory "pause" was prolonged. These apneic periods (greater than 5 seconds or about 3 times the normal nonperiodic postexpiratory pause) averaged about 11 seconds in length and occurred 145 times per hour, resulting in about equal time throughout hypoxic non-REM sleep being consumed by breathing versus not breathing. The potential exists for obstructive sleep apnea during sleep because hypoxia does cause some degree of airway narrowing at the laryngeal level in humans.[19] However, almost all of the apneas observed appeared to be of the so-called central or nonobstructed variety because there was a total cessation of all respiratory efforts as measured at the body surface when flow at the nose or mouth had stopped and no paradoxical motion of rib cage versus abdomen was observed. This is not to say that some "mixed" apneas with a minor obstructive component might not occur in hypoxic non-REM sleep. Indeed, in normal subjects at sea level, airway resistance increases and sometimes markedly so in non-REM sleep coincident with marked breath-by-breath reductions in inspiratory flow and tidal volume.[20,21] Some of these normal subjects do occasionally experience obstructive apneas during normoxic sleep (non-REM and/or REM) and these types of apneic episodes will carry over to sleep in hypoxia along with the episodic central apneas.[13]

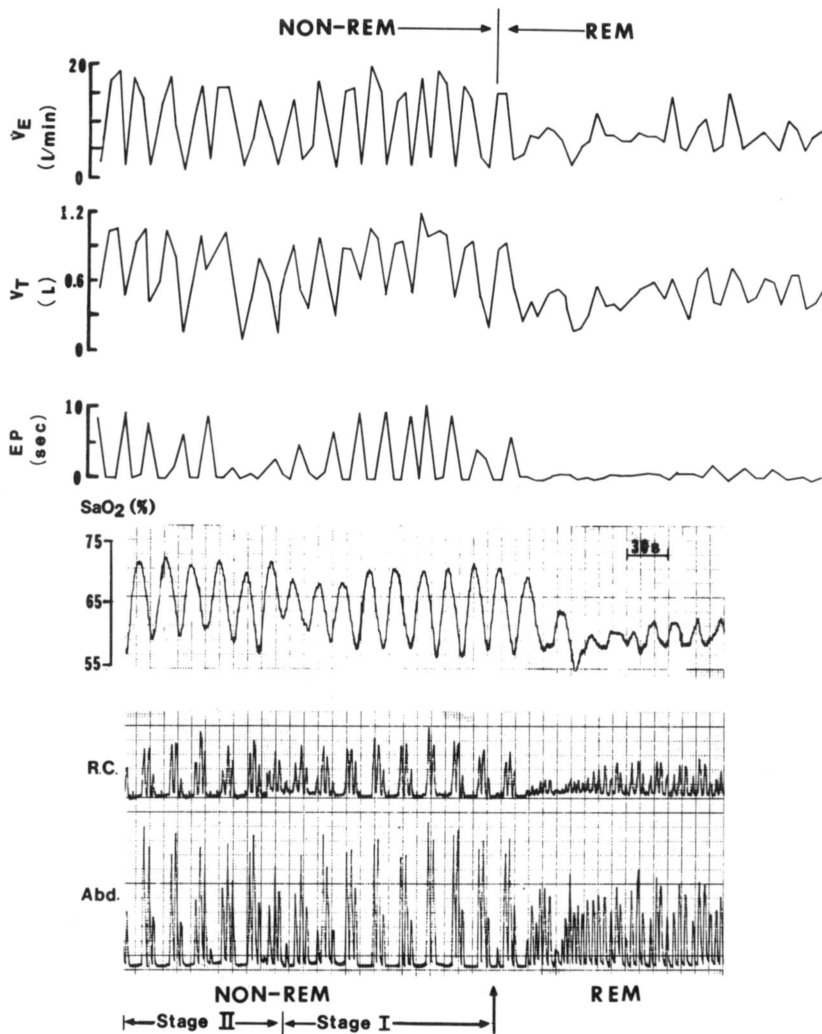

Fig. 5-4 Transition from non-REM to REM sleep showing breath-to-breath measurements of $\dot{V}_E$, V_T and apnea (expiratory pause) duration plus the corresponding polygraph tracing. The data were obtained from a single subject during the initial 4 hours of hypoxic exposure and are typical of the group of 6.[13] Note the apneas, periodicity and swings in $Sa0_2$ characteristic of hypoxic non-REM sleep. Major changes in REM sleep included the absence of significant postexpiratory pauses, the appearance of relatively low V_T's and $\dot{V}_E$'s with increased random variability and reduced mean SaO_2.

Changes in sleep state can have profound effects on ventilatory pattern. Within non-REM sleep, fluctuations in stage can cause instability of pattern in hypoxia or normoxia,[9,13] but variations in sleep stage within non-REM were not required to produce periodicity in hypoxia. We only rarely observed consistent periodicity with apneas during wakefulness in hypoxia, although Brusil et al. have reported "reinforcing oscillations" of $\dot{V}_E$ and frequency at 3000 m[18] and Waggener et al.[15] even report regularly occurring apneas during acute exposures at higher altitudes in normal sojourners who were apparently awake. Ventilatory pattern during hypoxic REM sleep appeared much like that obtained in normoxia (Fig. 5-4), i.e., random, erratic variations in breath volume and timing with no obvious cyclical waxing and waning. These data support the concept that dependence on classical respiratory afferent stimuli (such as vagal or chemoreceptor feedback) is suppressed during REM sleep and breathingrhythm is maintained by nonrespiratory neural events of the higher CNS.[22–25]

MEDIATION OF PERIODIC BREATHING DURING SLEEP IN HYPOXIA

Douglas et al.[12] originally noted the very abrupt ventilatory adjustments that occurred upon acute imposition and removal of hypoxia and drew an analogy to feedback control in an electric motor: "The (respiratory) center thus responds like an engine with a very sensitive governor but with no flywheel."[12] The work of Cherniack et al. in the past 20 years, using data obtained primarily in anesthetized or decerebrate animals, has provided a broad theoretical base for explaining and predicting many instabilities in ventilatory control.[26–31] A recent mathematical model by Khoo et al.[16] attempts to provide quantification of many of the parameters of periodic breathing in hypoxia. These authors emphasize that the feedback stimuli and pathways, which are so critical to homeostasis and error detection and correction in the steady-state of so many physiologic states, also cause instability and periodicity under certain circumstances. Key destabilizers here include:

1. Time delays in information transfer between the controller and the effector organ, so that the controller produces the wrong response at the wrong time (e.g., increased $\dot{V}_A$ at a time when P_ACO_2 is low) thereby reinforcing rather than dampening the effects of disturbances in feedback stimuli. This factor clearly plays a role in the Cheyne-Stokes respiration of congestive heart failure.[8] Experimentally, however, circulation times must be markedly prolonged (i.e., > three to five times normal) before this factor alone will cause significant instability in breathing pattern.
2. "Dampening" capabilities of the control system will determine both the magnitude of oscillation and its duration following a disturbance. For example, the larger stores of CO_2 than O_2 in blood means a ventilatory disturbance

will cause a faster, greater and more sustained oscillatory behavior in PO_2 than in PCO_2. Furthermore, changes in resting lung volume, functional residual capacity (FRC), with such factors as changes in posture will also play a role in dampening oscillations in alveolar gas following a ventilatory disturbance.

3. Controller gain appears to be the most critical determinant of oscillatory behavior in ventilatory control, as based on the analogy that when large forces are applied for very little current (i.e., high sensitivity), a mass would tend to oscillate for a long time following a disturbance. Since the ventilatory response to CO_2 is linear over a broad range (at least from eupnea upwards in awake humans—see below) changes in response gain would not be expected with changes in the magnitude of PCO_2; whereas with an alinear hypoxic ventilatory response, marked changes in gain over the range of PO_2 normally encountered in the normal person at high altitude would be expected.

The combination of alinear gain and reduced dampening characteristics seems to make hypoxia an ideal candidate for instability in ventilatory control and one would predict the occurrence of periodicity in these situations where the peripheral hypoxic drive—rather than the central CO_2 drive was dominant. Accordingly, when Cherniak et al.[26,29] obliterated medullary chemoreceptor activity (by cooling the ventral surface of the medulla), hypoventilation and hypoxemia occurred coincident with periodic breathing—and this periodicity was attenuated by either carotid body denervation or with hyperoxia.

4. Changes in "state" are also critical determinants of stability of ventilatory pattern—especially if the state change causes marked change in the gain of ventilatory responses. Thus, sleep may be likened to the inhibition of cortical influences associated with anesthesia or with higher CNS lesioning characteristic of certain neurologic diseases[32] where marked changes may occur in the response to hypercapnia or even more important to hypocapnia.

How might these various effectors of instability be applied to explain the breathing periodicity experienced in the healthy person during sleep in hypoxic environments? Two destabilizing mechanisms appear to be essential to this self-sustaining periodicity, namely, (1) a sleep-induced apneic threshold to small reductions in $PaCO_2$ whose sensitivity depends upon several kinds of background stimuli, and (2) a curvilinear ventilatory response to hypoxemia, especially when combined with hypercapnia.

The hypocapnic apneic "threshold" designates that P_ACO_2 below which inspiratory neural drive is sufficiently inhibited to cause a significant cessation of rhythmic breathing. In intact humans, this threshold may be estimated by passively inducing hyperventilation to gradually lower and lower levels of P_ACO_2 (below eupnea) and observing that P_ACO_2 at which a consistent and significant apnea (i.e., loss of at least one normal breath or an $\approx \times$ lengthening of T_E) occurs during the immediate posthyperventilation period.[33,34]

The apneic threshold was determined during constant stages of non-REM sleep by using many trials of positive pressure hyperventilation through a mask in two normal subjects and through an endotracheal tube in a patient.[33] The

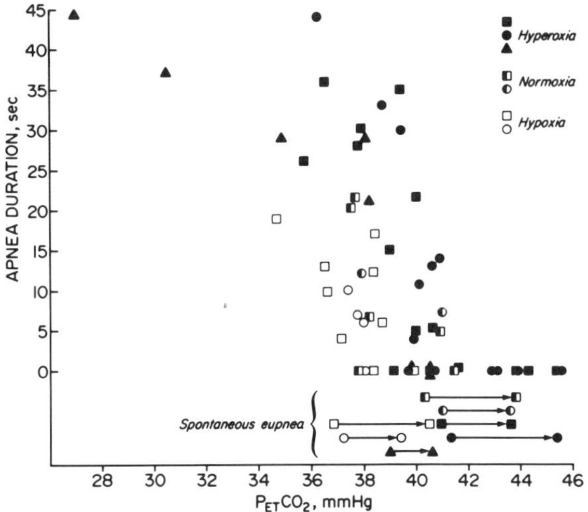

Fig. 5-5 Quantification of the hypocapnic apneic threshold during non-REM sleep in three human subjects with backgrounds of normoxia, acute hyperoxia and acute hypoxia (0.12 F_IO_2). $P_{ET}CO_2$ levels during spontaneous, eupneic breathing are shown at the bottom of the figure. Note that $P_{ET}CO_2$ increases from wakefulness to non-REM sleep (→). Multiple trials of 3 minutes of positive pressure hyperventilation were then superimposed. Points of zero apnea time represent $P_{ET}CO_2$ in trials that did not produce posthyperventilation apnea. The apneic "threshold" was defined as that $P_{ET}CO_2$ at which an apneic period of at least 5 seconds could be reproducibly obtained. In general, in all conditions, this threshold approximated the $P_{ET}CO_2$ obtained during eupneic breathing in wakefulness. Background hypoxia reduced this apneic threshold (relative to normoxia) and hyperoxia increased the threshold. (Skatrud J, Dempsey J: J Appl Physiol 55:813, 1983.)

individual data points are shown in Figure 5-5 and the following observations are most relevant:

1. $PaCO_2$ increases as a moderate but significant hypoventilation occurs from awake to non-REM sleep. Significant apnea (5 to 10 sec duration) occurred at slightly above the waking level of $P_{ET}CO_2$ achieved during eupnic breathing and as PCO_2 was lowered further, apnea duration increased in a fairly consistent and linear fashion. Posthyperventilation apnea may also occur on occasion in the awake state in normal subjects[33,34] especially after many trials and with distraction. But the hypocapnia-induced apnea during sleep is much more sensitive and reproducible and increases in duration in a fairly predictible fashion with magnitude of induced hypocapnia. Certain patients with higher CNS lesions who often exhibit Cheyne-Stokes type respiration also will rather consistently demonstrate posthyperventilation apnea in the awake state.[32]

2. Peripheral chemoreceptor activity is inhibited by systemic hypocapnia and T_E may be lengthened significantly;[35] however, given the relative gains of

the two chemoreceptor systems to changes in [H+],[3] medullary chemoreceptor inhibition must be the major contributor to the cessation of rhythm generation and apnea. Exactly how the cerebral alkalosis is produced may be important, as the pronounced effect of relatively small degrees of respiratory alkalosis (Fig. 5-5) contrasts with the maintenance of a normal, rhythmic breathing pattern and alveolar hypoventilation experienced by normal subjects during sleep in a background of marked, chronic metabolic alkalosis.[36] Even rather extreme levels of cerebral ECF pH achieved via cisternal perfusion of artificial cerebrospinal fluid (CSF) in the awake animal do not cause instability or periodicity of breathing pattern.[2]

3. The magnitude of the apneic threshold was reduced with a moderately hypoxic background and slightly increased with hyperoxia—with both thresholds remaining very close to the new, awake level of P_ACO_2 achieved in either hypoxia or hyperoxia. Recent evidence based on isolation of cerebral perfusate composition in anesthetized cats has shown that the apneic threshold may be as low as ≈5 to 10 mmHg cerebral PCO_2 so long as the level of carotid chemoreceptor stimuli is kept high.[37]

4. Some of the posthyperventilation apnea in sleep might emanate from inhibitory feedback effects of lung inflation secondary to the twofold increment in V_T achieved during passive hyperventilation. Indeed at least some level of a Hering-Brauer type of lung volume dependent inhibitory reflex appears to be operative in some anesthetized humans.[38] However this contribution is probably a minimal one because no apnea was obtained if P_ACO_2 was held constant (via increased F_ICO_2) during the 3 to 4 minutes of induced hyperventilation.[33]

This occurrence of a highly sensitive hypocapnic apneic threshold represents a very fundamental effect of sleep state on ventilatory control. This contrasts with the purely additive effects of most ventilatory stimuli such as inhaled CO_2, acute and chronic hypoxia, metabolic acidosis and various humoral stimuli, or most ventilatory inhibitions such as metabolic alkalosis or hyperoxia. With the acute and chronic perturbations, overall ventilatory minute volume and the level of $PaCO_2$ are affected in a predictable fashion and to about the same extent as they would be in the waking state; ventilatory output remains stable and rhythmic. There are some parallels between sleep and anesthetic effects in this regard.[39] Both non-REM sleep and varying depths of halothane or forane anesthesia in humans cause alveolar hypoventilation (+3 to 6 mmHg $PaCO_2$ in sleep and +10 to 20 mmHg with the anesthetics) and raise the apneic threshold to hypocapnia to within 3 to 5 mmHg of whatever level of $PaCO_2$ is achieved during eupnic, spontaneous breathing in sleep or anesthesia. This similarity between sleep and anesthesia in the markedly increased response to hypocapnia (relative to the waking state) is not consistent with the divergent ventilatory responses of these states to increased levels of added CO_2 (i.e., above eupnea). This response is markedly reduced (to as little as $\frac{1}{5}$ of the waking response) with increasing depth of anesthesia but is unchanged or only slightly reduced in non-REM sleep.[23,24]

Two problems remain here in applying these data and the sleep-induced apneic threshold to the concept of periodic breathing in hypoxic sleep. First, we used passively induced hyperventilation. But actively-induced hyperventilation in the anesthetized cat (i.e. such as by carotid sinus nerve stimulation or hypoxia) does not elicit apnea.[40] Secondly, hypocapnic apnea, per se, will not cause sustained periodic breathing because rhythmic breathing will return within a breath or two following the rise in CO_2 above the apneic threshold. This transient effect is commonly seen following a sigh or augmented breath in normal humans in normoxic sleep.

These questions were addressed by a series of experiments conducted during a few hours of hypoxic sleep in healthy subjects that quantitated the dual contributions of hypoxemia and hypocapnia to self-perpetuating periodic breathing during non-REM sleep. The basis of this is shown in the effect of sleep state on the ventilatory response to hypoxia and to CO_2 (Fig. 5-6). The major sleep effect here is on the CO_2 response gain not above but below eupneic $PaCO_2$. Sleep effects on the progressive hypoxic response are controversial—some studies claiming no effect and others showing a reduced response slope.[41,42] This controversy probably isn't relevant to the present discussion for two reasons: First, the dominant effect of sleep in hypoxia on ventilatory control is clearly breathing periodicity, but this effect is masked by any response test that artifically prevents hypocapnia from occurring. Secondly, it is likely (see below) that the nature of the hypoxic response will retain its critical role as a perpetuator of periodic breathing even if the response slope is changed somewhat so long as the basic characteristics of alinearity of response and gain stays intact over the range of PaO_2s encountered.

Four types of data point to the importance of the nature of these relative chemoreceptor responses and the presence of hypoxia and hypocapnia in combination during sleep in the production of periodicity.

1. The time-course data following onset of hypoxia shown in Fig. 5-1 demonstrates a clear relationship of a gradually declining P_ACO_2 to the development of periodicity. It was shown further[33] that the apneic periods in hypoxic sleep occurred coincidently with the reduction of P_ACO_2 to the predetermined apneic threshold. The "waning" of ventilation, or hypopneic periods, just preceeding the first apneic period also coincided with progressive reduction in P_ACO_2 to "near" the apneic threshold.

2. Why did the $PaCO_2$ finally reach the apneic threshold? With hypoxic hyperventilation a time-dependent excretion of CO_2 (and further increase in $\dot{V}_E$) might eventually be expected to lower $PaCO_2$ to the apneic threshold. In addition, it was very common to observe an augmented breath and ensuing hypocapnia immediately prior to the initial apneic episode. These breaths commonly appear as a sudden reinforcement at the crest of an otherwise normal inspiration and are viewed as a normal part of ventilatory control that occurs in normoxic sleep at the rate of about 2/hr in normal humans[43] and appear

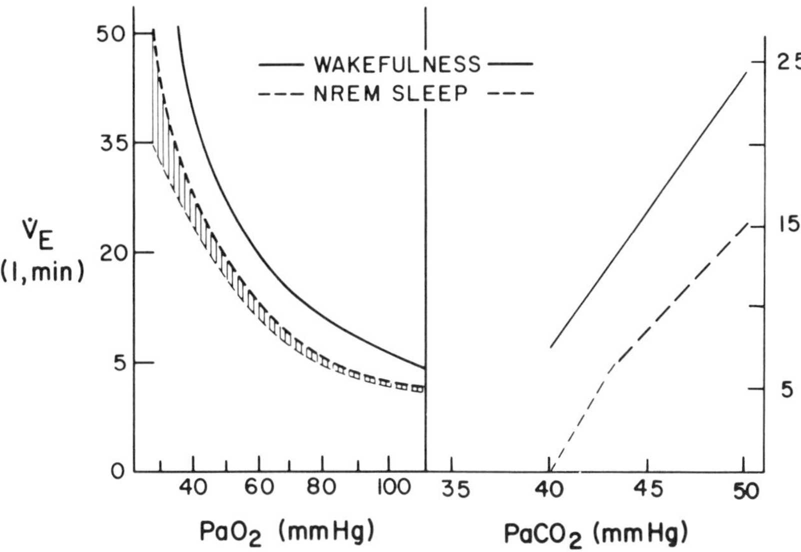

Fig. 5-6 Ventilatory response to progressive transient isocapnic hypoxia and hyperoxic hypercapnia and hypocapnia during wakefulness and non-REM sleep. The hatched area of the hypoxic response during non-REM sleep indicates the divergence of findings regarding sleep effects on hypoxic responsiveness. Either during wakefulness or sleep, the gain of the hypoxic response ($\triangle V_E/\triangle PaO_2$) increases progressively from an average of 0.3 to 0.4 L/mmHg (at ≈70 mmHg PaO_2) to 1.5 to 2.5 L/mmHg (at 40 mmHg PaO_2). The response to hypercapnia is fairly linear from eupnea upward during both wakefulness and non-REM sleep, with the slope of the hypercapnic response reduced ≈15 to 25 percent in sleep. We have not indicated a response slope for hypocapnia during wakefulness because the response following acute hyperventilation in wakefulness is too variable. During non-REM sleep we estimated the gain of the response to hypocapnia based on the $\triangle V_E$ and the $\triangle PaCO_2$ obtained between eupnea and the highest $P_{ET}CO_2$ at which significant apnea first occurred (i.e., the apneic "threshold") (see Fig. 5-5). The gain of the ventilatory response to CO_2 is shown to be slightly greater below versus above normocapnia, but this comparison is only an approximate one given the markedly different study conditions, i.e., progressive CO_2 rebreathing above normocapnia versus eupnea to posthyperventilation apnea below eupnea. The key point here is that a hypocapnic, apneic threshold was consistently manifested during sleep and at a $PaCO_2$ that was sufficiently high to be readily achieved in hypoxic sleep. At $P_{ET}CO_2$'s below the apneic threshold, the gain of the response in terms of apnea duration averaged ≈5 seconds per mmHg reduction in $P_{ET}CO_2$, so that at $PaCO_2$ ≈30 mmHg in hyperoxia the apneic period with approximate 1 minute.

especially strong in anesthetized animals and in the newborn human.[44,45] These augmented breaths have been associated most commonly with a vagally mediated deflation reflex necessary to avoid atelectasis. Some narrowing of small airways might occur in hypoxic sleep because of the relative hypopnea that occurs prior to apneic initiation (Fig. 5-1). Augmented inspirations have also been attributed to peripheral chemoreceptor mediated ventilatory stimulation and/or to transient changes in sleep stage (or arousals).[9,43,44,46–48]

3. Additional correlative data implicating the combination of hypoxemia with hypocapnia in the genesis of periodic breathing occurred with acute restoration of normoxia (in hypoxic sleep) (Figs. 5-1B and 5-8). Initially as SaO_2 rose, the periodicity "worsened" as apneic length increased, but then within 30 to 60 seconds at $SaO_2 > 90$ percent, the apneic periods were completely removed as was any noticeable cycling of ventilatory pattern and the frequency distribution of V_T (and of $\dot{V}_E$) was markedly reduced in variability. $PaCO_2$ also always rose 1 to 4 mmHg with this acute restoration of normoxia.

4. These correlative data are supported by more direct, experimental manipulations of $PaCO_2$. Note (in Fig. 5-7 to 5-9) that as little as 1 to 2 mmHg increments in $PaCO_2$ and 0.01 to 0.03 acidification of pHa—at maintained levels of hypoxemic SaO_2—removed periodic breathing during hypoxic sleep. The usual periodic pattern was readily restored when the elevated F_ICO_2 was discontinued. Clearly then, apnea and frank periodicity were dependent upon the prevailing level of $PaCO_2$—relative to the apneic threshold. However we cannot be sure that some more subtle oscillatory behavior in ventilatory pattern was not occurring even after CO_2 was raised above the apneic threshold. We doubt however, that this amount of periodicity was significant because hypoxia, per se, even at rather substantial levels did not precipitate periodic breathing or any evidence of cycling of breathing pattern beyond that obtained under normal normoxic conditions at sea level. This was demonstrated by holding $PaCO_2$ constant as hypoxia was initiated and maintained during non-REM sleep. $\dot{V}_E$ and V_T increased substantially, with this isocapnic hypoxemia but rhythmicity was maintained with no evidence of cycling.[13]

The critical importance of peripheral chemoreception and the interaction of hypoxemia and hypocapnia in the production of periodicity in hypoxic sleep is shown in the diagram summarizing the pathogenesis of periodic breathing (Fig. 5-10). Increased peripheral chemoreceptor drive initiates the sequence of events by causing hyperventilation, driving $PaCO_2$ toward the apneic threshold (and in so doing precipitating an unstable control system as manifested in a waxing and waning of tidal volume). The marked hyperpnea during the "waning" phases of this unstable period is then nudged into apnea—usually by a markedly augmented inspiration and coincident hypocapnia. During the apneic period the peripheral chemoreceptors again become critical to perpetuating periodicity as the hypercapnic–hypoxemic combination greatly increases chemoreceptor gain. The result is a marked augmentation of the first breath or two at the reinitiation of breathing and the apneic threshold is again exceeded and the periodic cycling is perpetuated and continues until chemoreceptor gains are reduced by changes in sleep state or arousal—or, of course, by restoring normoxia or slightly increasing $PaCO_2$.

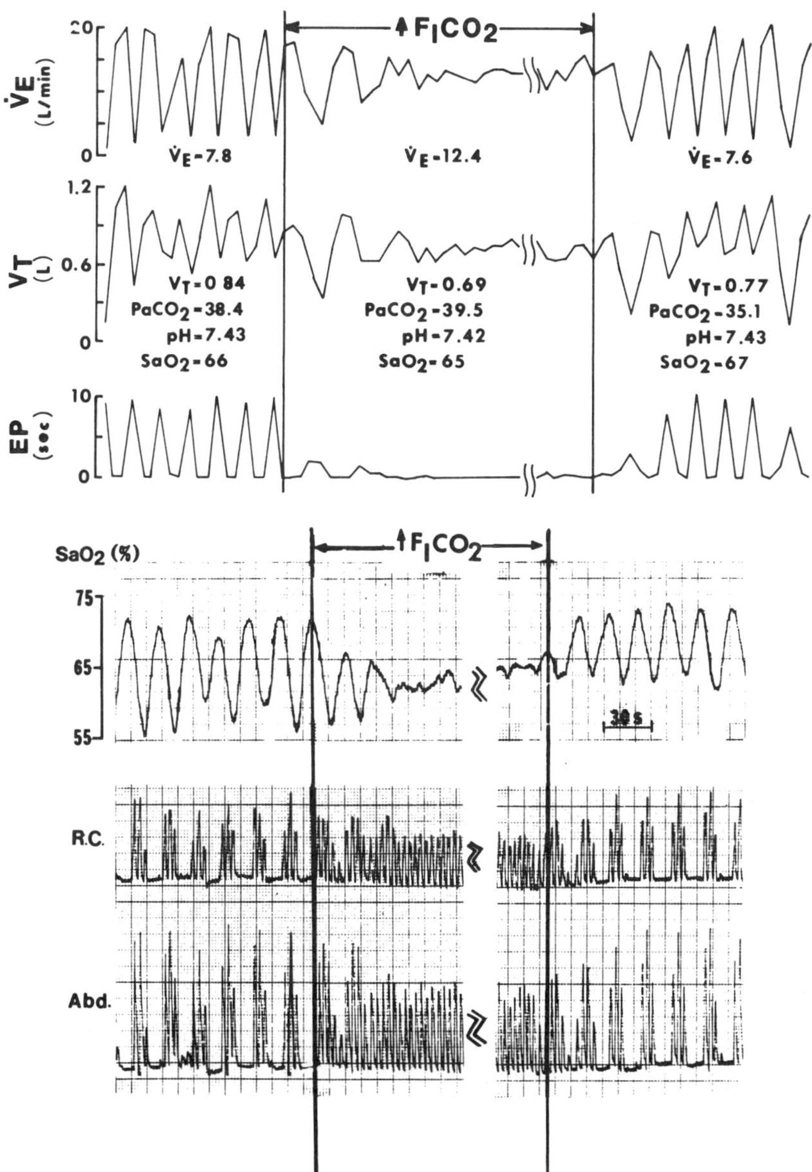

Fig. 5-7 Transition from ambient air breathing to elevated F_ICO_2 and return to ambient air, showing breath to breath measurements and the corresponding polygraph tracing during hypoxic non-REM sleep as in Figure 5-4. Mean SaO_2 was maintained when F_ICO_2 was elevated, by adding small amounts of N_2 to the inspired gas mixture. Note that a 1 to 2 mmHg increase in $PaCO_2$ resulted in an almost immediate (<20 sec) removal of all expiratory pauses, and V_E increased secondary to an increased breathing frequency.

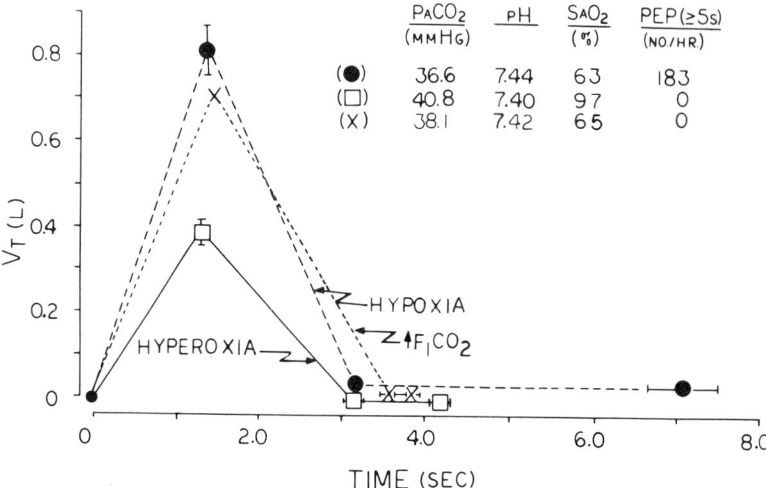

Fig. 5-8 Average spirograms obtained during non-REM sleep in hypoxia, upon acute restoration of normoxia (mean of eight trials in five subjects) and with elevated F_ICO_2 (mean of nine trials in four subjects). Both hyperoxia and mild hypercapnia removed expiratory pauses. V_T and V_T/T_I were reduced by hyperoxia but unchanged with increased $PaCO_2$.

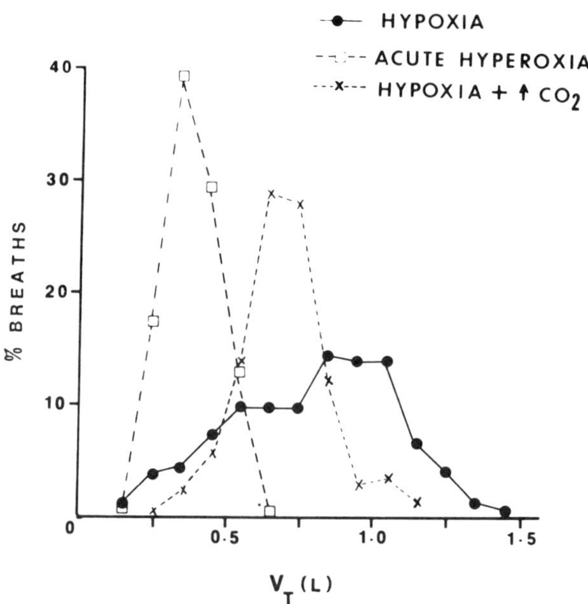

Fig. 5-9 Frequency distribution of V_T during non-REM sleep in hypoxia and upon acute increases in SaO_2 and $PaCO_2$ (from the data in Fig. 5-8). Note the marked reduction in variability induced by hyperoxia and mild hypercapnia.

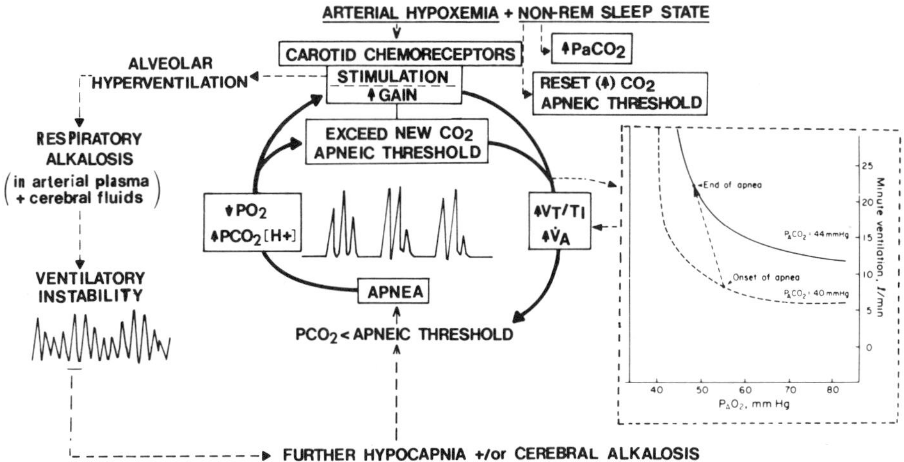

Fig. 5-10 Schema illustrating a possible mechanism for the pathogenesis of hypoxia-induced periodic breathing during non-REM sleep. See text for explanation. In essence: (1) non-REM sleep resets the apneic threshold to a level of $PaCO_2$ very close to that obtained in eupneic breathing; (2) peripheral chemoreceptor stimulation increases ventilation driving $PaCO_2$ down toward the apneic threshold (instability) and then below it (apnea); and (3) finally (see insert) the displacement of PaO_2 from a relatively low to very high gain on the peripheral chemoreceptor response curve by the end of the apneic period causes a marked increase in ventilatory drive following the apnea, again driving $PaCO_2$ below its apneic threshold.

FACTORS AFFECTING PERIODIC BREATHING DURING SLEEP IN HYPOXIA

The time required in hypoxic sleep to produce periodic breathing appears to be only that needed to insure that the $PaCO_2$ is reduced below the apneic threshold (i.e., ≈5 to 20 min). The degree of hypoxemia necessary to precipitate periodic breathing has also not been systematically studied, but Waggener et al.[15] have recently reported cyclical changes in breathing patterns in awake subjects after a few hours exposure to 9,000 ft altitude. This condition is roughly equivalent to PaO_2 levels of 55 to 65 mmHg (which are still in the mild hypoxemia category on the relatively flat portion of the HbO_2 dissociation curve). Short-term acclimatization to hypoxia over 4 to 12 days has generally been reported—usually with no documentation of sleep state—to result in less periodicity.[12,15,49] Sojourners studied after many weeks above 5000 m altitude clearly breathed periodically during sleep.[17] We found that between night 1 and night 4 at 4300 m the amount and frequency of periodic breathing remained essentially constant in two of five sojourners and in the remaining three apneic episodes were virtually eliminated by night four in hypoxia (see Fig. 5-11). The

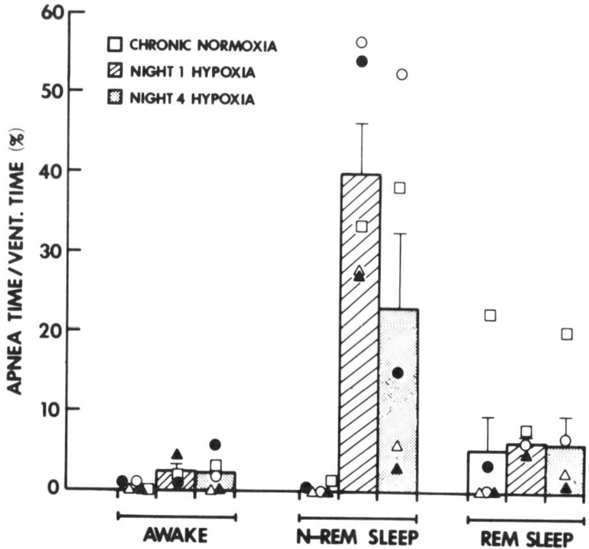

Fig. 5-11 Effects of sleep state and the duration of hypoxic exposure (at 4300 m altitude) on the proportion of time spent in apnea as a percent of total time in each sleep state. Apneas were not prevelant in REM sleep at any time of hypoxic exposure. In non-REM sleep three of the five sojourners showed marked reductions in the number of apneas per hour (113 to 145 apneas per hour on night 1 versus 17 to 55 per hour on night 4) with no change in the average apneic length.

occurrence of periodicity continued to be confined to non-REM sleep stages with acclimatization.

Hyperventilation progresses with time during the initial days of hypoxic exposure[3] and the magnitude and time course of this acclimatization is identical during wakefulness and all sleep stages.[13,14] Time-dependent change in the "gain" of peripheral chemoreceptors, which appear to be essential for normal acclimatization,[3] is possibly responsible for mediating ventilatory acclimatization to hypoxia.[87] The state of the higher CNS apparently plays no part. Despite these further reductions in $PaCO_2$ during the steady-state of eupneic breathing, the amount of periodic breathing was either unchanged or more often markedly reduced, meaning that with acclimatization $PaCO_2$ was driven below its apneic threshold less often.

This apparent paradox may be attributable to three influences. First the prevailing background of ventilatory stimuli influences the development of apnea. Alterations in ventilatory afferent stimuli such as metabolic acidosis in dogs,[50] acute hypoxia in humans (see Fig. 5-5) and peripheral chemoreception stimulation in anesthetized cats[37] decrease the CO_2 apneic threshold. It is likely, then, that ventilatory acclimatization as an additional stimulus to breathe also decreases the CO_2 apneic threshold. Thus, parallel reductions in both the new "set-point" $PaCO_2$ achieved during eupneic breathing with acclimatization relative to the mean apneic threshold would ensure that the amount of breathing periodicity would not increase with duration of hypoxic exposure. To use this same concept to explain the marked *reductions* in periodic breathing observed with acclimatization requires that the subjects must have reduced their apneic threshold to a *greater* extent than they reduced their eupneic level of $PaCO_2$. Secondly, the increase in arterial PO_2 coincident with ventilatory acclimatization may also contribute to the stabilization of breathing pattern by reducing peripheral chemoreceptor gain and thus attenuating the degree of ventilatory overshoot that occurs during apnea or hyperpnea; and may even have had some inhibitory effect on the number and/or magnitude of augmented breaths that were important in initiating apnea. Finally, another important stabilizing factor here is simply that dictated by the alveolar air equation, which relates $\dot{V}_A$ to P_ACO_2 at a fixed $\dot{V}CO_2$. That is, starting at a lower $PaCO_2$ (for example, during sleep onset in night 4 versus night 1) it follows from the parabolic shape of the $P_ACO_2 : \dot{V}_A$ relationship that a given transient increase in $\dot{V}_A$ will result in less of a reduction in P_ACO_2 than occurred at the relatively higher P_ACO_2 on night 1. Why some subjects and not others greatly reduce their periodicity with acclimatization is not attributable to any obvious differences in such factors as changes in arterial oxygenation *or* acid–base status *or* in sleep state during acclimatization. The general impression that acclimatization results in less arousals or changes in sleep state[49] (see below) needs further careful documentation and correlation with ventilatory changes, as these events are potentially important initial "destabilizers" of ventilatory pattern that might trigger augmented breaths, apneas and periodicity.

Administration of chronic ventilatory stimuli such as acetazolamide[51] or medroxyprogesterone acetate[52] reduced periodic breathing during sleep at high altitudes. Although sleep state was not measured and swings in oximeter SaO_2 were the only reported indices of periodicity in one study conducted above 18,000 ft.,[51] the effect of acetazolamide on diminishing oscillations in SaO_2 and the overall level of hypoxemia during sleep at this extreme altitude was indeed impressive. At least two factors might explain these findings. First, mean PaO_2 would be increased in both waking and sleeping states because of the attendant hyperventilation (via induced metabolic acidosis) plus the right-shifted HbO_2 dissociation curve, which would tend to reduce $AaDO_2$ and further elevate PaO_2.[53] Thus with arterial blood PO_2 on the less steep portion of the HbO_2 disassociation curve, observed oscillations in SaO_2 would be less for a given $\triangle PaO_2$ and the higher arterial PaO_2 would also produce less peripheral chemoreceptor drive and therefore lower gain. Secondly, just as with acclimatization, the "background" drive provided by the chronic stimuli might lower the CO_2 apneic threshold relative to eupneic $PaCO_2$, and would move $PaCO_2$ to a "less vulnerable" position on the $\dot{V}_A : PaCO_2$ relationship (see above).

Despite the rather striking effects of ventilatory stimulants on periodicity, their general use in the sojourner at high altitude for alleviating the periodic breathing in sleep may be ill-advised, given the chronic increase in ventilatory drive such agents would provide during the waking hours—especially while physically active. The combination of exercise, hypoxia and chronic metabolic acidosis may provide highly stressful levels of ventilatory drive and exertional dyspnea. The most logical remedy for the selective alleviation of periodic breathing during sleep would seem to be nocturnal administration of just sufficient oxygen to insure enough CO_2 retention to keep the high altitude sleeper above his apneic threshold and at a high enough arterial PO_2 to significantly reduce peripheral chemoreceptor gain.

Some data are available to suggest that periodic breathing in hypoxic sleep may be inversely related to hypoxic ventilatory response. Lahiri et al.[17] observed that most sojourners after even 4 weeks at 5400 m altitude experience periodic breathing in sleep, whereas most of the Sherpa guides on the same expedition experienced no or little apnea. A major drawback in these studies is the absence of sleep stage documentation. However the data are impressive in demonstrating that when the transient, progressive, hypoxic response (in wakefulness) was nearly flat, virtually no sleep apneas occurred. Among sojourners with about a fourfold range of hypoxic response to isocapnic or hypocapnic hypoxia, no correlation was evident with periodic breathing during hypoxic sleep.[13,17,52] Further, Kryger et al.[54,55] reported that most of a sample of 10 natives of 3100 m altitude showed "irregular" and often "periodic" breathing patterns during sleep in hypoxia as defined by oscillations in SaO_2. These natives all had blunted ventilatory responses to transient isocapnic hypoxia that averaged about $\frac{1}{2}$ that found in a normal sea-level population and there was no correlation within the group between the magnitude of hypoxic response and the amount of sleep-induced "disordered" breathing or arterial hypoxemia. We caution here that the many types of "disordered" breathing described for these high altitude residents[54,55] may not actually mimic the characteristics of (and mechanisms responsible for) the "periodic" breathing we are describing for the sojourner to high altitude.

Obviously, the question is unresolved at this time. Theoretically a nonexistent (or extremely blunted) hypoxic response (obtained over the range of PaO_2's experienced in hypoxic sleep) will remove at lease some source of the hyperventilation required to drive $PaCO_2$ below or at least very close to the apneic threshold; and will most certainly prevent the necessary increase in hypoxic response gain and hypoxic–hypercapnic interaction at the end of the apneic period that is so necessary to the perpetuation of periodicity. However this reasoning does not explain the coexistence of a normal (or even high) ventilatory response to hypoxia in some acclimatized sojourners at high altitude who show relatively little discernable periodic breathing (Fig. 5-11). More subtle effects of this acclimatization might be uncovered and more discerning correlations with response tests may be drawn if breathing pattern "instability" was analyzed with more sensitive and quantitative techniques for assessing oscillatory behavior.[15,18]

This question bears on the physiologic significance of the blunted hypoxic response in the native or long-term resident of high altitude. This blunted response is also manifested in the ventilatory response to exercise in hypoxia. Quite different from the tachypneic, hyperventilatory response achieved at high mechanical cost to the lung and respiratory muscles in the exercising sojourner at high altitudes,[3,4] the native shows an isocapnic or even mildly hypercapnic hyperpnea. Arterial oxygenation is not sacrificed because alveolar to arterial gas transport is greatly enhanced by the resident's markedly enhanced alveolar-capillary surface area. Perhaps the additional manifestation of this blunted hypoxic response in the avoidance of periodic breathing during sleep in hypoxia also provides the healthy native with the luxury of uninterrupted sleep states and some tightly regulated arterial blood gases and acid–base status, cerebral blood flow and pulmonary vascular pressures. Such potential benefits of the blunted response in these two dominant physiologic states—exercise and sleep—clearly point to a significant role for this adaptation in the quality of life and even for survival in chronic hypoxia. An apparent paradox here is that the capability to complete a more transient, highly demanding event in hypoxia such as reaching the summit of Mt. Everest clearly requires a marked hyperventilatory response to hypoxia at least during exhausting exercise.[5] It seems more likely that this last-mentioned response is probably determined by more varied and complex mediators than those that dictate the relatively simple response to acute isocapnic hypoxia in the resting state.

CONSEQUENCES OF PERIODIC BREATHING IN HYPOXIC SLEEP

Sleep Quality

The quality of sleep suffers in hypoxia. Barcroft clearly documented this insomnia in 1925 when he commented on the divergence of opinion between observers of his sleeping habits in hypoxia (who thought it to be normal) and his own experience of the same night in hypoxia.[56] "The two opinions can only be reconciled on the hypothesis that while I spent most of the night in sleep, the slumber was very light and fitful with incessant dreams. The night seemed long and we awoke unrefreshed".

More objective measurements of the electroencephalograph (EEG) generally confirm these early impressions: that is, on the first night or two in hypoxia, proportionately more time is spent in lighter versus deeper stages of non-REM sleep, less time in REM sleep and the number of arousals increases about twofold from normoxia to hypoxia.[13,49] In the nocturnal rat, daily sleeping habits are changed markedly from 5 to 15 minute periods of non-REM sleep at sea level to 2 to 3 minute episodes of "incompletely developed" non-REM sleep at a simulation of 18,000 feet altitude.[57] Patients with chronic hypoxemia because of chronic obstructive pulmonary disease (COPD) also experience many arousals during non-REM sleep.[58]

Why should hypoxemia affect the quality of sleep? There are many apparently logical links here. CNS neurotransmitters, especially serotonin, have been strongly linked with neurochemical "sleep factors"[59] and along with most CNS monoamines, its metabolism is especially sensitive to even mild levels of hypoxemia, especially acute hypoxemia.[60] Associations of ventilatory events to sleep stage changes may also be realized via carotid body stimulation or lung inflation, with appropriate excitation of respiratory center and/or reticular activating system neurons via sinus nerve or vagal afferents. Unfortunately, the available data provides no clearcut support for these seemingly logical interrelationships. Arousal thresholds to HbO_2 desaturation seemed to be very low in normal humans, requiring about 70 to 75 percent SaO_2 (or $PaO_2 < 35$ to 40 mmHg) in non-REM and sometimes even less in REM sleep.[41] Clearly, during sleep at altitudes above 3500 m, hypoxemia approaches these levels of desaturation and will certainly be a factor, but sleep disturbances in hypoxia are also known to occur at much higher levels of HbO_2 saturation. This apparent insensitivity of arousal to hypoxemia is also indicated in the sleeping COPD patient in whom acute hyperoxia was shown to be ineffective in reducing arousals.[58] Hypercapnia, on the other hand, is thought to be a potent stimulus to arousal in humans.[61]

A species difference in susceptibility to hypoxia seems to exist, as dogs need little HbO_2 desaturation relative to cats to stimulate arousal.[62,63] Further, arousal sensitivity is greatly affected by carotid body denervation in dogs but remains unaffected in the denervated cat. Several other potential pulmonary-related arousal factors have been tested in dogs, including lung inflation that frequently causes apnea but not arousal in non-REM sleep, and tracheal smooth muscle stimulation, to which the cough reflex is removed during sleep, and which causes arousal only during non-REM (but not in REM sleep[64]).

Mechanical loads including increased inspiratory resistance[65] and complete airway occlusion[66] also cause arousal in human adults and infants. This arousal response becomes an important consideration even in the healthy individual where airway resistance may increase many times the waking level during all stages of sleep.[20] The sensitivity of the arousal response to "loading" is highly variable among normal subjects, i.e., $\approx$ 4 to 60-fold differences exist among subjects in the time to arousal following load imposition.[65,66] While upper airway, pulmonary and/or chest wall receptors may all be involved to some extent, chemoreceptor stimuli must also be considered because of the sustained hypoventilation that commonly results from the sluggish ventilatory compensation to loads imposed during non-REM sleep.[65,67] Carotid body denervation in the dog greatly dampens the arousal response to this type of loading.[64] The likely humoral stimulus here is the powerful combination of a progressive hypercapnia and hypoxemia.

Clearly, the arousal response is important physiologically as a pulmonary-related event. For example, occlusion in the upper airway is not terminated until arousal restores airway muscle tone[68] and hypoventilation will persist with increased airway resistance until ventilatory load compensation is activated by arousal.[65,67] In patients with (obstructive) sleep apnea syndrome, periodic breathing occurs during sleep and each apnea-ventilation cycle is usually associated with a lightening of sleep state or an arousal.[69,70] In hypoxia, the rationale for frequent arousals is not as clear. On the one hand, arousal will eliminate most of the periodic breathing patterns and normal gas exchange would be restored. On the other hand, transient changes in sleep state, especially between light and deep sleep and wakefulness, promotes even more unstable breathing.[9] Perhaps no link does exist here. That is, in the sojourner at 4500 m or in the native of high altitude[54,55] arousals were not significantly correlated with the severity of periodic breathing; and the sojourner at high altitude was reported to reduce periodic breathing during acclimatization without markedly affecting the proportion of time spent in each sleep state.[14,49] Certainly arousal may be perceived as a ventilatory event or one intimately related to powerful ventilatory stimuli such as hypoxic hypercapnia and especially to load compensation. However, these pulmonary-related factors may also be overridden in extremely complex situations pathophysiologically, such as occurs in acute hypoxia where insomnia is just one manifestation of a whole range of symptoms experienced with acute mountain sickness. These overriding factors may at least partially explain why we generally noted that normal subjects appeared to sleep much more soundly and with fewer arousals when the sleep period was begun within an hour of entering the hypoxic environment (in a hypobaric chamber) versus initiating the sleep period at the end of the initial day in hypoxia.

Pulmonary Gas Exchange

Disorders of ventilatory control during sleep, which include both frank periodic breathing and transient hypopnea, may have profound effects on arterial oxygenation during sleep—even in health. Simple alveolar hypoventilation with CO_2 retention during sleep may cause substantial hypoxemia in patients with COPD at sea level as PaO_2 falls coincident with the reduction in PAO_2. However, with periodic breathing and apnea the steady-state condition requirements for application of the alveolar air equation no longer apply. Thus in nonsteady states such as the obstructive sleep apnea syndrome at low altitudes, hypoxemia often occurs with no measurable CO_2 retention[69] and during periodic breathing at high altitudes arterial O_2 desaturation exceeds that predicted from corresponding changes in $PaCO_2$.

Why might periodic breathing cause such extreme transient hypoxemia? One explanation relates to the aforementioned differences in body stores of O_2 versus CO_2, which would cause much more rapid changes in PaO_2 than $PaCO_2$ following an apneic period. Findley et al.[71] have recently investigated the effect of various types of breath-holding on oxygenation revealing that, whereas Valsalva or Mueller maneuvers during the breath-hold made little difference to oxygenation, any reduction in FRC caused marked desaturation following a 30 seconds breath-hold, especially if lung volume was reduced to or below airway closing capacity. This hypoxemia far exceeded that predicted from simple CO_2

retention alone. Sleep effects on FRC appear to be minimal in normal subjects when measured under steady-state conditions in normoxia[72]; however in the transition from non-REM to REM, some substantial reductions in end-expiratory lung volume have been observed in patients with cystic fibrosis[73] and have been implicated as a major cause of the accompanying hypoxemia in these patients.

The depressed inspiratory neural drive inherent in much of the cycle of periodic breathing may also lead to further hypoventilation and hypoxemia if sensory input to upper airway muscles is reduced sufficiently to cause increased airway resistance (also see section below). Certainly normal subjects may experience significant and sometimes marked increases in airway resistance during sleep. Given the relative absence of mechanical load compensation in sleep, substantial hypoventilation would be expected to ensue. If this effect on reducing tidal volume was combined with even relatively small reductions in FRC, then narrowing of small airways with abnormal ventilation distribution and the creation of areas of low ventilation to perfusion would surely follow.

The intermittent hypoxemia induced by periodic breathing in sleep may have long-term consequences on pulmonary-vascular resistance and on red cell production. Alveolar hypoxia, especially when combined with a restrictive pulmonary-vascular bed, causes marked increases in pulmonary arterial pressure; indeed these effects have been noted in sleeping COPD patients with transient bouts of hypoxemia secondary to hypoventilation and obstructive apneas.[74] Whether this intermittent hypoxemia can cause *chronic* pulmonary hypertension with right ventricular hypertrophy has not been documented in humans although these long-term effects have been found in otherwise normal rats and dogs who have been exposed to intermittent hypoxemia.[75] In long-term residents of high altitude with "chronic" mountain polycythemia, some degree of lung disease was common but daytime SaO_2 was within the normal range (for 3100 m altitude). More severe hypoxemia was present in these subjects during sleep coincident with "irregular" breathing patterns and large swings in SaO_2.[54,55] Administration of a chronic ventilatory stimulant (medroxy progesterogerone acetate) lessened the duration and severity of nocturnal hypoxemia in these subjects and lessened their polycythemia.[54,55]

Clinical Correlates

Some aspects of the periodic breathing pattern in the newborn, especially preterm infant, are analogous—with some interesting exceptions—to that seen in the healthy adult in high altitudes. Sleeping newborns will readily demonstrate periodic breathing when made hypoxic, as observed either with acutely induced hypoxia at sea level[76,77] or in infants born at high altitudes. The premature infant may manifest periodic breathing even at PaO_2s in the 70 to 80 mmHg range.[78] An interesting contrast here, however, is that the infant's overall ventilatory response to hypoxia is a "biphasic" one with initial stimulation followed within minutes by ventilatory depression. This secondary depression may be true alveolar hypoventilation (i.e., CO_2 retention)[76] or may be secondary to a hypoxic-induced reduction in metabolic rate (i.e. isocapnia at reduced $\dot{V}_A$).[77] Further, preterm infants in the first few weeks of life, and especially in the first hours after delivery, commonly show a highly irregular and often periodic breathing pattern in all sleep stages and even wakefulness when significant hypoxemia is not apparent.[76,79] Like hypoxic adults, low levels of inspired CO_2 and increases of only ≈2 mmHg in $P_{ET}CO_2$ will reduce T_E and regularize breathing pattern in these infants. Acute hyperoxygenation also regularizes breathing pattern in premature infants[78,79]—an effect that might also be explained by the combined effects of reduced peripheral chemoreceptor activity and elevated $PaCO_2$ above the apneic threshold.

The mechanisms of increased chemoreceptor gain during sleep may also contribute significantly to some types of obstructive sleep apneas, especially those of the "mixed" variety, i.e., central plus occlusive. The link may be found in the commonality in nervous innervations of skeletal muscles that regulate upper airway calibre on the one hand, and inspiratory chest wall muscle activity on the other.

If even moderate hypoxemia is already existent in the waking state then any transient hyperventilation and hypocapnia in the sleeping state—secondary to spontaneous, augmented inspirations, sleep state changes, or even slightly more hypoxemia—will initiate oscillatory periods of waxing and waning of V_T. These oscillations further augment peripheral chemoreceptor activity, ventilatory overshoots, and eventually with sufficient hypocapnia, central apnea. This occurrence is like that described in the healthy person in hypoxic sleep, who then terminates his central apnea with an augmented ventilatory response. However, in the predisposed patient with an already hypotonic, narrowed upper airway the negative tracheal pressure generated by his inspiratory effort during the (central) apneic period will cause occlusive apnea. Another recent model emphasizes the importance of a differential temporal activation of upper airway versus chest wall muscles[80] as the final precipitating event in converting ventilatory instability into occlusive apnea.[81]

Some limited experimental support of this link between chemoreceptor-induced instability of breathing pattern and obstructive apnea does exist. First, parallel reductions in EMG activity of the genioglossus versus diaphragm were observed during the hypoventilation period obtained just prior to the onset of obstructive apnea.[82,83] Secondly, 30 minutes of hyperoxia were shown to markedly reduce the number and length of obstructive apneas in some adults with sleep apnea syndrome who were moderately hypoxemic in the waking state.[84] This effect differs substantially from that found in other obstructive apnea patients in whom hyperoxia only markedly prolonged the duration of their apneic episodes, often causing marked respiratory acidosis.[85,86] In this latter group, which probably comprises the majority of occlusive sleep apnea patients, hypoxemia's role was only that of increasing inspiratory drive during the apneic period. With the former group, their apnea was in part caused by hypoxemic-induced hypocapnia, and hyperoxia removed both increased peripheral chemoreceptor gain and gradually increased central chemoreceptor PCO_2 (via decreased $\dot{V}_A$ and reduced cerebral blood flow) to eventually exceed the apneic threshold.

SUMMARY

Non-REM sleep in hypoxia presents an ideal combination for destabilization of ventilatory control. The key destabilizers are to be found in the alteration of characteristics of both types of chemoreception during hypoxic sleep. Thus, the sleeping state, per se, causes a marked nonlinearity in the medullary chemoreceptor response to reduced [H+], as manifested in the appearance of an apneic threshold; high peripheral chemoreceptor gain occurs because of the hypoxemia secondary to the hypoxic environment.

Non-REM sleep may be viewed then as being highly vulnerable to instability. The primary reason is the absence of the stabilizing influences of wakefulness and thus the overwhelming dependence of ventilatory regulation on CO_2 during sleep. Therefore, variation in sleep state and/or (upper) airway resistance cause fluctuations in CO_2 and corresponding ventilatory "disturbances", usually secondary to inhibiting feedback. These events are usually transient and are of little consequence to homeostasis—of sleep state or gas transport—unless hypoxemia is superimposed as yet another very potent feedback influence to "destabilize" PCO_2.

Why would the control system be designed to permit periodic breathing? Clearly, the same elements of the system that cause instability in hypoxic sleep are essential to stability and homeostasis in other physiologic states. Negative feedback via chemoreception is an essential means of error detection and for quick restoration of homeostasis in a wide variety of transient, acute and chronic perturbations in health and disease in different postures, during exercise, etc. The major change between these conditions and the sleeping state is the susceptability of chemoreceptor output to CO_2 loss; even this is not a major problem unless hypoxemia occurs as the perpetuating agent.

It is difficult to rationalize the occurrence of periodic breathing in hypoxic sleep. The overall regulation of alveolar ventilation and $PaCO_2$ is not significantly affected by the periodic pattern; it is the marked temporal fluctuations in ventilation, which epitomize this state. On the one hand, the fact that the apneic threshold does constrain the amount of continuous hyperventilation, and hypocapnia in hypoxic sleep may permit hypoxic cerebral vasodilation not to be overridden by too severe a level of arterial hypocapnia. On the other hand, this potentially protective mechanism seems relatively minor in the face of marked temporal fluctuations in pulmonary vascular pressures, oxygen transport and acid–base status and the likely contributions of breathing pattern instability to sleep state disturbance and as a precursor to obstructive apnea. It seems fortunate, then, that these destabilizers may at least be overridden by augmented drives to breathe, in the case of the apneic threshold, or may even be substantially dampened by chronic hypoxia, as may be the case with adaptive influences on peripheral chemoreceptor gain.

REFERENCES

1. Musch TI, Dempsey JA, Smith CA et al: Metabolic acids and [H+] regulation in brain tissue during acclimatization to chronic hypoxia. J Appl Physiol 55:1486, 1983
2. Smith CA, Jameson LC, Mitchell GS et al: Central-peripheral chemoreceptor interaction in the awake CSF-perfused goat. J Appl Physiol 56:1541, 1984
3. Dempsey JA, Forster HV: Mediation of ventilatory adaptations. Physiol Rev 62:262, 1982
4. Dempsey JA, Gledhill N, Reddan WG et al: Pulmonary adaptation to exercise: Effects of exercise type and duration, chronic hypoxia, and physical training. Ann NY Acad Sci 301:243, 1977
5. West JB: Human physiology at extreme altitudes on Mount Everest. Science 223:784, 1984
6. Karp HR, Sieker HO, Heyman A: Cerebral circulation and function in Cheyne–Stokes respiration. Am J Med 30:861, 1961
7. Schwartz BA, Eprinchard MF: Cheyne–Stokes respiration and sleep: A diurnal polygraphic study. Electroencephalogr Clin Neurophysiol 39:575, 1975
8. Dowell AR, Buckley CE, Cohen R et al: Cheyne–Stokes respiration. Arch Intern Med 127:712, 1971
9. Bulow K: Respiration and wakefulness in man. Acta Physiol Scand (Suppl 209) 59:1, 1963
10. Webb P: Periodic breathing during sleep. J Appl Physiol 37:899, 1974
11. Webber CL, Speck DF: Experimental biot periodic breathing in cats: Effects of changes in PI_{O_2} and PI_{CO_2}. Respir Physiol 46:327, 1981
12. Douglas CG, Haldane JS, Henderson Y, Schneider EC: VI. Physiological observations made on Pike's Peak, Colorado, with special reference to adaptation to low barometric pressures. Philos Trans R Soc Lond [Biol] 203:185, 1913
13. Berssenbrugge A, Dempsey JA, Iber C et al: Mechanisms of hypoxia-induced periodic breathing during sleep in humans. J Physiol (London) 343:507, 1983
14. Berssenbrugge A, Dempsey JA, Skatrud J: Effects of sleep state on ventilatory acclimatization to chronic hypoxia. J Appl Physiol 57:1089, 1984
15. Waggener TB, Brusil PJ, Kronauer RE et al: Strength and cycle time of high-altitude ventilatory patterns in unacclimatized humans. J Appl Physiol 56:576, 1984
16. Khoo MCK, Kronauer RE, Strohl KP, Slutsky AS: Factors inducing periodic breathing in humans: A general model. J Appl Physiol 53:644, 1982
17. Lahiri S, Maret K, Sherpa MG: Dependence of high altitude sleep apnea on ventilatory sensitivity to hypoxia. Respir Physiol 52:281, 1983
18. Brusil PJ, Waggener RE, Kronauer RE, Gulesian P: Methods for identifying respiratory oscillations disclose altitude effects. J Appl Physiol 48:545, 1980
19. England SJ, Bartlett D: Comparison of human vocal cord movements during isocapnic hypoxia and hypercapnia. J Appl Physiol 53:81, 1982
20. Hudgel DW, Martin RJ, Johnson B, Hill P: Mechanics of the respiratory system and breathing pattern during sleep in normal humans. J Appl Physiol 56:133, 1984
21. Tabachnik E, Muller NL, Bryan AC, Levison H: Changes in ventilation and chest wall mechanics during sleep in normal adolescents. J Appl Physiol 51:557, 1981

22. Orem J, Montplaiser J, Dement WC: Changes in the activity of respiratory neurons during sleep. Brain Res 82:309, 1974
23. Remmers JE: Effects of sleep on control of breathing. In Widdicombe JG (ed): Respiratory Physiology III. Vol. 23. University Park Press, Baltimore, 1981
24. Phillipson EA: Control of breathing during sleep. Am Rev Respir Dis 118:909, 1978
25. Parmeggiani PL, Sabattini L: Electromyographic aspects of postural respiratory and thermoregulatory mechanisms in sleeping cats. Electroencephalogr Clin Neurophysiol 33:1, 1972
26. Cherniack NS, von Euler C, Homma I, Kao F: Animal models of Cheyne–Stokes Breathing. p. 417. In von Euler C, Logercrantz H (eds): Central Nervous Control Mechanisms in Breathing, Pergamon, London 1979
27. Cherniack NS: Respiratory dysrhythmias during sleep. N Engl J Med 305:325, 1981
28. Cherniack NS, Longobardo GS: Cheyne–Stokes breathing: An instability in physiologic control. N Engl J Med 288:952, 1973
29. Cherniack NS, von Euler C, Homma I, Kao FF: Experimentally induced Cheyne–Stokes breathing. Respir Physiol 37:185, 1979
30. Cherniack NS, Longobardo GS, Levine OR et al: Periodic breathing in dogs. J Appl Physiol 21:1847, 1966
31. Cherniack NS, von Euler C, Homma I, Kao FF: Effects of increased respiratory controller gain during hypoxia and hypercapnia on periodic breathing in cats. p. 423. In Fitzgerald R, Lahiri S, Gautier H (eds): Regulation of Respiration During Sleep and Anesthesia. Plenum, New York, 1978
32. Brown HW, Plum F: The neurologic basis of Cheyne–Stokes respiration. Am J Med 30:849, 1961
33. Skatrud J, Dempsey J: Interaction of sleep state and chemical stimuli in sustaining rhythmic ventilation. J Appl Physiol 55:813, 1983
34. Bainton CR, Mitchell RA: Posthyperventilation apnea in awake man. J Appl Physiol 21:411, 1966
35. Bowes G, Audrey SM, Kozar L, Phillipson EA: Carotid chemoreceptor regulation of expiratory duration. J Appl Physiol 54:1195, 1983
36. Skatrud J, Berssenbrugge A: Effect of sleep state and chemical stimuli on breathing. p. 87. In Sutton JR, Houston CS, Jones NL (eds): Hypoxia, Exercise, and Altitude: Progress in Clinical and Biological Research, Vol. 136. Alan R. Liss, New York, 1983
37. Berkenbosch A, Van Beek JHG, Olievier CN et al: Central respiratory CO_2 sensitivity at extreme hypocapnia. Respir Physiol 55:95, 1984
38. Polacheck J, Strong RS, Arens J et al: Phasic vagal influence on inspiratory motor output in anesthetized human subjects. J Appl Physiol 49:609, 1980
39. Hickey RF, Fourcade HE, Eger EI et al: The effects of ether, halothane, and forane on apneic thresholds in man. Anesthesiology 35:32, 1971
40. Eldridge FL: Posthyperventilation breathing: Different effects of active and passive hyperventilation. J Appl Physiol 34:422, 1973
41. Berthon-Jones M, Sullivan CE: Ventilatory and arousal responses to hypoxia in sleeping humans. Am Rev Respir Dis 125:632, 1982
42. Douglas NJ, White DP, Weil JV et al: Hypoxic ventilatory response decreases during sleep in normal men. Am Rev Respir Dis 125:286, 1982
43. Perez-Padilla R, West P, Kryger MH: Sighs during sleep in adult humans. Sleep 6:234, 1983

44. Reynolds LB: Characteristics of an inspiration augmenting reflex in anesthetized cats. J Appl Physiol 17:683, 1962
45. Thach BT, Taeusch HW: Sighing in newborn human infants: Role of inflation augmenting reflex. J Appl Physiol 41:502, 1976
46. Cherniack NS, von Euler C, Glogowska M, Homma I: Characteristics and rate of occurrence of spontaneous and provoked augmented breaths. Acta Physiol Scand 111:349, 1981
47. Glogowska M, Richardson PS, Widdicombe JG, Winning AJ: The role of the vagus nerves, peripheral chemoreceptors and other afferent pathways in the genesis of augmented breaths in cats and rabbits. Respir Phys 16:179, 1972
48. Bartlett D: Origin and regulation of spontaneous deep breaths. Respir Physiol 12:230, 1971
49. Reite M, Jackson D, Cahoon R, Weil JV: Sleep physiology at high altitude. Electroencephalogr Clin Neurophysiol 38:463, 1975
50. Mitchell R, Bainton C, Edelist G: Posthyperventilation apnea in awake dogs during metabolic acidosis and hypoxia. J Appl Physiol 21:1363, 1966
51. Sutton JR, Houston CS, Mansell AL et al: Effects of acetazolamide on hypoxemia during sleep at high altitude. N Engl J Med 301:1329, 1979
52. Weil JV, Kryger MH, Scoggèn CH: Sleep and breathing at high altitude. p. 119. In Guilleminault C, Dement WC (eds): Sleep Apnea Syndromes. Allan R. Liss, New York, 1978
53. Skatrud J, Dempsey J: Relative effectiveness of acetazolamide versus medroxyprogesterone acetate in correction of chronic CO_2 retention. Am Rev Respir Dis 127:405, 1983
54. Kryger M, Glas R, Jackson D et al: Impaired oxygenation during sleep in excessive polycythemia of high altitude: Improvement with respiratory stimulation. Sleep 1:3, 1978
55. Kryger M, McCullough R, Doekel R et al: Excessive polycythemia of high altitude: Role of ventilatory drive and lung disease. Am Rev Respir Dis 118:659, 1978
56. Barcroft J: The respiratory function of the blood. Part II, Lessons from high altitudes. Cambridge University Press, Cambridge 1925
57. Pappenheimer JR: Sleep and respiration of rats during hypoxia. J Physiol 266:191, 1977
58. Fleetham J, West P, Mezon B et al: Sleep, arousals, and oxygen desaturation in chronic obstructive pulmonary disease. Am Rev Respir Dis 126:429, 1982
59. Jouvet M: Biogenic amines and the states of sleep. Science 163:32, 1969
60. Olson EB, Vidruk EH, McCrimmon DR, Dempsey JA: Monoamine neurotransmitter metabolism during acclimatization to chronic hypoxia. Respir Physiol 54:79, 1983
61. Phillipson EA, Sullivan CE: Arousal: The forgotten response to respiratory stimuli. Am Rev Respir Dis 118:807, 1978
62. Bowes G, Townsend ER, Bromley SM et al: Role of the carotid body and of afferent vagal stimuli in the arousal response to airway occlusion in sleeping dogs. Am Rev Respir Dis 123:644, 1981
63. Neubauer JA, Santiago T, Edelman N: Hypoxic arousal in intact and carotid chemodenervated sleeping cats. J Appl Physiol 51:1294, 1981
64. Sullivan CE, Kozar LF, Murphy E, Phillipson EA: Arousal, ventilatory and airway responses to bronchopulmonary stimulation in sleeping dogs. J Appl Physiol 47:17, 1979

65. Iber C, Berssenbrugge A, Skatrud JB, Dempsey JA: Ventilatory adaptations to resistive loading during wakefulness and non-REM sleep. J Appl Physiol 52:607, 1982
66. Issa FG, Sullivan CE: Arousal and breathing responses to airway occlusion in healthy sleeping adults. J Appl Physiol 55:1113, 1983
67. Wilson PA, Skatrud JB, Dempsey JA: Effects of slow wave sleep on ventilatory compensation to inspiratory elastic loading. Respir Physiol 55:103, 1984
68. Remmers JE, DeGroot WJ, Sauerland EK, Anch AM: Pathogenesis of upper-airway obstruction during sleep. J Appl Physiol 44:931, 1978
69. Tilkian AG, Guilleminault C, Schroeder JS: Hemodynamics in sleep-induced apnea. Ann Intern Med 85:714, 1975
70. Guilleminault C, Tilkian A, Dement WC: The sleep apnea syndromes. Ann Rev Med, 27:465, 1976
71. Findley LJ, Ries A, Tisi G, Wagner PD: Hypoxemia during apnea in normal subjects: Mechanisms and impact of lung volume. J Appl Physiol 55:1777, 1983
72. Hudgel DW, Devadatta P: Decrease in functional residual capacity during sleep in normal man. J Appl Physiol 57:1319, 1984
73. Muller NL, Francis PW, Gurwitz D: Mechanism of hemoglobin desaturation during REM sleep in normal subjects and patients with cystic fibrosis. Am Rev Respir Dis 121:463, 1980
74. Wynne JW, Block AJ, Hemenway J et al: Disordered breathing and oxygen desaturation during sleep in patients with chronic obstructive lung disease (COLD). Am J Med 66:573, 1979
75. Nattie EE: Pulmonary hypertension and RVH caused by intermittant drop in PO_2 and rise in PCO_2 in the rat. Am Rev Resp Dis 118:653, 1978
76. Rigatto H, Brady JP: Periodic breathing and apnea in preterm infants. II. Hypoxia as a primary event. Pediatrics 50:219, 1972
77. Haddad GG, Schaeffer JI, Bazzy AR: Postnatal maturation of the ventilatory response to hypoxia. p. 39. In Sutton JR, Houston CS, Jones NL (eds): Hypoxia, Exercise, and Altitude: Progress in Clinical and Biological Research, Volume 136, Alan R. Liss, New York, 1983
78. Lagercrantz H, Ahlström H, Jonson B: A critical oxygen level below which irregular breathing occurs in premature infants. p. 161. In von Euler C, Lagercrantz H (eds): Central Nervous Control Mechanisms in Breathing. Pergamon, London 1979
79. Kalapesi Z, Durand M, Leahy FN et al: Effect of periodic or regular respiratory pattern on the ventilatory response to low inhaled CO_2 in preterm infants during sleep. Am Rev Respir Dis 123:8, 1981
80. Weiner D, Mitra J, Salamone J, Cherniack NS: Effect of chemical stimuli on nerves supplying upper-airway muscles. J Appl Physiol 48:500, 1980
81. Longobardo GS, Gothe B, Goldman MD, Cherniack NS: Sleep apnea considered as a control system instability. Respir Physiol 50:311, 1982
82. Onal E, Lopata M: Periodic breathing and the pathogenesis of occlusive sleep apneas. Am Rev Respir Dis 126:676, 1982
83. Onal E, Lopata M, O'Connor T: Pathogenesis of apneas in hypersomnia-sleep apnea syndrome. Am Rev Respir Dis 125:167, 1982
84. Martin RJ, Sanders MH, Gray BA, Pennock BE: Acute and long-term ventilatory effects of hyperoxia in the adult sleep apnea syndrome. Am Rev Respir Dis 125:175, 1982

85. Motta J, Guilleminault C: Effects of oxygen administration in sleep-induced apneas. p. 137. In Guilleminault C, Dement W (eds): Sleep apnea syndrome. Alan R. Liss, New York, 1978
86. Garay SM, Rapoport D, Sorkin B et al: Regulation of ventilation in the obstructive sleep apnea syndrome. Am Rev Respir Dis 124:175, 1981

6 Control of the Upper Airway During Sleep

Kingman P. Strohl

The physiology described in this chapter concerns the conducting airway from the nose and mouth to the larynx.[1–3] Although the upper airway does not participate in gas exchange, changes in its flow-resistive properties or in the response of upper airway mechanoreceptors may influence respiratory rate and tidal volume and consequently affect gas exchange. One example of the importance of the upper airway in breathing is the occurrence of obstructive apneas during sleep.

This chapter will consider three areas of the upper airway physiology relating to sleep: sensory feedback of respiratory events from upper airway receptors; the mechanical characteristics of the airway itself; and upper airway muscle function. At present, more information is available from studies in animals than in humans. This chapter will not comprehensively review upper airway physiology as it relates to deglutition, speech and song, or to senses such as smell or taste, except to illustrate some respiratory issues. I will attempt to provoke thinking on factors that affect upper airway function during sleep and which may lead to the pathogenesis of apneas during sleep in humans.

ANATOMY

Under ordinary conditions, including sleep, airflow moves through the nose on its way into and out of the pharynx, larynx, trachea, and lungs (Fig. 6-1). The nose is well designed to be a heat exchanger, having a highly developed vascular mucosa overlying curved turbinates, which allows air to be warmed and humidified on inspiration and heat and water to be retained on expiration.[1–3] The narrowest portion of the nose and, consequently, its site of major resistance, lies within the first few centimeters of the external nares and has been termed the "nasal valve."[1] Vascular factors greatly affect the mucosa and, consequently, the size of the nasal valve.[1] In addition, the caliber of the nasal valve can be altered by action of muscles on cartilages forming the external nares. The result is to decrease nasal resistance, particularly inspiratory resistance, by flaring the walls of the nasal vestibule.[4] Besides changing resistance, the nasal valve may work as a nozzle and change flow direction to optimize heat exchange.

The nasopharynx is a secondary region of narrowing. Structures surrounding the airway at this point include (1) the cranial ethmoid roof, (2) the lateral and posterior adenoidal lymphoid tissues, (3) the soft palate, and (4) the various muscles inserting into the soft palate and surrounding the airway. The uvula has no known role in humans and simple uvulectomy apparently does not affect upper airway function. The palate is important in directing airflow through the mouth.[5,6] Studies of cleft palate and cleft palate repair have demonstrated that palatal incompetence results in an inability to breathe exclusively through the mouth.[6] During "pursed lip breathing," the position of the palate is a major factor preventing expiratory airflow through the nose.[5] Changes in the position of the palate may also be important in the transition from nose to mouth breathing with exercise.[7] A surgically narrowed nasopharynx can precipitate upper airway obstruction during sleep.[8]

The oronasal pharynx is a region less well studied because of its seeming lack of importance during quiet breathing or other respiratory maneuvers performed while awake and in the upright posture. During sleep, when the supine position is assumed and/or when its negative intraluminal pressures are greater, the contribution of the pharynx to upper airway resistance may increase. Posteriorly, the constrictor muscles wrap around the pharyngeal airway. In the anterior pharyngeal wall the hyoid bone is positioned by 12 pairs of muscles and by connective tissue attachments from the hyoid to the epiglottis, the tongue, the thyroid cartilage and the sternum. In the nonprimate mammal, from the main arch of the hyoid two jointed cartilages, the superior cornu, project on either side of the airway and attach to the styloid process of the skull. Two inferior cornu project from the main body of the hyoid and attach to the sides of thyroid cartilage. Thus the hyoid apparatus forms a cartilagenous, flexible cage around the pharynx in the nonprimate. This structure is not present in the primate, giving the airway apparently less external structural stability.

Mouth breathing is accomplished by lowering the mandible, lifting the palate and probably by forward movement of the base of the tongue and hyoid apparatus. Mouth breathing occurs commonly during periods where high inspiratory flows (during speech), high expiratory flows (cough) and/or increased ventilation (exercise) are required. Predominant mouth breathing in humans occurs at exercise levels greater than 65 to 70 percent of maximal oxygen consumption.[7] The mouth is less efficient in heat exchange than the nose.

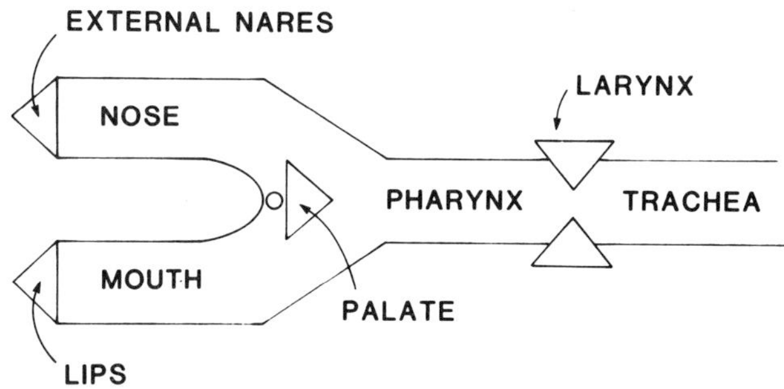

Fig. 6-1 This schematic diagram identifies the major intraluminal anatomic regions. Air moves in and out of the lungs through the nose and/or mouth, pharynx, and larynx. Valvular regions of the external nares, lips, palate, and larynx are identified by the triangle symbols.

For breathing purposes the larynx can be thought to act as a choke valve in a rigid tube. Its position in the airway is ideally suited for modifying expiratory airflow.[1] Of the parts of the upper airway, laryngeal action has been most extensively studied. Changes in the shape as well as size of the laryngeal orifice occur as the result of a coordinated activation of muscles and movement of structures anterior and posterior to the vocal folds.[9–14]

RESPIRATORY REFLEXES FROM THE UPPER AIRWAY

In addition to the sensation of taste and smell, the upper airway contains a number of different receptors that respond to a variety of mechanical and chemical agents. Histologically, exposed nerve endings are found in the mucosa and submucosa from the nose to the trachea. The sensory information from these upper airway receptors travels to the central nervous system through cranial nerves V, VII, IX, X, XI, and XII. It is likely that proprioceptive information is also mediated by receptors in muscles, tendons, and joints. For instance, muscle spindles in the tongue project to other upper airway motor centers and can mediate changes in heart rate and vascular resistance.[15]

Experiments in anesthetized animals employing electrical stimulation of cranial nerves have shown powerful effects on respiratory rate and rhythm. Stimulation of the superior laryngeal nerve can completely inhibit respiration and lead to death of the animal.[16] Stimulation of the glossopharyngeal nerve alters respiratory frequency and depth.[17] Newborn rabbits respond to mechanical stimulation at the external nares and to the larynx with a fatal apnea but in response to similar stimuli adult animals will resume breathing.[18,19] Thus, there is a developmental feature of receptor function that is currently of interest.

One dramatic response elicited from the upper airways is the diving reflex. Cold water applied intranasally or to the face in the distribution of the maxillary division of the trigeminal nerve will elicit apnea, bradycardia, and peripheral vascular constriction.[20] The input/output characteristics of the diving response has been extensively studied although it is not known where or how the response is coordinated in the central nervous system.

The remainder of this section will focus on mucosal mechanoreceptors from each region of the upper airway.

Nose and Nasopharynx

Mechanical stimulation of the nasopharynx mucosa alters breathing frequency. Small negative pressures applied to the nasopharynx increase inspiratory time and decrease the rate of diaphragmatic activity, but increase the amount of dilator muscle activation not only in the alae nasi but also in the genioglossus and posterior cricoarytenoid as well.[21,22] Absence of these reflexes after application of topical anesthesia to the nasopharynx suggests that the receptors lie at or near the mucosal surface.

Recent studies in man found that breath-holding time is prolonged when air is blown through the nose.[23] This study did not identify either the site or mechanism of the effect of airflow or temperature stimuli but did demonstrate that in awake humans there exist potential influences on respiration rising from nasal receptors.

Mouth and Pharynx

Unlike the responses found in the isolated nasopharynx or larynx, negative pressures applied to the oropharynx do not appreciably alter respiratory timing.[22] Mechanoreceptors lying in the mucosa are presumably involved with deglutination and protection of the tracheorespiratory tree from aspiration.[2] Effects of airflow or temperature on oropharynx receptors have not been studied.

Larynx

The internal branch of the superior laryngeal nerve provides sensory fibers to regions above the cords and to a lesser extent below the cords as well. In the isolated larynx, frequency and amplitude response curves can be constructed for discretely applied sinusoidal indentations of the mucosa.[24] These studies have suggested interaction of multiple stimuli on the tonic and elicited firing pattern observed in afferent fibers from laryngeal receptors.

Negative pressures applied to the larynx elicit respiratory responses qualitatively similar to negative pressures to the nasopharynx; namely, breathing frequency falls and rate of rise of chest wall muscle activation decreases while activation of upper airway dilator muscles is increased[20,21] (Fig. 6-2). The effects of negative pressures applied to the larynx are abolished by topical anesthesia or by superior laryngeal nerve block. Stimulation of the superior laryn-

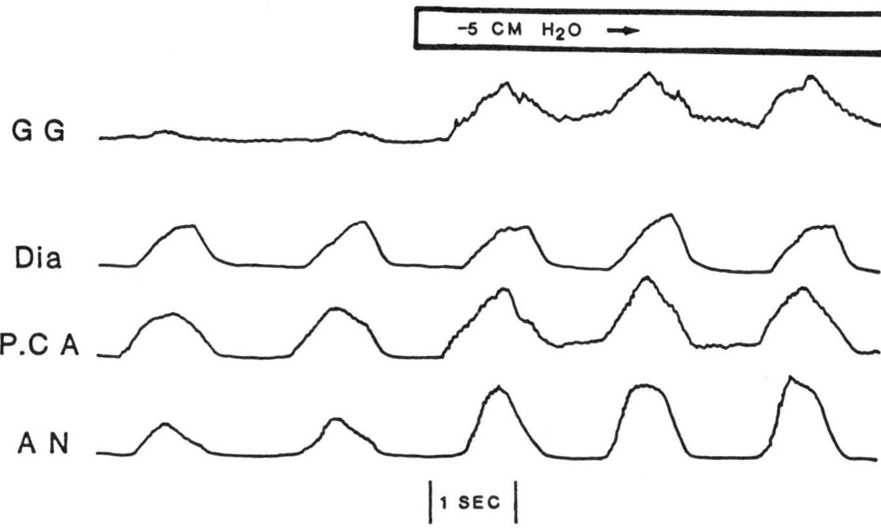

Fig. 6-2 The effect of statically applied negative pressure (-5 cmH_2O) applied intraluminally to the larynx in an anesthetized dog. Note the changes in breathing frequency as well as changes in the amount and duration of the upper airway (GG = genioglossus; PCA = posterior cricoarytenoid; AN = alae nasi) and diaphragm (DIA) muscle activation. (van Lunteren E, van de Graaff WB, Parker DM et al: Reflex effects of negative pressure in the upper airway. J Appl Physiol 56:746, 1984.)

geal nerve depresses respiratory activity in upper airway as well as chest wall muscles, and therefore does not mimic the effects of statically applied negative pressures to the larynx.[21] Negative pressures applied only to the larynx appear to increase posterior cricoarytenoid activity more than alae nasi activity; with negative pressures applied to the nose, alae nasi activity appears to respond more.[21] These findings suggest that collapsing forces applied intraluminally to the upper airway elicit greater responses in muscles locally surrounding that part of the airway than in muscles more distant from the stimulus.

Changes in afferent information in phase with the respiratory cycle has been observed and studied in the superior laryngeal nerve. Sant'Ambrogio et al.[25] have found firing patterns that appear to conform to the presence of inspiratory flow, to changing pressure, or to the presence of respiratory efforts ("drive related").[25] Phasic afferent feedback related to upper airway flow and pressure may have relevance in the initiation, restoration, or maintenance of upper airway patency.

The recurrent laryngeal nerve supplies sensory fibers to the laryngeal region below the vocal cords. Experiments using statically applied pressures have shown reflex effects on laryngeal aperture.[14,27] Conceivably, these same receptors could modulate expiratory flow.

Trachea

Slowly adapting receptors, in series with trachealis smooth muscle, and rapidly adapting receptors in the mucosa and submucosa discharge in relation to airway transmural pressure and flow, respectively.[28]

MECHANICAL CHARACTERISTICS OF THE UPPER AIRWAY

General

The trachea is of sufficient size and stiffness to cause minimal inspiratory and expiratory resistance to airflow, yet compliant enough to be effective in helping clear material from the lungs and to avoid mechanical problems during postural changes or large respiratory excursions. In contrast, the upper airway above the trachea serves several purposes besides just being an air passage. The upper airway serves as a heat exchanger and as a filter for particulate matter or soluable gases. In addition, to allow speech, swallowing, taste and smell, the upper airway is flexible, equipped with valves, and responsive to muscular forces exerted on it. In the upper airway, muscles also alter the route of airflow from the nose to the mouth or to both nose-and-mouth breathing. Mechanical elements in the pharynx and larynx act in series with either the nose or mouth or both.

Upper Airway Caliber

In the nineteenth century the inspiratory nasal air currents were studied using ammonia fumes and litmus paper and it was demonstrated that airflow was greatest at sites of constriction at the nasal valve near the external nares and at the nasopharynx.[29] Later studies using casts of the entire human upper airway obtained postmortem have found that the narrowest regions of the upper airway lie at the external nares and at the larynx, although turbulent flow regimens could also be observed at the nasopharynx and epiglottis at flow rates approximating resting breathing.[1,29]

These in vitro geometrical observations were confirmed to a large extent by in vivo studies of pressure-flow relationships across the different regions of the upper airway. Sites of proportionately greater flow resistance during resting breathing are the nose and across the glottis.[30,31] Opening the mouth resulted in a decrease in upper airway resistance, and resistance during exclusive mouth breathing was less than during exclusive nose breathing during both inspiration and expiration.[31] In humans, values for inspiratory resistance are usually lower than expiratory resistance.[31] Recent studies in humans have also found postural differences in upper airway resistance. An increase in supraglottic resistance in the supine posture is largely attributed to increases in vascular volume in the nasal cavity.[32] (Even in the upright posture the nasal mucosa substantially effects nasal resistance.) Positional differences of upper airway resistance could also reflect a shift in soft tissue or a reflex change in neuromuscular tone.

Nasal resistance is affected by activation of muscles at the external nares. Muscle activation flares the nares, widening the opening to the nose.[4] Changes in nasal caliber may affect flow regimes in the nose either in disrupting laminar flow patterns in order to filter out particulate matter or in dispersing airstreams over wider areas in order to facilitate heat exchange in the nose.[1,29]

Rigidity of the Airway Wall

Geometric factors are dependent upon changes in airway stiffness. Few studies have attempted to control for factors of airway stiffness either in the casting of models of the airway or in measurements of resistance during airflow.

Recent studies suggest that the pharyngeal region closes at very low levels of negative pressure.[33] Closing pressures in the pharynx of the anesthetized rabbit are more negative than those found postmortem, suggesting that an active neuromuscular process exists during life that maintains some degree of airway rigidity.[34,35] Phrenic nerve pacing produces a high grade upper airway resistance, particularly if applied during expiration[33] (Fig. 6-3). Some of the increase in resistance is due to passive collapse of the upper airway. In anesthetized dogs, collapse occurs at the level of the hyoid apparatus.[33] In awake humans, the vocal cords appear to approximate with negative intraluminal pressures.[36] These studies imply that factors related to airway stiffness may be an important element in evaluating upper airway mechanical function.

Valves in the Upper Airway

Three distinct valves exist in the upper airway. The nasal valve at the anterior nares is not capable of complete airway closure, at least not in the human, but can change size and shape of the narrow external nares.[1,4] The soft palate and epiglottis alter the route of airflow between nose and mouth breathing.[5,7] Coordinated muscular events can close off either the nose or mouth or, in the case of deglutition, close off the nose and with the arytenoid structures close off the larynx.[1] The larynx is a variable orifice.[13] The larynx is widest during panting maneuvers.[37] Complete closure of the larynx will occur only when both the superior and recurrent laryngeal nerves are cut.[1] Dilatation or closure of the larynx from its normal mid-position occurs primarily as the consequence of muscular activation. During resting breathing in the cat and lamb, and with bronchoconstriction in humans, slowing or "braking" of expiratory flow often occurs as the result of an active closure of the larynx.[38–40] Since the larynx is the first resistor encountered in the upper airway during

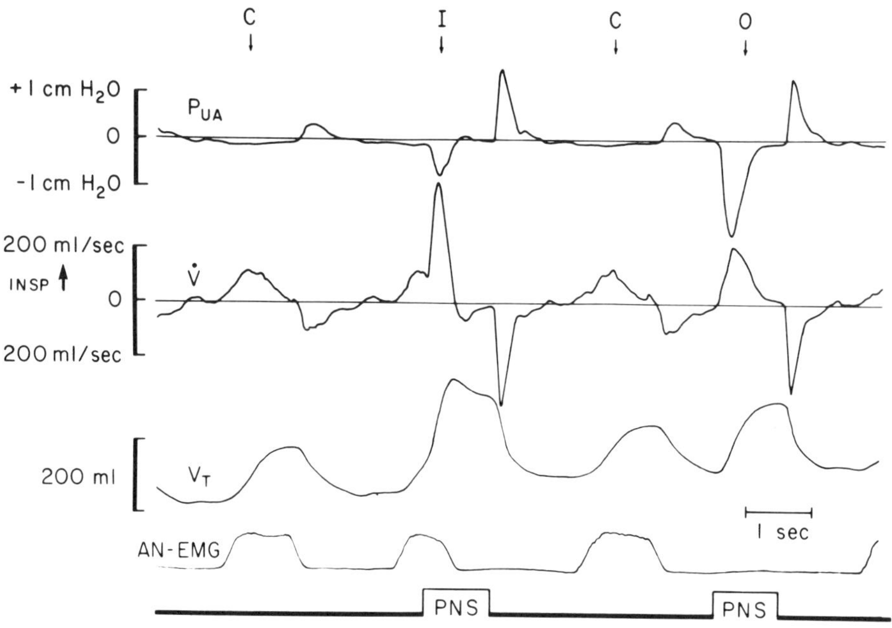

Fig. 6-3 This tracing from an anesthetized dog preparation shows the effect of phrenic nerve pacing (PNS) on upper airway pressure (P_{ua}), airflow ($\dot{V}$), tidal volume (V_T), and the moving average of alae nasi (AN) EMG activation. Spontaneous (control) inspirations (C) precede an instance when PNS occurred in-phase (I) and an instance when PNS occurred out-of-phase (O) with AN activation. Note that between I (AN present) and O (AN absent), flow is less and negative upper airway pressures are greater indicating a substantial increase in flow resistance. (Gottfried SB, Strohl KP, van de Graaff WB et al: Effects of phrenic stimulation on upper-airway resistance in the anesthetized dogs. J Appl Physiol 55:419, 1983)

expiration, active constriction of this structure seems to be a simple and efficient way to decrease the rate of fall in lung volume.

UPPER AIRWAY MUSCLE ACTIVATION

Analysis of muscle function involves consideration of the motor innervation, of the developed force or tension during contraction, and of the resultant action on the structure(s) to which the muscle is attached.[41] In the upper airway, assessment of muscle function is complicated by the multiple functions of the muscles, their complex geometric arrangement, and their interdependence. In general, airway patency seems to be maintained by active neuromuscular mechanisms.[42,43] The occurrence of airway occlusion is documented by the failure of the airway to transmit flow, but this is too crude a measurement of upper airway muscle function. For instance, muscles may function quite normally in a physiological sense but not be able to maintain flow due to changes in the passive characteristics (size or stiffness) of the airway itself. Alternatively, inadequate neuromuscular activation may reduce airway patency even if the airway itself is normal.

Methods

Recordings of electromyographic (EMG) activation of upper airway muscles can be made from electrodes placed on the body surface over or near specific muscles or muscle groups or by inserting pairs of fine wire electrodes directly into an individual muscle. Electromyographic activity can be analyzed for its relationship to airflow or to other respiratory EMG signals. In addition, the electromyographic signal can be processed to obtain an estimate of the amount of activity over time.[44] In the diaphragm, this moving average of EMG activity correlates well with isometric force.[45] Results among different subjects may not be comparable due to differences in electrode placement, muscle position, or gain of the signal. Electromyographic techniques are most useful for comparing different interventions in the same subject or in recognizing patterns rather than for comparing the amount of activation during respiration in different subjects. In Figure 6-4, the moving average of three upper airway muscles

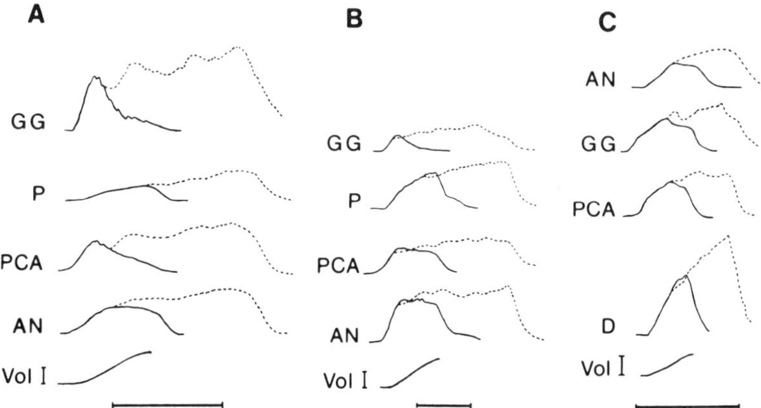

Fig. 6-4 Tracings from three anesthetized dogs (A,B, and C) of the moving average of upper airway and diaphragm muscle activity during a spontaneous breath and a subsequent inspiratory effort when the trachea is occluded at end-expiration. The amount and duration of EMG activity increases during the occluded effort and is the result of absence of vagal feedback associated with lung expansion. This effect occurs earlier and to a greater degree in upper-airway muscles (GG = genioglossus; AN = alae nasi; PCA = posterior cricoarytenoid) than in the phrenic nerve (P) or diaphragm (D). (van Lunteren E, Strohl KP, Parker DM et al: Phasic volume related feedback on upper-airway muscle activity. J Appl Physiol 56:730, 1984.)

and the diaphragm are shown before and during end-expiratory airway occlusion in three anesthetized dogs. The moving averages can allow quantitative analysis of differences in electromyographic activity. In Figure 6-4, it is apparent that airway occlusion increases the amount of activation in upper airway muscles more than in the diaphragm.[55]

Airflow and the pressure drop across the entire upper airway give estimates of flow resistance. Different regions of the upper airway can be isolated by differential pressures. For example, nasal resistance is determined from the pressure drop between the front of the nose and nasopharynx.[4]

Recently, a pulse flow method of estimating the resistive properties of the respiratory system has been described.[48] Applied through a facemask, the pressure resulting from a step change in flow will in part be dependent on the nose and mouth. An elevated pulse flow resistance may indicate an anatomically abnormal upper airway. The test can be performed during wakefulness to detect subjects with obstructive sleep apnea.

In animals, the upper airway can be surgically isolated from the rest of the tracheobronchial tree.[46,47] Flow can be directed in one direction and maintained constant. Pressure drop across structures will then be directly proportional to resistance (Fig. 6-5). In Figure 6-5, airway occlusion is accompanied

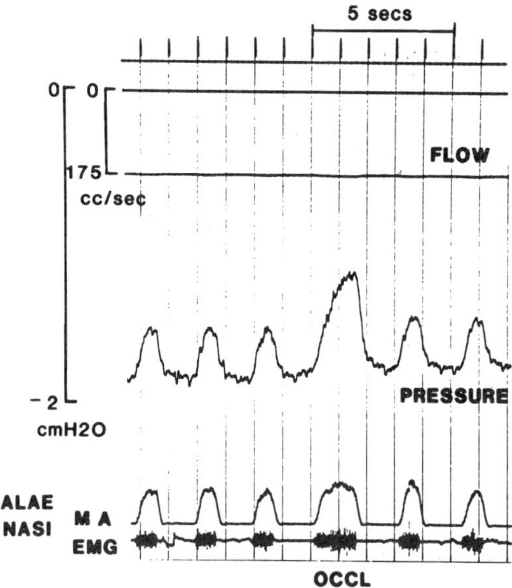

Fig. 6-5 Shown are the changes in pressure across the entire upper airway under conditions when a constant flow of 175 cc/sec is pulled through the airway in an inspiratory direction. Also shown are alae nasi EMG activity in the form of the moving average and the raw signal. Shown are three unimpeded breaths before and two breaths after an effort (OCCL) when the trachea is occluded at end-expiration. Note that the fall in pressure, and therefore, resistance occurs in phase with alae nasi activation patterns and is greater during the occluded effort.

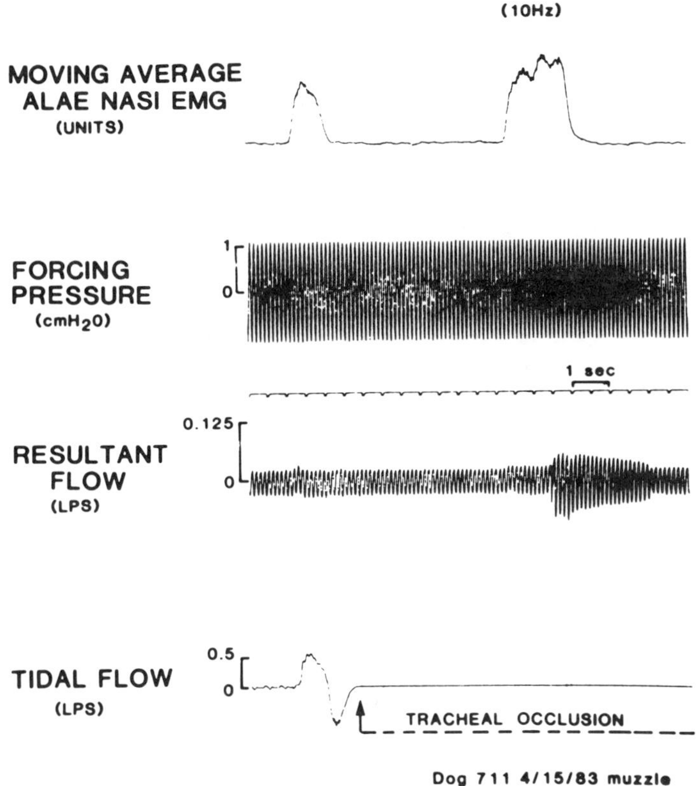

Fig. 6-6 A small sinusoidal forcing pressure at a discrete frequency of 10 Hz was applied to the isolated sealed upper airway of an anesthetized dog. Shown are changes in the moving average of alae nasi activity and the resultant flow during a spontaneous breath and the successive effort when the trachea was occluded at end expiration. The technique of forced oscillation may be a useful way to detect changes in the mechanical properties of the upper airway resulting from contraction of muscles around the upper airway. (Courtesy of C.E. Hafer and J.M. Fouke, Dept. of Biomedical Engineering, Case Western Reserve University, Cleveland, Ohio.)

by a larger inspiratory fall in pressure and, consequently, resistance when compared to the unoccluded breaths.

The method of forced oscillation[49] involves applying small sinusoidal pressure fluctuations to an isolated sealed upper airway and monitoring resultant flow. By noting differences in the magnitude and phase of pressure and flow across a frequency spectrum, one can construct models for the mechanical properties of the upper airway and changes with the respiratory cycle. Using this technique one may be able to assess changing size and stiffness as the result of upper airway muscle activation. An example of forced oscillation at a discrete frequency of 10 Hz is shown in Figure 6-6. Forced oscillatory measurements, however, are not specific for regional variations in upper airway function.

Changes in upper airway geometry can be assessed using radiographic methods. Lateral radiographs provide anterior-posterior views of the airway and several fluoroscopic studies have recorded changes in airway size during cycles of obstructive apnea.[50] Computerized axial tomography can give an estimate of cross-sectional area at specific sites in the upper airway;[51,52] however, currently tomograms take 1 to 2 seconds and, therefore, cannot be used to detect changes within the normal respiratory cycle. Area–distance measurements have been made of the trachea using high frequency sound wave analysis[53] and may be useful in making measurements of the upper airway as well.

Neurophysiological Factors

Phasic changes in upper airway activation coincident with respiratory rate and depth have been recognized for many years. The time course of activation, however, is different from that seen in chest wall muscles.[54,55] Studies of airway dilator muscles such as the alae nasi, genioglossus, and posterior cricoarytenoid show on earlier onset and peak of activation in the upper airway muscles when compared to that observed in the diaphragm. Often activity declines and disappears before expiratory airflow begins. This pattern of activation correlates with mechanical events associated with inspiratory airflow rather than with chest wall expansion. Some upper airway muscles, like the anterior cricothyroid, are active in early expiration and are thought to break expiratory flow.[9–14] A tonic activation can be demonstrated in some muscles, which will change with muscle length and position and with chemical drive.[54]

Contraction of an upper airway muscle will depend upon the firing of its motoneurons. Upper airway motoneurons receive synaptic inputs from at least three major systems of the central nervous system: (1) respiratory drive from medullary brainstem regions; (2) nonrespiratory motor drive from the brainstem and extrabulbar motor systems for deglutition, singing, etc., (3) and reflex drive.

Since the motoneuron is the final common pathway for muscle activation, any nonrespiratory inputs could be a factor in determining whether upper airway motoneurons are sufficiently depolarized to reach firing thresholds in response to changing central respiratory input.

Excitatory and inhibitory bulbar reflex responses have been described in anesthetized and unanesthetized animals. Lung inflation reflexes and chest wall reflexes affect the time course and amount of upper airway muscle activation in a manner similar to but not identical to that of chest wall muscles. For example, lung inflation reflexes inhibit upper airway dilator muscle activation earlier and to a greater degree than chest wall diaphragm muscle activation (Fig. 6-5).[55]

THE UPPER AIRWAY DURING SLEEP

The phenomenon of snoring is used theatrically as an indicator of sleep; this the association of the two is sufficiently common as to be universally recognized. Snoring represents a substantial increase in flow resistance in the upper airway. Obstructive apneas are an infinite resistance, i.e., a functional obstruction in the upper airway. Recent demonstration of the adverse cardiorespiratory effects of both snoring and obstructive apneas have changed attitudes of both laymen and clinicians from bemusement to concern.

Current studies of upper airway function have measured flow resistance or electromyograms in animals or in patients with obstructive apneas during wakefulness or sleep. Basic issues of how the structure changes geometry, shape, and stiffness often remain to be addressed. In spite of these limitations, four general areas of interest seem to emerge. Although they are interrelated, they will be treated independently.

Influence of Posture

Changing from the upright posture to the supine posture increases upper airway resistance by at least two mechanisms. First, gravity moves the mandible and hypopharyngeal structures posteriorly compromising the size of the airway.[56,57] Secondly, supraglottic resistance increases, probably due to a large degree by increased blood in the nasal mucosa.[32]

Part of the increase in upper airway resistance produced by posture may be offset by increased activation of dilator muscles. Genioglossal electromyographic activity, both tonic activity and that phasic with inspiration, increases with the change from upright to supine posture.[58]

The position of the head relative to the rest of the body also seems an important postural factor governing airway patency. Studies in anesthetized adults and unanesthetized infants show that passive neck flexion can cause complete obstruction of the upper airway.[59] In infants, airway obstruction caused by neck flexion is restored after a few respiratory efforts presumably by increasing upper airway muscle activation[43]; in anesthetized adults it is not.[56,57]

Influence of Chemical Drive

Most studies in animals and humans have demonstrated that hypoxia or hypercapnia increase upper airway muscle activation. The proportionate change with a change in drive may differ not only between upper airway muscles and the chest wall but also among upper airway muscles. In both anesthetized and unanesthetized animals motor output to the genioglossus and to the diaphragm show different patterns of recruitment with increasing chemical drive, resulting in a potential mismatch of forces at low to moderate levels of chemical drive.[54] These findings support the concept that alinearities in the response of upper airway and chest wall muscles to changing drive may contribute the occurrence of obstructive apneas during sleep.[60] That is, there may be generation of negative airway pressure by the major inspiratory muscles without appropriate concomittant activation of upper-airway dilator muscles.

Studies in humans have not wholly confirmed these results in animals. In adults during wakefulness[61–64] and sleep,[63] genioglossus responses are proportional to diaphragm responses. In the preterm infant, however, although genioglossal EMG has not been studied, the alae nasi which usually parallels genioglossal activity increases its activity in response to high levels of added CO_2 and chest wall EMG activity increases proportionately.[65] The differences between the studies in animals and humans may be explained by differences in the recruitment of muscle activation at certain regions of the upper airway. In addition, it is uncomfortable and potentially dangerous to produce the range of hypoxia or hypercapnia in humans as one can in animals.

Besides the amount of recruited phasic activation, three other elements of neuromuscular drive may be important in considering how changing chemical drive might affect upper airway function. First, the level of tonic (or expiratory) activation may affect airway size or stiffness. Tonic activity is modulated by chemical drive.[54] Changes in tonic activity could affect the force generated during inspiration by altering expiratory airway size and, consequently, muscle length or, if the airway is allowed to close at end-expiration, add to the force required to overcome surface tension of the occluded airway, a significant factor promoting airway occlusion. Secondly, the threshold of phasic activation may be different for different muscles. The genioglossus begins to show activity at higher levels of PCO_2 than the diaphragm, while the posterior cricoarytenoid muscle manifests phasic activity at lower levels.[54] Alae nasi activation, which lowers nasal resistance, occurs only 30 percent of the time with inspiratory efforts in quiet sleep in the sleeping human infant,[65] while in the adult alae nasi activation is present 99 percent of the time in NREM sleep.[61] These differences in the threshold of activation may be important to understanding the increased number of respiratory disturbances during sleep in infants. Finally, a change in the timing of upper airway muscle activation relative to inspiratory activation of chest wall muscles will result in changes in the balances of forces acting to open and close the airway. Timing appears to change with chemical drive with the result that the interval between the onset of alae nasi activation and the onset of inspiratory airflow is greater at higher levels of drive.[33]

Recently, Bruce et al.[66] found evidence that central and peripheral chemoreceptor function might differently affect respiratory drive to the diaphragm and genioglossal muscles. They found that carotid sinus nerve section decreased hypoglossal nerve respiratory activation more than phrenic nerve activation, but with central medullary cooling the reverse was found. These findings suggest that carotid body input has proportionately greater effects on airway dilator muscle activation while central chemosensitivity has greater effects on inspiratory activation of chest wall muscles.

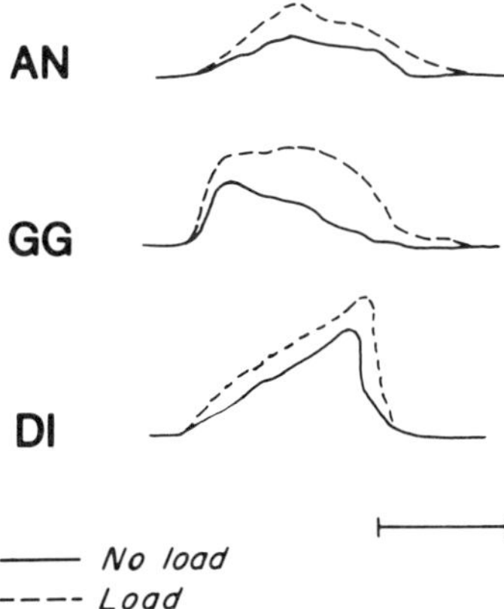

Fig. 6-7 Shown are comparisons of the moving average of alae nasi (AN), genioglossus (GG) and esophageal diaphragm (DI) EMG activity at PCO_2 = 61 mmHg during successive CO_2 rebreathing trials, one without a load (solid line) and a load of 15 $cmH_2 0.1^{-1}$ sec^{-1}. The onset of activation in each signal are aligned to appear identical. Imposition of a load increases the amount of activity in each signal independent of the level of chemical drive. (See Patrick, et al.[64] for further details.)

Influence of Nonchemical Drive

Studies in awake humans have shown that external inspiratory resistive loading increases alae nasi and genioglossal activation in a manner similar to that seen in the diaphragm even when the level of chemical drive is held constant[64] (Fig. 6-7). These results show that nonchemical factors can influence the amount of upper airway muscle activity in humans. Studies in animals where greater isolation of receptor input can take place have shown that lung inflation, chest wall distortion, negative pressures applied to the larynx and/or nose, blood pressure, and visceral afferent stimulation can all alter the amount of upper airway muscle activity.[54,55,67–69] In addition, the timing and amount of upper airway muscle activation relative to that for the chest wall muscles can change during these maneuvers. The specific relevance of these reflexes in the deterioration of upper airway function during sleep in humans is unknown.

Influence of Sleep State

With the transition from wakefulness to sleep, there is a major change in the intensity of postural and nonrespiratory behavioral drive to muscles. Central respiratory chemical and nonchemical drive appear to change, but are less well described for upper airway than for chest wall muscles. The effects of rapid eye movement (REM) sleep and non-rapid eye movement (NREM) sleep on upper airway function are different. During REM sleep, afferent input is diminished and postsynaptic inhibition of motoneuron activity occurs. Sullivan et al. demonstrated that responses to laryngeal stimulation were diminished during NREM sleep; these responses, including arousal were further diminished in REM sleep.[70]

A decrease in upper airway muscle activation would decrease upper airway patency. The state of nasal resistance is important since it is the first resistance pathway on inspiration. Loss of alae nasi EMG activation or withdrawal of sympathetic tone from nasal mucosa would increase nasal resistance at the nose and produce greater narrowing in downstream from the nose in the less stiff pharynx.

Although one does not need to invoke anatomic abnormalities to explain loss of upper airway function during sleep, anatomic abnormalities could help compromise upper airway airflow by making the airway smaller or more compliant. Several clinical studies suggest that airway size, particularly in the region of the hypopharynx and nasopharynx, is compromised in patients with obstructive apnea syndrome. Radiographs and computerized axial tomography of the upper airway show small nasopharyngeal channels during wakefulness.[51,52] Using a pulse flow method, Suratt et al.[36] have shown that resistance of the upper airway is greater in patients with sleep apnea syndrome. Although these studies are not controlled for normal variation in the population, flow resistance, or state of respiratory or nonrespiratory drive, the apparent incidence of a narrowed airway in the sleep apnea patient is impressive. The clearest demonstration of the importance of anatomic narrowing in airway function is the beneficial effect of tonsillectomy and adenoidectomy in relieving obstructive apneas in children.[71] Abnormalities in airway stiffness in the pathogenesis of upper airway obstruction during sleep have only recently been addressed. A large proportion of patients with obstructive apneas during sleep show during wakefulness a "saw-toothing" in the inspiratory limb of a flow-volume loop.[72] The site and mechanism of this fluttering is probably in the nasopharynx. Fluttering suggests the presence of dynamic narrowing (the so-called Starling resistor) where the walls of a resistor are known to abruptly alter flow rate.[73]

Two separate studies have demonstrated that nasal obstruction by itself will provoke upper airway obstruction.[74,75] Nasal resistance is rarely studied in patients but anatomic obstruction may contribute to the onset of obstructive apnea by increasing intrapharyngeal pressures.

When symptomatic, laryngeal obstruction usually is apparent as much during wakefulness as during sleep. Bilateral recurrent laryngeal nerve paralysis does not necessarily result in obstructive apneas; rather patients awaken frequently at night apparently with aspiration of oropharyngeal contents (N.T. Feldman, unpublished observations).

THE UPPER AIRWAY IN THE PATHOGENESIS OF APNEAS DURING SLEEP

Central Nonobstructive Apneas

Central or "arrhythmic" apneas are characterized by the absence of respiratory efforts. Upper airway muscles show diminished tonic and absent phasic EMG activation during central apneas. The upper airway may close in

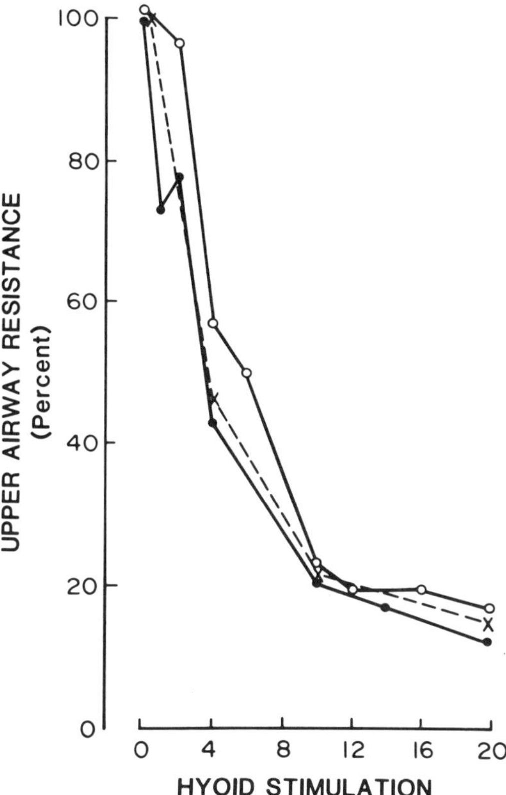

Fig. 6-8 Shown are the changes in upper airway resistance expressed as percent of values obtained during phrenic stimulation alone during trials in three dogs where simultaneous hyoid muscle stimulation (40 Hz) was varied from no stimulation to 20 mA. Resistance fell as the amount of hyoid stimulation increased, indicating restoration of upper-airway patency during phrenic pacing. Study is from an anesthetized dog. (Gottfried SB, Strohl KP, van de Graaff WB et al: Effects of phrenic stimulation on upper-airway resistance in anesthetized dogs. J Appl Physiol 55:419, 1983.)

some cases, but the site of occlusion is not known. When respiratory efforts of the chest wall muscles resume, occasionally a first obstructed or partially obstructed breath can be observed. This may be the result of an uneven distribution of activation between upper airway and chest wall muscles; alternatively, if the airway is closed or mucosal surfaces touch during a central apnea, surface tension forces must be overcome before airway patency is restored.

One treatment of central apneas is phrenic nerve pacing; however, since upper airway respiratory activity is absent, pacing the phrenic-diaphragm unit often creates obstructive apneas.[76,77] Restoration of activation of upper airway muscles, either voluntarily in humans[36] or by electrical stimulation in anesthetized dogs,[33] will restore upper airway patency under conditions of diaphragm pacing (Fig. 6-8).

Since afferent feedback can evoke powerful inhibitory effects on respiratory rate and depth, the importance of upper airway sensory input should not be overlooked in the pathogenesis of central apnea. In adult dogs laryngeal stimulation can produce a central apnea of brief duration during sleep but more often produces arousal or cough.[70] Responses are sleep-state dependent. Recent studies in unanesthetized young animals have found apneas during sleep

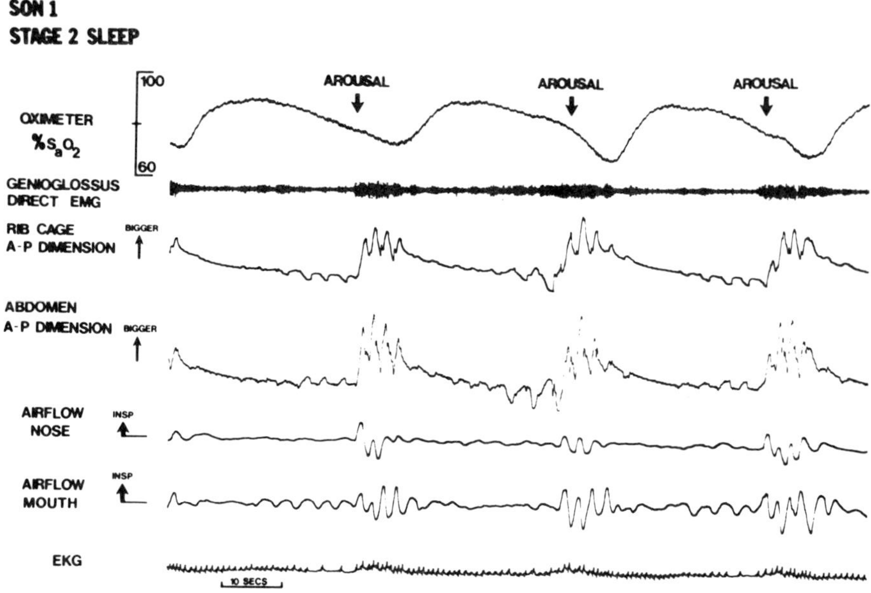

Fig. 6-9 Three consecutive apneas are shown during sleep in one patient with obstructive sleep apnea syndrome. Shown are changes in oxygen saturation, genioglossal EMG from wire electrodes, anterior-posterior (A-P) dimensions of the rib cage and abdomen, airflow at the nose and mouth, and the EKG. Arousals terminated each apneic period. Note that the amount of genioglossal EMG activity is greater during ventilatory periods than during apnea. (Strohl KP, Feldman NT, Saunders NA, Hallett M: Obstructive sleep apnea syndrome in family members. N Engl J Med 299:969, 1978.)

associated with increased cricothyroid muscle activity.[38] These findings suggest that some events during sleep might trigger a prolonged phase of postinspiratory neural activity and arrest the respiratory rhythm.[78]

Flow through the upper airway can augment respiratory drive;[25] therefore, absent flow potentially may diminish afferent feedback and decrease respiratory cycling at the level of the motoneuron. Topical anesthesia to the upper airway mucosa in anesthetized rabbits produces obstructive apnea and can lead to death.[26]

Obstructive and Mixed Apneas

Obstructive apneas are characterized by the presence of respiratory efforts but the absence of airflow at the nose and mouth. In mixed apneas, a combination of central and obstructive events are found. Most commonly a period of central apnea will precede obstructive events; however, obstructed efforts have been shown to bracket a period of central apnea (Fig. 6-9).

Obstructive apneas occur because of occlusion of the upper airway. The occurrence of apneas only during sleep implicates changes in motoneuron activation but it is not clear whether this is the result of normal respiratory or nonrespiratory suppression of upper airway muscle activation.

Anatomic deformity, either acquired (e.g., macroglossia due to acromegaly) or congenital (e.g., micrognathia) is associated with obstructive apneas. Anatomic abnormalities could alter the orientation of muscles, decrease airway caliber, or decrease airway stiffness. Nasal obstruction, as previously discussed, probably acts indirectly to narrow the pharyngeal aperture by increasing negative intraluminal pressures. Even when anatomic factors are recognizable, however, the onset of obstructive apneas are characterized by a decrease in electromyographic activity in numerous upper airway muscles and relief of obstruction is accompanied by increased EMG activation.[79,80] Consequently, anatomic narrowing of the upper airway may increase the importance of neuromuscular control mechanisms in the maintenance of upper airway patency.

At the onset of obstructive apneas, there is decreased neuromuscular activation of upper airway muscles. In the patient with repetitive, periodic obstructive apneas in NREM sleep, the decrease in tonic and phasic activation occurs following the previous hyperpnea. There is a substantial amount of evidence that obstructive apneas start in the context of a decrease in respiratory drive. Respiratory frequency, diaphragmatic electromyographic activity, and pleural pressure swings all are decreasing at the onset of the obstructive apneas.[81] The changes in upper airway muscle electromyographic activation appear to parallel these events. Therefore, in both NREM and REM sleep, obstructive apneas occur in the context of decreased drive to upper airway muscles.

In NREM sleep, changing drive to the upper airway is perhaps best explained by changes in respiratory drive to the motoneuron; in REM sleep, nonrespiratory input may also change abruptly in upper airway motoneurons as it does in postural muscles and result in intermittent absence of upper airway respiratory activation. Sleep-related inputs or withdrawal of stimuli during wakefulness also may influence the threshold of activation of the upper airway.

Whether a decrease in neuromuscular activation results in functional occlusion of the upper airway will depend upon the size and stiffness of the upper airway relative to the driving pressure for airflow generated by the chest wall muscles. A mismatch of forces promoting airway occlusion could occur if there is unequal drive to the muscle groups or unequal mechanical effects of the drive to each muscle group resulting in a greater collapsing force present in the upper airway.

ACKNOWLEDGMENTS

I thank Drs. M.D. Altose, N.S. Cherniack, J.M. Fouke, M.J. Hensley, D.F. Proctor, and N.A. Saunders for their helpful critique. The author thanks Sandy Shaft for helping prepare the manuscript. This review was supported in part by the National Institutes of Health (HL29726 and HL25830). Dr. Strohl is a recipient of an NIH Clinical Investigator Award (HL01067).

REFERENCES

1. Proctor DF: The upper airways, I. Nasal physiology and defense of the lungs. Am Rev Respir Dis 155:97, 1977
2. Proctor DF, Swift DL: Temperature and water vapor adjustment. p. 95. In Brain JD, Proctor DF, Reid LM (eds): Respiratory Defense Mechanisms Part I. Marcel Dekker, New York, 1977
3. Proctor DF: The naso-oro-pharyngo-laryngeal airway. Eur J Respir Dis 64(Suppl. 128):89, 1983
4. Strohl KP, O'Cain CF, Slutsky AS: Alae nasi activation and nasal resistance in healthy subjects. J Appl Physiol 52:1432, 1982
5. Rodenstein DO, Staunescu DC: Absence of nasal airflow during pursed lips breathing. Am Rev Respir Dis 128:716, 1983
6. Greene MCL: Speech analysis of 263 cleft palate cases. J Speech Dis 25:144, 1960
7. Niinimaa V, Cole P, Mintz S, Shepard RJ: Oronasal distribution of respiratory airflow. Resp Physiol 43:69, 1981
8. Kravath RE, Pollack CP, Borowiecki B, Weitzman ED: Obstructive sleep apnea and death associated with surgical correction of velopharyngeal incompetence. Pediatrics 96:645, 1980
9. Dixon M, Szereda-Przestaszewska M, Widdicombe JG, Wise JCM: Studies on laryngeal caliber during stimulation of peripheral and central chemoreceptors, pneumothorax and increased respiratory loads. J Physiol (London), 239:347, 1974
10. Bartlett, Jr D: Effects of vagal afferents on laryngeal responses to hypercapnia and hypoxia. Respir Physiol, 42:189, 1980
11. Bartlett, Jr D, Remmers JE, Gautier H: Laryngeal regulation of respiratory airflow. Respir Physiol 18:194, 1973
12. England SJ, Bartlett, Jr D, Daubenspeck JA: Influence of human vocal cord movements on airflow and resistance during eupnea. J Appl Physiol 52:773, 1982
13. Megirian D, Sherry JH: Respiratory functions of the laryngeal muscles during sleep. Sleep 3:289, 1980
14. Szereda-Przestaszewska M, Widdicombe JG: Reflex effects of chemical irritation of the upper airways on the laryngeal lumen in cats. Respir Physiol 18:107, 1973
15. Tomori Z, Widdicombe JG: Muscular, bronchomotor, and cardiovascular reflexes evoked from stimulation of the respiratory tract. J Physiol (London) 200:25, 1969
16. Long WA, Lawson EE: Maturation of the superior laryngeal nerve inhibiting effect. Am Rev Respir Dis 123:166, 1981
17. Barron DH: A note on the course of proprioceptive fibers from the tongue. Anat Rec 66:11, 1936
18. Sauerland EK, Mizuno N: Hypoglossal nerve afferents: Elicitation of a polysynaptic hypoglosso-laryngeal reflex. Brain Res 10:256, 1968
19. Teitelbaum HA, Ries FA: A study of the comparative physiology of the glossopharyngeal nerve - respiratory reflex in the rabbit, cat and dog. Am J Physiol 112:684, 1935
20. Donald DE, Shepherd JT: Autonomic regulation of the peripheral circulation. Annu Rev Physiol 42:429, 1980

21. Mathew OP, Abu-Osba YK, Thach BT: Genioglossus muscle responses to upper airway pressure changes: afferent pathways. J Appl Physiol 52:445, 1982
22. van Lunteren E, van de Graaff WB, Parker DM et al: Reflex effects of negative pressure in the upper airway. J Appl Physiol 56:746, 1984
23. McBride B, Whitelaw WA: A physiological stimulus to upper airway receptors in humans. J Appl Physiol 51:1189, 1981
24. Nail BS, Sterling GM, Widdicombe JG: Epipharyngeal receptors responding to mechanical stimulation. J Physiol (London) 204:91, 1969
25. Sant'Ambrogio G, Mathew OP, Fisher JT, Sant'Ambrogio FB: Laryngeal receptors responding to transmural pressure, airflow, and local muscle activity. Resp Physiol 54:317, 1983
26. Abu-Osba YK, Mathew OP, Thach BT: Animal model for airway sensory deprivation producing obstructive apneas with postmortem findings of sudden infant death syndrome. Pediatrics 68:796, 1981
27. Sasaki CT, Fukuda H. Kirchner JA: Laryngeal abductor activity in response to varying ventilatory resistance. Trans AAOO 77:403, 1973
28. Sant'Ambrogio G: Information arising from the tracheobronchial tree in mammals. Physiol Rev 62:531, 1982
29. Proetz AW: Essays on the applied physiology of the nose. 2nd Ed, Annals Publishing Co, St. Louis, 1953
30. Hyatt RE, Wilcox RE: Extra thoracic airway resistance in man. J Appl Physiol 16:326, 1961
31. Ferris, Jr BG, Mead J, Opie LH: Partitioning of respiratory flow resistance in man. J Appl Physiol 19:653, 1964
32. Anch AM, Remmers JE, Bunce H III: Supraglottic resistance in normal and patients with airway occlusion during sleep. J Appl Physiol 53:1158, 1982
33. Gottfried SB, Strohl KP, van de Graaff WB et al: Effects of phrenic stimulation on upper airway resistance in anesthetized dogs. J Appl Physiol 55:419, 1983
34. Brouillette RT, Thach BT: A neuromuscular mechanism maintaining extrathoracic airway patency. J Appl Physiol 46:772, 1979
35. Reed WR, Roberts JL, Thach BT: Role of inspiratory suction and muscle hypotonia in obstructive sleep apnea. Pediatric Res 16:360A, 1982
36. Scharf SM, Feldman NT, Goldman MD: Vocal cord closure: A cause of upper airway obstruction during controlled ventilation. Am Rev Respir Dis 117:391, 1978
37. Butler J, Caro CG, Alvola R, DuBois AB: Physiological factors affecting airway resistance in normal subjects and in patients with obstructive respiratory disease. J Clin Invest 39:584, 1960
38. Harding R, Johnson P, McClelland MC: Respiratory function of the larynx in developing sheep and the influence of sleep state. Respir Physiol 40:165, 1980
39. Gautier H, Remmers JE, Bartlett, Jr D: Control of the duration of expiration. Respir Physiol 18:205, 1973
40. Orem J, Netick A, Dement WC: Increased upper airway resistance to breathing during sleep in the cat. Electroenceph Clin Neurophysiol 43:14, 1977
41. Derenne J-Ph, Macklem PT, Roussos CH. The respiratory muscles: Mechanics, control, and pathophysiology. Part 1. Am Rev Respir Dis 118:119, 1978
42. Brouillette RT, Thach BT: Control of genioglossus muscle inspiratory activity. J Appl Physiol 49:801, 1980
43. Wilson SL, Thach BT, Brouillette RT, Abu-Osba YK: Upper airway patency in

the human infant: Influence of airway pressure and posture. J Appl Physiol 48:500, 1980
44. Evanich MJ, Lopata M, Lourenco RV: Analytical methods for the study of electrical activity in respiratory nerves and muscles. Chest 70:158, 1960
45. Eldridge F: Relationship between respiratory nerve and muscle activity and muscle force output. J Appl Physiol 39:567, 1975
46. McCaffrey TV, Kern EB: Response of nasal airway resistance to hypercapnia and hypoxia in the dog. Acta Otolaryngol 87:545, 1979
47. McCaffrey TV, Kern EB: Laryngeal regulation of airway resistance. I. Chemoreceptor reflexes. Ann Otol 89:209, 1980
48. Suratt PM, Wilhoit SC, Atkinson RL: Elevated pulse flow resistance in awake obese subjects with obstructive sleep apnea. Am Rev Respir Dis 127:162, 1983
49. Strohl KP, Mazza FG, Hafer CE et al: Geometric and elastic properties of the upper airway in supine anesthetized dogs. Proc Int Union Physiol Sci XV:307, 1983
50. Feldman AH, Loughlin GM, Leftridge CA, Cassinsi NJ: Upper airway obstruction during sleep in children. AM J Radiol 133:213, 1979
51. Haponik EF, Smith PL, Bohlman ME et al: Computerized tomography in obstructive sleep apnea. Am Rev Respir Dis 127:221, 1983
52. Suratt PM, Dec P, Atkinson RL et al: Fluoroscopic and computed tomographic features of the pharyngeal airway in obstructive sleep apnea. Am Rev Respir Dis 127:478, 1983
53. Brooks LJ, Castile RG, Glass GM et al: Reproducibility and accuracy of airway area by acoustic reflection. J Appl Physiol 57:777, 1984
54. Weiner D, Mitra J, Salamone J, Cherniack NS: Effect of chemical stimuli on nerves supply upper airway muscles. J Appl Physiol 52:530, 1982
55. van Lunteren E, Strohl KP, Parker DM et al: Phasic volume related feedback on upper airway muscle activity. J Appl Physiol 56:730, 1984
56. Safar P: Failure of manual respiration. J Appl Physiol 14:84, 1959
57. Safar P, Escarraga LA, Chang F: Upper airway obstruction in the unconscious patient. J Appl Physiol 14:760, 1959
58. Harper RM, Sauerland EK: The role of the tongue in sleep apnea. p. 219. In Guilleminault C, Dement WC (eds): Sleep Apnea Syndrome. Alan R. Liss, New York, 1978
59. Tonkin SL, Partridge J, Beach D, Wither S: The pharyngeal effect of partial nasal obstruction. Pediatrics 63:261, 1979
60. Cherniak NS: Respiratory dysrythmias in sleep. N Engl J Med 305:325, 1981
61. Strohl KP, Hensley MJ, Hallett M et al: Activation of upper airway muscles before onset of inspiration in normal humans. J Appl Physiol 49:638, 1980
62. Onal E, Lopata M, O'Connor TD: Diaphragmatic and genioglossal electromyogram responses to CO_2 rebreathing in humans. J Appl Physiol 50:1052, 1981
63. Onal E, Lopata M, O'Connor T: Diaphragmatic and genioglossal electromyogram responses to isocapnic hypoxia in humans. Am Rev Respir Dis 124:215, 1981
64. Patrick GB, Strohl KP, Rubin SB, Altose MD: Upper airway and diaphragm muscle responses to chemical stimulation and loading. J Appl Physiol 53:113, 1982
65. Carlo WA, Martin RJ, Bruce EN et al: Alae nasi activation (nasal flaring) decreases nasal resistance in preterm infants. Pediatrics 2:76, 1983
66. Bruce EN, Mitra J, Cherniack NS: Central and peripheral chemoreceptor inputs in phrenic and hypoglossal motoneurons. J Appl Physiol 53:1504, 1982

67. Cohen MI: Phrenic and recurrent laryngeal discharge patterns and the Hering–Breuer reflex. Am J Physiol 228:1489, 1975
68. Salamone JA, Strohl KP, Weiner DM et al: Comparison of cranial and phrenic nerve responses to changes in systemic blood pressure. J Appl Physiol 55:61, 1983
69. Cherniack NS, Haxhiu MA, Mitra J et al: Responses of upper airway, intercostal, and diaphragm muscle activity to stimulation of oesophageal afferents in dogs. J Physiol (London) 349:15, 1984
70. Sullivan CE, Murphy E, Kozar LF, Phillipson EA: Waking and ventilatory responses to laryngeal stimulation in sleeping dogs. J Appl Physiol 45:681, 1978
71. Mangat D, Orr WC, Smith RO: Sleep apnea, hypersomnolence and upper airway obstruction secondary to adenotonsillar enlargement. Arch Otolaryngol 103:383, 1977
72. Sanders MH, Martin RJ, Pennock BE, Rogers RM: The detection of sleep apnea in the awake patient. JAMA 245:2414, 1981
73. Miller RD, Hyatt RE: Evaluation of obstructing lesions of the trachea and larynx by flow-volume loops. Am Rev Respir Dis 108:475, 1973
74. Zwillich CE, Pickett C, Hanson FN, Weil JV: Disturbed sleep and prolonged apnea during nasal obstruction in normal men. Am Rev Respir Dis 124:158, 1981
75. Tonkin SL, Stewart JH, Withey S: Obstruction of the upper airway as a mechanism of sudden infant death: Evidence for a restricted nasal airway contributing to pharyngeal obstruction. Sleep 3:375, 1980
76. Glenn WL, Gee JB, Cole DR et al: Combined central alveolar hypoventilation and upper airway obstruction. Am J Med 64:50, 1978
77. Hyland RH, Hutcheon MA, Perl A et al: Upper airway occlusion induced by diaphragm pacing for primary alveolar hypoventilation: Implications for the pathogenesis of obstructive sleep apnea. Am Rev Respir Dis 124:180, 1981
78. Lawson EE: Prolonged central respiratory inhibition following reflex-induced apnea. J Appl Physiol 50:874, 1981
79. Remmers JE, DeGroot WJ, Sauerland EK, Anch AM: Pathogenesis of upper airway occlusion during sleep. J Appl Physiol 44:931, 1978
80. Strohl KP, Feldman NT, Saunders, NA, Hallett M: Obstructive sleep apnea syndrome in family members. N Engl J Med 299:969, 1978
81. Martin RJ, Pennock BE, Orr WC et al: Respiratory mechanics and timing during sleep in occlusive sleep apnea. J Appl Physiol 48:432, 1980

7 Diagnostic Methods in Adults

Barbara Gothe

Breathing during sleep can be evaluated in numerous ways. Apneas can be often detected by watching a patient breathe while sleeping; it may also be possible to differentiate between central and obstructive apneas. Changes in oxygen saturation, however, one of the most important determinants in the outcome of patients with sleep apnea, cannot be detected by observation alone, and qualitative as well as quantitative measurements are necessary to direct therapeutic efforts.

In the evaluation of a patient with a suspected breathing disorder during sleep a detailed medical history regarding sleep behavior is necessary. Questions should be asked about usual bedtime, length of sleep, number and cause of awakenings during the night, snoring, morning headaches, and daytime sleepiness. The physical examination must include a detailed examination of the upper airway to look for anatomic narrowing, which may predispose to a greater than normal increase in upper airway resistance during sleep. Pulmonary function tests, arterial blood gases, and tests of respiratory muscle function serve to recognize patients with compromised ventilatory capacity during wakefulness who may develop hypoventilation and desaturation during sleep. The flow-volume loop is often abnormal in patients with structural and functional airway narrowing. Related information about the circulatory system may be obtained by measurements of blood pressure, and a 24-hour monitoring of the electrocardiogram (ECG) for rhythm disturbances; in addition, echocardiography or radioisotopic gated blood pool scans may be useful noninvasive tests to detect abnormalities in left or right ventricular ejection fractions. An elevated hematocrit may provide a clue that chronic intermittent hypoxemia is present.

Sleep studies are used to detect and determine possible causes and degree of severity of hypoventilation and oxygen desaturation during sleep, to detect and characterize apneas during sleep, and to evaluate possible relationships between disordered breathing, oxygen desaturation, and disrupted sleep. Sleep studies are also used to evaluate different modes of therapy by serial studies.

Measurements include those of sleep stages, changes in gas exchange, detection and quantification of apneas and other abnormal respiratory events, and monitoring of heart rate and rhythm. Ideally, measurements are made without interrupting sleep, cause no discomfort to the sleeping subject, are reliable and stable over several hours, and are easy to use.

METHODS

Measurement of Sleep

Stages of sleep are by convention divided into quiet (NREM) sleep, which consists of stages I, II, III and IV, and active (REM) sleep. The distribution of sleep stages follows a typical pattern. From wakefulness subjects go through a short period of stage I into stages II, III, and IV quiet sleep, successively, which is interrupted approximately every 90 minutes by a period of REM sleep. The REM episodes tend to lengthen from a few minutes at first to between 20 and 30 minutes or more in the early morning hours. In normal young or middle aged adults, approximately one quarter of time asleep is spent in REM sleep. Stages III and IV quiet sleep seem to occur early in the night, and the amount of sleep in these sleep stages decreases with age.

In order to evaluate primary and secondary disorders of sleep, all-night recordings are considered necessary, with monitoring of the electroencephalogram (EEG), electromyogram of the chin (EMG), electrocardiogram (ECG), and some measurement of ventilation and gas exchange.[1–3] Sleep stages are scored using accepted criteria.[1,2,4,5] During stage I quiet sleep the alpha waves (6 to 8 Hz) of drowsy wakefulness disappear and the EEG shows a mixed frequency mixed voltage. Stage II quiet sleep is characterized by appearance of sleep spindles. In stage III high voltage, low-frequency electrical activity is present approximately half of the time, and in stage IV the high voltage, low frequency pattern is predominant. Muscle tone diminishes with onset of sleep progressively from stages I to IV. In REM sleep the EEG resembles that of stage I sleep showing mixed voltage and frequency, but muscle tone is absent and random bursts of rapid eye movements or sporadic bursts of muscle activity are seen. In analyzing the sleep profile, the total time in bed is recorded, as well as total sleep time; the ratio of the two is the sleep efficiency. Sleep latency is the time from beginning of the recording (lights out) to sleep onset, defined as the first of three consecutive epochs of stage I NREM sleep or any other sleep stage. REM latency is the time in minutes from sleep onset to the first appearance of REM. The total number of awakenings and the length is noted. The time spent in each sleep stage can be reported in minutes or as percentages of total sleep time. In research studies or in difficult diagnostic settings, two nights are monitored in the laboratory to account for internight variability and in order to give subjects a chance to get accustomed to the recording equipment and the different environment of a sleep laboratory. On the other hand, in many subjects with the fully developed obstructive sleep apnea syndrome, a few hours of good quality recording may be all that is necessary to establish the diagnosis.

Scoring sleep may be difficult in the presence of apneas or periodic breathing as the EEG often shows an arousal response at the end of an apnea. If sleep is present by EEG criteria for more than 50 percent of each epoch between arousals associated with hyperventilation terminating an apnea, the epoch is scored as sleep. If the time of arousal is more than 50 percent of the epoch, no sleep is scored for that epoch.[6] Another adjustment to classical scoring criteria applies to the scoring of the sleep EEG in older subjects.[7] Frequently the amplitude of the EEG during slow wave sleep (SWS) decreases with age. SWS can more easily be recognized in older subjects by applying frequency criteria only.

A recent survey of the results of polysomnographic recordings in a national cooperative study of the Association of Sleep Disorders Centers has shown that of nearly 5,000 patients referred for sleep evaluation 51 percent had disorders of excessive sleepiness (hypersomnias), and sleep apnea syndrome was the most prevalent diagnosis in this group of patients.[8] From this and from other studies, it is estimated that disordered breathing during sleep is a very common disorder, and the requirement for overnight studies for evaluation of possible sleep and breathing disorders requiring much time and personnel has been criticized as being costly, cumbersome, and not readily accessible at a community hospital level.

Several other methods have been proposed that may fall into the category of screening procedures for possible sleep apnea. Daytime nap studies for evaluation of patients with suspected sleep apnea syndrome have shown that it is possible to diagnose sleep apnea syndrome. In one study as little as 20 minutes of recordings during mid-day sleep were considered satisfactory for diagnostic purposes.[9] A comparison between the information gathered from nap recordings versus all-night recordings was not made in this study and, therefore, final conclusions cannot be drawn regarding the validity of day-time recordings in the overall evaluation of patients with sleep apnea syndrome. It has been suggested that a polysomnogram without appearance of REM sleep must be considered incomplete ecause the severe decreases in oxygen saturation and disturbance of breathing patterns may be restricted to REM sleep.[6] REM sleep may not occur during daytime nap studies.[10] Another approach to decrease the number of overnight studies in the laboratory and yet evaluate more patients with suspected sleep disorders has been proposed by Mullaney et al.,[11] who described a method of estimating sleep time by monitoring movements of the wrist. A spring-loaded wire and a piezoceramic element sensitive to movement were attached to the wrist. During sleep, as muscular activity decreased, move-

Table 7-1. Commonly Used Methods to Evaluate Breathing during Sleep

Method	Measurement	Advantage	Disadvantage
EMG (diaphragm or intercostal)	Respiratory rate and effort	Accurate, if properly used	Difficult to standardize.
Thermistors	Respiratory rate; airflow	Noninvasive	Qualitative results only. False negative reading not uncommon.
Analysis of thoracoabdominal movements strain gauges magnetometers inductive plethysmograph (Respitrace)	Respiratory rate; estimate of tidal volume	Noninvasive	Qualitative or semiquantitative. Validity of tidal volume estimates not firmly established, particulary in patients with COPD or sleep apneas
Mask	Respiratory rate; tidal volume	Accurate	May influence breathing pattern. May prevent sleep in some subjects due to discomfort.
Canopy	Respiratory rate; tidal volume	Accurate	May cause some discomfort.
Arterial blood gases	Gas exchange	Accurate	Invasive
Ear Oximetry	Gas exchange	Noninvasive	Not accurate below oxygen saturation of 50 percent.
Transcutaneous blood gases	Gas exchange	Noninvasive	Validity of results not firmly established in adults.

ments of the wrist also decreased, and the authors found a good correlation between wrist activity and EEG activity for total sleep time in normal subjects. Most investigators agree that at least two nights are necessary for a more accurate assessment of a patient's sleep disorder; however, in some patients fairly complete information can be obtained during one night only. A first-night effect is not always seen.[12]

Measurement of Ventilation

There are a number of ways to measure breathing during sleep (Table 7-1).

Direct Quantitative Measurements of Air Flow (Mask, Mouthpiece, Canopy). Breathing can be measured directly by analyzing the airflow at the mouth quantitatively using a mouthpiece or tight fitting mask attached to a pneumotachograph. Mouthpieces and noseclips or facemasks have been used in the earlier studies involving normal subjects.[13–16] It is difficult to measure breathing over prolonged periods of time because secretions accumulate in the mouth; the increased dead space may stimulate breathing; the mask or mouthpiece may become uncomfortable with time; and only selected subjects can be studied during sleep, since many normal subjects cannot fall asleep wearing masks or mouthpieces. In addition, breathing patterns may be changed by breathing through a mouthpiece.[17–19] Subjects usually breathe more and with higher tidal volume and lower respiratory rate with a mouthpiece.[17] Early studies in normal volunteers found that with sleep ventilation falls, metabolic rate decreases, PO_2 falls, and PCO_2 rises.[13,14] It is not known whether or not the presence of a mouthpiece or mask continues to have an influence on breathing pattern during sleep as it has been shown to have during wakefulness, but it seems likely that the hyperventilation induced by the measurement is related to conscious wakefulness. Measurements made with mouthpieces or masks therefore may overestimate the awake ventilation.

Another approach to measuring airflow at the mouth quantitatively is by the use of a ventilated facemask[20] or a canopy.[21,22] The canopy consists of an airtight rigid structure that encloses the subject's head and seals around the neck. The canopy is flushed with air, and flow in and out of the system is balanced. Room air or gas of any composition suitable for study or treatment of a subject can be used. Attached to the canopy is a pneumotachograph that measures changes in airflow within the canopy produced by the subject's breathing pattern. The canopy is well tolerated, and its accuracy in measuring tidal volume compared with direct pneumotachograph measurements was 96 percent.[22] The disadvantage of the method is that subjects have to lie on their back and cannot move freely in their sleep. It has been used successfully to assess breathing during sleep in patients with sleep apnea syndrome.[23]

Although the methods to measure airflow at the mouth are uncomfortable to the subject, may overestimate ventilation during wakefulness, and may by the stimulation of the face alter apnea behavior during sleep, it is generally believed that the direct measurement of airflow or tidal volume is the only wholly accurate method to detect lung volume changes during tidal breathing during sleep. Direct airflow measurements are usually the standard against which other methods that claim to measure tidal volume have to be compared.[24]

Indirect Qualitative or Semiquantitative Methods (Thoracoabdominal Movement Analysis, EMG, Pleural Pressure). There are numerous indirect qualitative methods that are used to assess respiratory effort and respiratory rate during sleep. Thermistors are temperature-sensitive devices that sense changes in temperature as air at environmental temperature (usually 18 to 20°C) is inhaled and air at body temperature (37°C) is exhaled. Thermistors can be calibrated over a desired temperature range. Usually one or two thermistors are placed at the nostrils and another thermistor is placed at the corner of the mouth. Meticulous placement in the midstream of inhaled or exhaled air is necessary for optimal airflow recordings. Airflow can also be measured qualitatively by sampling end-tidal CO_2 either from nasal prongs or by catheters attached to a loosely fitting facemask. Exhaled air is drawn at rates of 0.5 L/min through an infrared CO_2 analyzer. This method may give information not only regarding the presence or absence of airflow but also regarding PCO_2 levels during sleep as long as respiratory efforts are slow and deep enough to produce a clear alveolar plateau at the end of each breath. The disadvantage of this method is that the sampling catheter has to be short to avoid damping of the signal. Over a prolonged period of recording water may accumulate in the catheter and render the reading inaccurate. Desiccating filters have to be used and changed frequently or a water trap has to be placed in the line.

Respiratory Thoracoabdominal Movements. Analysis of rib cage and abdominal movements during breathing and estimating tidal volume from measuring the sum of rib cage and abdominal respiratory movements is rapidly becoming the most popular method of measuring breathing during sleep. Respiratory movements of the trunk have been measured for a long time. Belts or pneumographs have long been used to measure respiratory rate and relative variations of chest wall movements.[25–31]

The interest in a more detailed analysis of respiratory rib cage movement initially was generated by the desire to understand the action of the diaphragm in moving the thorax. Wade measured the circumference of the rib cage by strain gauges while assessing diaphragm excursions radiographically.[26] Shapiro and Cohen measured rib cage as well as abdominal excursions with strain gauges and provided a theoretical analysis of respiratory thoracoabdominal movements.[27] They also showed that rib cage movement as well as abdominal movement decreased during REM sleep. Respiratory movements of the rib cage and abdomen are of interest for at least two reasons. The signals can be calibrated to obtain estimates of tidal volumes and, therefore, can be used to obtain quantitative measurement of ventilation; and rib cage and abdominal movements during breathing can also be used to detect discoordination or nonuniformities in respiratory movements; and thus indirectly the function of various groups of respiratory muscles in causing normal and abnormal respiratory movements of the chest and abdomen can be assessed. The principle in analyzing rib cage and abdominal respiratory movements was outlined by Konno and Mead.[28] During breathing the rib cage and abdomen can be considered as a system with two parts (rib cage and abdomen) arranged in series, separated by the diaphragm. The content of the abdomen is not considered affected by breathing, and any configurational change of the rib cage and abdomen are proportional to changes in lung volume during breathing. With the airway open the system has two degrees of freedom. When the airway is closed any volume change in the rib cage compartment is equal to the change of volume in the abdominal compartment; overall volume does not change; the system now has only one degree of freedom. By determining the volume motion coefficients of the system operating at one degree of freedom, the behavior of the system having two degrees of freedom can be predicted, assuming that the overall functional and mechanical properties of the system are similar in the two conditions. Therefore, movements of the rib cage and abdomen during breathing can be translated into tidal volume estimates. Changes in configuration and, proportionally, volume of the rib cage and abdomen can be measured by assessing a change in diameter. Most commonly used are the anterior diameters of the rib cage and abdomen and sometimes, in addition, the lateral diameter of the rib cage or a change in cross section or in circumference. Methods that have been used to measure configurational changes are strain gauges,[26,27] magnetometers,[28,29] and the inductive plethysmograph.[30]

Magnetometers are usually placed anteriorly and posteriorly at the level of the fourth intercostal space on the chest and 1 inch above the umbilicus and the corresponding place over the spine on the abdomen. They can be calibrated in terms of lung volume change by having the subject perform an isovolume maneuver. Subjects are asked to hold their breath and move their abdomen in and out rapidly at the end of a breath several times before resuming normal breathing. This maneuver can be repeated at end inspiration. The gains of the rib cage and abdominal amplifiers are displayed on a storage oscilloscope with the rib cage signal on the vertical and the abdominal signal on the horizontal axis. The gains are adjusted so that the signals are equal and opposite producing a line with the slope of -1 during an isovolume maneuver. The sum of the two signals is then related to a tidal volume signal obtained by spirometry or a pneumotachograph attached to a mouthpiece for 10 to 20 spontaneous breaths. The tidal volume and sum signals are plotted and a linear regression is obtained by least-square analysis. Other methods of calibration have been published that may be of use in subjects who cannot perform an isovolume maneuver.[30] The magnetometers are sensitive to changes in posture, and it is felt they cannot be used to estimate tidal volume with the subject lying in the lateral position.

Analysis of chest wall and abdominal movements have revealed that normal subjects increase the thoracic diameter more than the abdominal diameter in the upright position than in the supine posture; in the supine posture the abdominal diameter increases more than that of the thorax.[32] Patients with chronic obstructive lung disease show more variability and significantly more distortion in rib cage abdominal configuration during breathing than normal subjects.[33,34] Distortion of either rib cage or abdominal signal may influence the sum of the two and, therefore, the correlation between tidal volume measured at the mouth and the estimation of tidal volume from the sum signal may show greater variability in patients with chronic obstructive pulmonary disease than in normal subjects.

The *inductive plethysmograph* consists of two coils of wire sewn into bands that can be placed across the chest and abdomen or glued on an elastic garment.[31] Changes in position of the wires induced by movements of the subject seem to affect the garment less than the bands.[35] The expansion and contraction of the wires during breathing causes changes in an oscillator that are demodulated to produce output voltage signals. The device can be calibrated by using the isovolume maneuver/spirometer method or by using a least-square method assuming that rib cage/spirometer + abdomen/spirometer = 1. The calibration is validated by relating the sum of the rib cage and abdominal respiratory movements to tidal volumes obtained with a spirometer for a 20 second period.[36]

Quantitative results obtained by inductive plethysmography on ventilation at rest and during exercise in normal subjects and in patients with different lung disease have been published.[37,38]

Qualitative measurements of ventilatory patterns in patients with sleep apnea syndrome indicated the usefulness of this device in the diagnosis and classification of apneas and hypopneas.[38,39] Quantitative comparison of tidal volume measurements and tidal volume estimates during sleep have not yet been reported in large enough numbers or in different disease states.

Pleural pressure measured by esophageal balloons has long been used to differentiate central from obstructive apneas. The disadvantage of this method is the relative discomfort of having to swallow an esophageal balloon; and although patients with sleep apnea who are chronically sleepy can be studied relatively easily with this device during sleep, normal subjects may not always be able to sleep due to relative discomfort. The value of the measurement is that it provides a highly reliable estimate of the force generated by the respiratory muscles.

A noninvasive device that reflects changes in pleural pressure has been described.[38] The surface inductive plethysmograph consists of a loop of insulated wire taped to the skin of the suprasternal fossa. As negative pressure is developed within the chest during breathing and transmitted to the larynx, there are corresponding inward and outward motions of laryngeal structures that reflect, qualitatively, pleural pressure changes with respiratory efforts. This device senses these movements. Monitors detecting airflow or apneas acoustically have also been described.[40]

All techniques currently in use can be applied to sleep studies, particularly in patients with sleep apnea.[41,42,43] In order to understand the pathophysiologic mechanisms of sleep apnea, it is often necessary to obtain simultaneous information of the electrical activity of the muscles, the movements of the rib cage and abdominal compartments and corresponding lung volume changes as well as pressures developed by the respiratory muscles.[44] On the other hand a variety of relatively simple methods can confirm a diagnosis of sleep apnea syndrome in clinical practice.[45]

Electrical Activity of Respiratory muscles (EMG). Ventilatory activity can also be assessed by measuring the electrical activity of the respiratory and related muscles. At present this is largely a research technique. The EMG signal can be analyzed qualitatively and quantitatively. The moving average of the EMG activity can also be obtained and the rate of rise can be determined as well as the peak activity from the processed signal. The signal is affected by the techniques used in applying the electrodes, the size of the electrodes, conducting characteristics of the tissues between muscle and electrode, and the amplifying and recording apparatus. Signals cannot be easily compared among subjects, but the EMG can be very useful in defining changes in respiratory muscle activity in a given individual under various conditions.

The electrical activity of upper airway muscles can be recorded from the chin,[46] and there seems to be a good correlation between the signal recorded from needles inserted into the tongue and the surface EMG. Respiratory muscle activity can be obtained by applying electrodes on the surface of the thorax to measure the EMG. The second and third intercostal spaces are often used to assess intercostal muscle activity and the fifth and seventh intercostal spaces to assess activity of the diaphragm. Surface measurements of diaphragm activity are probably not very accurate because other muscles of the chest wall may be recorded as well.

Measurement of Oxygenation

In early studies blood gases during sleep were measured by sampling from arterial catheters.[47–49] The presence of a catheter and sampling from it interferes with sleep.[50] Ear oximetry was initially difficult due to instability of the instrument requiring frequent recalibrations thus interrupting sleep, but ear oximetry has long been used to document desaturation in patients with lung disease.[51] Oximetry measures spectrophotometrically the amount of oxygenated hemoglobin flowing through the ear at a constant temperature. In most instances the accuracy is adequate and reflects changes in oxygenation reliably.[52] Anemia or dark pigment in the skin may influence the reading, and it is felt that accuracy significantly drops off at oxygen saturations of less than 50 percent. Many reports have confirmed the clinical usefulness of ear oximetry.[53–55] Transcutaneous measurements of PO_2 (PtO_2) and PCO_2 ($PtCO_2$) are also possible by applying heated electrodes directly to the skin.[56–58] The electrode used to measure transcutaneous oxygen is a small light-weight modified Clark electrode. The response time in vitro is less than 10 seconds, however, the response time in vivo is longer. In part the response time is related to skin thickness. In adults response time is usually 45 to 60 seconds. Age also appears to be a major determinant of the relationship between transcutaneous and arterial PO_2. With increasing age the correlation becomes worse and PtO_2 is less than arterial PO_2. Certain drugs may affect arterial pressure or the distribution of blood flow to the periphery and therefore influence the reading. Currently PtO_2 measurements are most useful in infants in whom arterial blood gases are not readily available. In contrast to the PO_2 electrode, which can be calibrated with air, the PCO_2 electrode has to be calibrated with a known calibration gas mixture. The feasibility of using transcutaneous PO_2 and PCO_2 measurements in adults during sleep awaits further study.

Analysis of Data

Breathing Pattern. Analysis of breathing during sleep has focused on determining the number and type of apneas and the associated change in oxygen saturation. An apnea has been defined as cessation of airflow at the nose and mouth lasting at least 10 seconds.[1–3] For a full study, the sleep apnea syndrome is judged to be present if during nocturnal recording of 360 minutes at least 30 apneas are identified both in NREM and REM sleep. Criteria are scaled accordingly for briefer or "nap" studies. Central apneas are defined as absent airflow accompanied by cessation of respiratory effort measured from thoracoabdominal respiratory movements or from recordings of pleural pressure. Obstructive apneas are defined as absence of airflow associated with respiratory effort, and in mixed apneas both a central and obstructive component are present, the central portion usually preceding the obstructive portion. In a given patient one type of apnea usually predominates although all three types may be present in a given patient in a single night. In addition to apneas, ventilation can fall and the occurrence of both apnea and hypopnea has been termed an abnormal respiratory event. The severity of sleep apnea can be assessed by expressing the number of apneas and hypopneas per hour of sleep: Abnormal respiratory event during sleep index = Apnea + Hypopnea × 60 (A + H)/total sleep time (in minutes).[59] The average duration of various apneas has not been reported widely although this may be an important variable determining in part the degree of desaturation occurring with apneas. Chokroverty et al.[60] have reported a mean duration of central apneas of 17.9 seconds, obstructive apneas were longer (22.9 seconds) and mixed apneas were 27.2 seconds long in patients with primary sleep apnea syndrome. These authors also calculated the total apnea time in minutes per hour of sleep and determined the contribution of central, obstructive, and mixed events on total apnea time in percent.

However, if only apneas and hypopneas are considered in analyzing breathing patterns during sleep valuable information may be lost. Patients with cystic fibrosis may show oxygen desaturation without apneas or clear hypopneas.[61,62] Patients with asthma may show worsening of their pulmonary function associated with changes in breathing pattern during sleep, requiring modification of their therapeutic regimen based on analysis of breathing and oxygenation during sleep.

Respiratory dysrhythmias during sleep can be considered as an instability of respiratory control.[63] The breathing pattern seen in patients with sleep apnea resembles that of Cheyne-Stokes breathing, complicated by upper airway obstruction; and mathematical models have been developed that seem to explain some of the features seen in these patients.[64] Data analysis of respiratory patterns, therefore, should include an analysis of the apneas in context with the hyperventilatory periods that are often associated with the apneas. A standardized approach is not yet available.

Possibilities of quantitative analysis of ventilation during sleep include: (1) assessment of the strength of the respiratory cycle by comparing the maximal amplitude of the hyperventilatory portion to the minimal amplitude or apnea of the cycle; (2) comparison of the level of ventilation obtained noninvasively awake and in different sleep stages quantitatively with different lung diseases; (3) evaluation of relative contribution of rib cage and abdominal movements to tidal volume during wakefulness and sleep;[65,66] (4) frequency distributions (histograms) of tidal volume and respiratory rate under various conditions;[67,68] (5) determination of variability of respiratory parameters in different disease states;[69,70] and (6) analysis of number and causes of arousal, perhaps associated with or induced by falls in oxygen saturation or rises in PCO_2.

To assess the possible effects of therapeutic intervention requires unequivocal quantitative data and agreement about data analysis among different laboratories.

Oxygenation. With sleep oxyhemoglobin saturation decreases. A decrease of more than 4 percent has been considered abnormal.[53,54] To describe clinically significant decreases in oxygen saturation several methods have been proposed: the lowest oxygen saturation observed, the mean high and mean low oxygen saturation, the time spent at oxygen saturation of less than 80 percent,[71] and more recently a cumulative percent time oxygen saturation plot to evaluate levels of oxygen saturation over time.[72] The effects of various therapeutic regimens in sleep apnea syndrome or other disorders causing falls in oxygen saturation at night can be conveniently followed by comparing the change in position of the oxygen profile curve in serial studies.

APPENDIX: OUTLINE OF APPROACH TO EVALUATE PATIENTS WITH SUSPECTED BREATHING DISORDER DURING SLEEP

Indications:

1. Clinically suspected sleep apnea syndrome.
2. Other clinical signs and symptoms suggesting a breathing disorder during sleep, i.e., shortness of breath or choking at night, nocturnal asthma, restless sleep in the presence of lung or neuromuscular disease.
3. Unexplained hypoxemia or erythrocytosis.
4. Evaluation of patients with lung disease for nocturnal oxygen therapy.
5. Nocturnal cardiac arrhythmia.

We schedule the sleep study to roughly coincide with a patient's usual bedtime, and we ask him or her to avoid stimulating beverages at least 6 hours before the study.

We monitor the eye movements, the EEG, EMG of the chin, and the ECG by applying surface electrodes using standard techniques. Airflow at the nose and mouth is monitored by thermistors. We set the gain of the thermistors to read ± 20 mm deflection during normal breathing without a mouthpiece and to show no deflection during a breath-hold maneuver. Respiratory movements of the rib cage and abdomen are recorded using the inductive plethysmograph. We calibrate the plethysmograph by isovolume maneuvers and a spirometer or pneumotachograph signal[73] (Fig. 7-1). The gain of the rib cage and abdominal signal are set to read zero during an isovolume maneuver. Subsequently the subject breathes with a pneumotachograph or into a spirometer. Tidal volume and the sum signal of the rib cage are then recorded simultaneously for 10 to

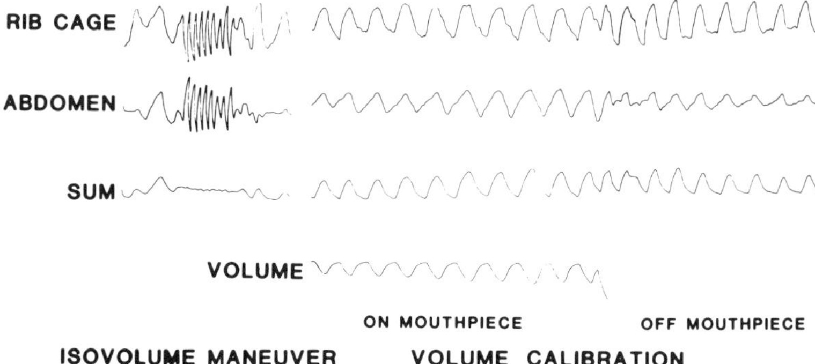

Fig. 7-1 The procedure of calibrating the inductive plethysmograph is shown in one subject. During the isovolume maneuver, on the left, rib cage and abdominal excursions are equal and opposite while the sum of both signals shows no significant deflection. The sum signal is then calibrated with a known airflow signal during tidal breathing on a mouthpiece.

20 breaths and the correlation between the two signals determined by least-square linear regression analysis. If subjects change position during sleep to lateral, another set of calibrations is obtained for the new position. Oxygen saturation is measured by ear oximetry, and end-tidal CO_2 is sampled from nasal prongs and analyzed with an infrared CO_2 analyzer. To apply the electrodes and monitors and to calibrate the signals requires approximately 30 minutes.

Figure 7-2 shows an example of central apneas; Figure 7-3, an example of obstructive apneas; and Figure 7-4, breathing during sleep in a patient with chronic obstructive lung disease. All measurements are noninvasive and well tolerated by patients and normal volunteers.

We usually observe a patient until we have seen and recorded all stages of sleep including REM sleep. If we do encounter significant desaturation during sleep (falls in oxygen saturation below 70 percent or a mean oxygen saturation of less than 85 percent), we apply supplemental oxygen with a loosely fitting facemask to evaluate the effect of oxygen on oxygen saturation, heart rate, and rhythm and breathing pattern during sleep.

Analysis of Data

We determine onset of sleep, duration and distribution of sleep stages, and REM sleep latency using standard technique. Oxygen saturation during sleep is analyzed using the method described by Slutsky.[72] Figure 7-5 shows the cumulative percent time oxygen saturation curve for the same patient as shown

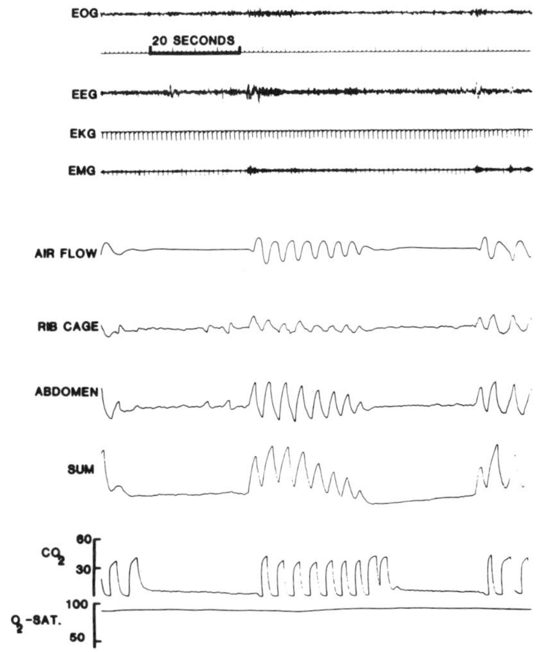

EOG
20 SECONDS
EEG
EKG
EMG
AIR FLOW
RIB CAGE
ABDOMEN
SUM
CO_2
60
30
100
O_2-SAT.
50

Fig. 7-2 An example of central apneas during NREM sleep without significant oxygen desaturation is shown.

EOG
20 SECONDS
EEG
EKG
EMG
AIR FLOW
RIB CAGE
ABDOMEN
SUM
60
CO_2
30
100
O_2-SAT.
50

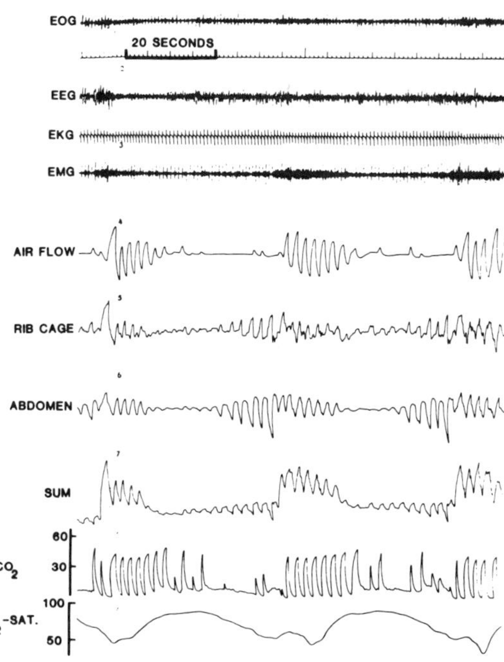

Fig. 7-3 An example of obstructive apneas with significant oxygen desaturation is shown.

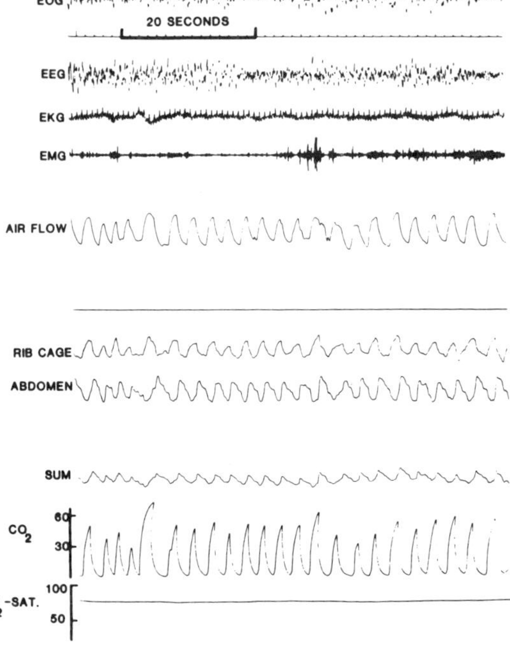

Fig. 7-4 An example of irregular breathing pattern with paradoxical movements of rib cage and abdomen but preserved airflow is shown in a patient with chronic obstructive pulmonary disease. Oxygen saturation is reduced.

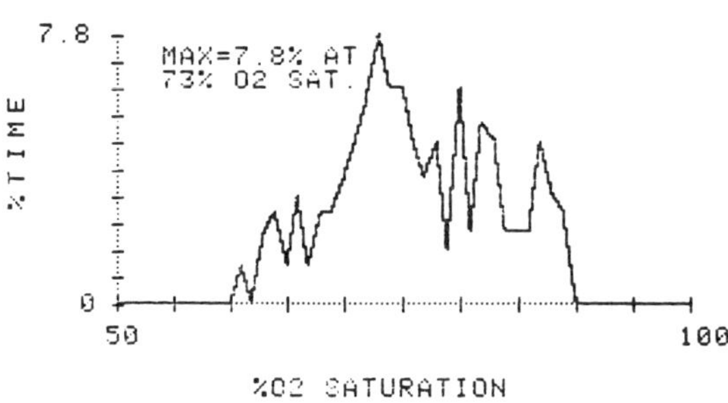

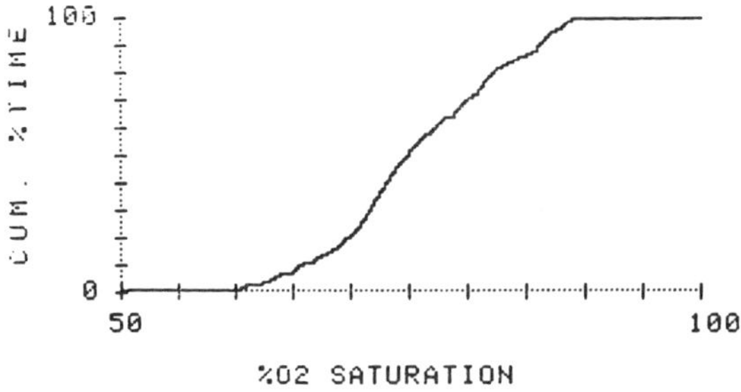

Fig. 7-5 The cumulative percent time oxygen saturation curve during sleep is shown for the same patient as in Fig. 7-4.

in Figure 7-3. Although this patient showed no apneas, oxygen saturation during sleep was markedly reduced. We analyze breathing during sleep by determining the coefficient of variability for tidal volume, respiratory rate, and instantaneous minute ventilation. We also count the apneas and report them as number of apneas per hour of sleep. We measure the central and obstructive portion of apneas and determine the total central and obstructive apnea time per hour of sleep for different sleep stages, in order to obtain some measure of how much percent of the time asleep a patient spends in central versus obstructive apneas. This differentiation is important to estimate how much benefit a patient might gain from relief of upper-airway obstruction during sleep. Treatment efforts in predominantly central apneas might be quite differrent compared to those used in predominantly obstructive sleep apneas. Variability in the type, duration and number of apneas can occur from night to night, and more than one recording may be necessary in the clinical management of patients with breathing disorders during sleep.

REFERENCES

1. Guilleminault C, Eldridge FL, Simmons B, Dement WC: Sleep apnea syndrome: Can it induce hemodynamic changes? West J Med 123:7, 1975
2. Guilleminault C, Tilkian A, Dement WC: The sleep apnea syndromes. Annu Rev Med 27:465, 1976
3. Guilleminault C, Cummiskey J, Dement WC: Sleep apnea syndrome: Recent advances. Adv Int Med 26:347, 1980
4. Rechtschaffen A, Kales A: A Manual of Standardized Terminology, Techniques and Scoring system for Sleep Stages of Human Subjects. National Institutes of Health Publication #204, Washington, D.C., 1968
5. Agnew HW, Webb WB: Sleep stage scoring. Journal supplement abstract service, American Psychological Association, MS. #293, May 1972
6. Bornstein SK: Respiratory monitoring during sleep: Polysomnography. p. 183. In Guilleminault C (ed): Sleeping and Waking Disorders: Indications and Techniques, Addison-Wesley, Menlo Park, 1982
7. Webb WB, Dreblow LM: A modified method for scoring slow wave sleep of older subjects. Sleep 5:195, 1982
8. Coleman RM, Roffwarg HP, Kennedy SJ et al: Sleep-wake disorders based on a polysomnographic diagnosis. A national cooperative study. JAMA 247:997, 1982
9. Browne-Goode G, Slyter HM: Daytime polysomnogram diagnosis of sleep disorders. J. Neur Neurosurg Psych 46:159, 1983
10. Guilleminault C: Sleep and breathing. p. 155. In Guilleminault C (ed): Sleeping and Waking Disorders, Indications and Techniques, Addison-Wesley, Menlo Park, 1982
11. Mullaney DJ, Kripke DF, Messin S: Wrist-actigraphic estimation of sleep time. Sleep 3:83, 1980
12. Kader GA, Griffin PT: Reevaluation of the phenomena of the first night effect. Sleep 6:67, 1983
13. Robin ED, Whaley RD, Crump CH, Travis DM: Alveolar gas tensions, pulmonary

ventilation and blood pH during physiologic sleep in normal subjects. J Clin Invest 37:981, 1958
14. Birchfield RL, Sieker HO, Heyman A: Alterations in respiratory function during natural sleep. J Lab Clin Med 54:216, 1959
15. Buelow K: Respiration and wakefulness in man. Acta Physiol Scand 59 (Suppl. 209):1, 1963
16. Snyder F, Hobson JA, Morrison DF, Goldfrank F: Changes in respiration, heart rate and systolic blood pressure in human sleep. J Appl Physiol 19:417, 1964
17. Gilbert R, Auchincloss JH, Brodinsky J, Boden W: Changes in tidal volume, frequency and ventilation induced by their measurement. J Appl Physiol 33:252, 1972
18. Askanazi J, Silverberg PA, Foster RJ et al: Effects of respiratory apparatus on breathing pattern. J Appl Physiol 48:577, 1980
19. Hirsch JA, Bishop B: Human breathing patterns on mouthpiece or facemask during air, CO_2 or low O_2. J Appl Physiol, 53:1281, 1982
20. Webb P, Troutman, Jr SJ: An instrument for continuous measurement of oxygen consumption. J Appl Physiol 28:867, 1970
21. Spencer JL, Zirkia BA, Kinney JM et al: A system for continuous measurement of gas exchange and respiratory functions. J Appl Physiol, 33:523, 1972
22. Sorkin B, Rapoport DM, Falk DB, Goldring RM: Canopy ventilation monitor for quantitative measurement of ventilation during sleep. J Appl Physiol 48:724, 1980
23. Garay SM, Rapoport D, Sorkin B, et al: Regulation of ventilation in the obstructive sleep apnea syndrome. Am Rev Respir Dis 124:451, 1981
24. Krieger J, Turlot JC, Mangin P, Kurtz D: Breathing during sleep in normal young and elderly subjects: Hypopneas, apneas and correlated factors. Sleep 6:108, 1983
25. Heaf P, Scott P, Smith WDA, Williams KG: A jerkin plethysmograph. Lancet 11:317, 1961
26. Wade OL: Movements of the thoracic cage and diaphragm in respiration. J Physiol 124:193, 1954
27. Shapiro A, Cohen HD: The use of mercury capillary length gauges for the measurement of the volume of thoracic and diaphragmatic components of human respiration: A theoretical analysis and a practical method. Trans New York Acad Sci 27:634, 1965.
28. Konno K, Mead J: Measurement of the separate volume changes of rib cage and abdomen during breathing. J Appl Physiol 22:407, 1967
29. Mead J, Peterson N, Grimby G: Pulmonary ventilation as measured from body surface movements. Science 156:1383, 1967
30. Stagg D, Goldman M, Newsom-Davis J: Computer aided measurement of breath volume and time components using magnetometers. J Appl Physiol 44:623, 1978
31. Cohn MA, Watson H, Weisshaut R, et al: A transducer for noninvasive monitoring of respiration. p. 119. In Stott FD, Raffery EB, Sleight P, Goulding L (eds): Proceedings of the Second International Symposium on Ambulatory Monitoring (ISAM 1977). Academic Press, London, 1978
32. Sharp JT, Goldberg NB, Druz WS, Danon J: Relative contributions of rib cage and abdomen to breathing in normal subjects. J Appl Physiol 39:608, 1975
33. Sharp JT, Goldberg NB, Druz WS et al: Thoracoabdominal motion in chronic obstructive pulmonary disease. Am Rev Respir Dis 115:47, 1977
34. Ashutosh K, Gilbert R, Auchincloss JH, Peppi D: Asynchronous breathing movements in patients with chronic obstructive pulmonary disease. Chest 67:553, 1975

35. Spier S, England S: The respiratory inductive plethysmograph: Bands vs. jerkins. Am Rev Respir Dis 127:784, 1983
36. Chadha TS, Watson H, Birch S et al: Validation of respiratory inductive plethysmography using different calibration procedures. Am Rev Respir Dis 125:644, 1982
37. Tobin MJ, Chadha TS, Jenouri G et al: Breathing patterns. 1. Normal subjects. Chest 84:202, 1983
38. Tobin MJ, Chadha TS, Jenouri G et al: Breathing patterns. 2. Diseased subjects. Chest 84:286, 1983
39. Tobin MJ, Cohn MA, Sackner MA: Breathing abnormalities during sleep. Arch Int Med 143:1221, 1983
40. Krumpe PE, Cummiskey JM: Use of laryngeal sound recordings to monitor apnea. Am Rev Respir Dis 122:797, 1980
41. Onal E, Lopata M, Ginzburg AS, O'Connor TD: Diaphragmatic EMG and transdiaphragmatic pressure measurements with a single catheter. Am Rev Respir Dis 124:563, 1981
42. Martin RJ, Pennocck BE, Orr WC et al: Respiratory mechanics and timing during sleep in occlusive sleep apnea. J Appl Physiol 48:432, 1980
43. Littner MR, McGinty DJ, Arand DL: Determinants of oxygen desaturation in the course of ventilation during sleep in chronic obstructive pulmonary disease. Am Rev Respir Dis 122:849, 1980
44. Grimby G, Goldman M, Mead J: The action of respiratory muscles inferred from rib cage and abdominal volume-pressure partitioning. J Appl Physiol 41:739, 1976
45. Reidy RM, Hulsey R, Bachus BF et al: Sleep apnea syndrome: Practical diagnostic method. Chest 75:81, 1979
46. Sauerland EK, Sauerland BAT, Orr WC, Hairston LE: Noninvasive electromyography of human genioglossal (tongue) activity. Electromyogr Clin Neurophysiol 21:279, 1981
47. Koo KW, Sax DS, Snider GL: Arterial blood gases and pH during sleep in chronic obstructive pulmonary disease. Am J Med 58:663, 1975
48. Leitch AG, Clancy LJ, Leggett RJE et al: Arterial blood gas tensions, hydrogen ion and electroencephalogram during sleep in patients with chronic ventilatory failure. Thorax 31:730, 1976
49. Pierce AK, Jarrett ChE, Werkle Jr G, Miller WF: Respiratory function during sleep in patients with chronic obstructive lung disease. J Clin Invest 45:631, 1966
50. Adam K: Sleep is changed by blood sampling through an indwelling venous catheter. Sleep 5:154, 1982
51. Trask ChH, Cree EM: Oximeter studies on patients with chronic obstructive emphysema, awake and during sleep. N Engl J Med 266:639, 1962
52. Saunders NA, Powles AGP, Rebuck AS: Ear oximetry: Accuracy and practicability in the assessment of arterial oxygenation. Am Rev Respir Dis 113:745, 1976
53. Flick MR, Block AJ: Continuous in vivo monitoring of arterial oxygenation in chronic obstructive lung disease. Ann Int Med 86:725, 1977
54. Block AJ, Boysen PG, Wynne JW, Hunt LA: Sleep apnea, hypopnea and oxygen desaturation in normal subjects. N Engl J Med 300:513, 1979
55. Wynne JW, Block AJ, Hemenway J et al: Disordered breathing and oxygen desaturation during sleep in patients with chronic obstructive pulmonary disease. Chest (Suppl) 73:301, 1978

56. Gothgen I, Jacobsen E: Transcutaneous oxygen tension measurement. 1. Age variation and reproducibility. Acta Anaesthesiol Scand 67:66, 1978
57. Gregory GA: Transcutaneous oxygen measurement. p. 74. In Spence AA (ed): Respiratory Monitoring in Intensive Care. Churchill Livingstone, Edinburgh, 1982
58. Severinghaus JW: Transcutaneous monitoring of arterial PCO_2. p. 85. In Spence AA (ed): Respiratory Monitoring in Intensive Care. Churchill Livingstone, Edinburgh, 1982
59. Guilleminault C, Cummiskey J, Motta J: Chronic obstructive airflow disease and sleep studies. Am Rev Respir Dis 122:397, 1980
60. Chokroverty S, Sharp JT: Primary sleep apnoea syndrome. J Neurol Neurosurg Psych 44:970, 1981
61. Stokes DC, McBride JT, Wall MA et al: Sleep hypoxemia in young adults with cystic fibrosis. Am J Dis Child 134:741, 1980
62. Muller NL, Francis PW, Gurwitz D et al: Mechanism of hemoglobin desaturation during rapid eye movement sleep in normal subjects and in patients with cystic fibrosis. Am Rev Respir Dis 121:463, 1980
63. Cherniack NS: Respiratory dysrhythmias during sleep. N Engl J Med 305:325, 1981
64. Cherniack NS, Longobardo GS, Gothe B, Weiner D: Interactive effects of central and obstructive apnea. p. 553. In Hutas I, Debreczeni LA (eds): Advances in Physiological Sciences, Vol. 10: Respiration, Pergamon Press, Oxford, 1981
65. Mortola JP, Anch AN: Chest wall configuration in supine man: Wakefulness and Sleep. Respirat Physiol 35:201, 1978
66. Tusiewicz K, Moldofsky H, Bryan AC, Bryan MH: Mechanics of the rib cage and diaphragm during sleep. J Appl Physiol 43:600, 1977
67. Priban IP: Breathing patterns in man at rest. J Physiol (London) 166:425, 1963
68. Newsom DJ, Stagg D: Interrelationships of volume and time components of individual breaths in resting man. J Physiol (London) 225:481, 1975
69. Askanazi J, Silverberg PA, Hyman AI et al: Patterns of ventilation in postoperative and acutely ill patients. Crit Care 7:41, 1979
70. McNicholas WT, Rutherford R, Grossman R et al: Abnormal respiratory pattern generation during sleep in patients with autonomic dysfunction. Am Rev Respir Dis 128:429, 1983
71. Weil JV, Kryger MH, Scoggin CH: Sleep and breathing at high altitude. p. 119. In Guilleminault C, Dement WC (eds): Sleep Apnea Syndromes. Alan R. Liss, New York, 1978
72. Slutsky AS, Strohl KP: Quantification of oxygen saturation during episodic hypoxemia. Am Rev Respir Dis 121:893, 1980
73. Gothe B, Altose MD, Goldman MD, Cherniack NS: Effect of quiet sleep in humans on resting and CO_2 stimulated breathing. J Appl Physiol 50:724, 1981

8 Diagnostic Methods and Clinical Disorders in Children

Martha J. Miller
Richard J. Martin
Waldemar A. Carlo

The past 20 years have seen great progress in the care of premature infants. These babies are born incompletely adapted to extrauterine life, and the majority of their medical problems, such as respiratory distress syndrome (RDS), intraventricular hemorrhage (IVH), patent ductus anteriosus (PDA), and recurrent apnea derive from this physiological immaturity. Apnea appears to be a basic disorder of respiratory control during sleep, which may be intensified by a wide variety of pathophysiologic problems in the premature infant.

Apneic episodes requiring respiratory support or pharmacologic intervention occur in at least 50 percent of surviving infants weighing less than 1500 g. The incidence of apnea in these babies is inversely correlated with gestational age and weight,[1,2] and may begin at 1 to 2 days of life in preterm infants without respiratory disease. Interestingly, the peak occurrence of apnea is not until 3 to 7 days in babies who initially manifest RDS, thus coinciding with resolution of their lung disease.[3,4] Thereafter, as the infant matures, apnea generally decreases in incidence. As will be discussed in more detail, the frequency of neonatal apnea may be increased by a multiplicity of disorders of the premature infant (Fig. 8-1). Often, when these are corrected, the apnea resolves. Apnea may, however, occur as an isolated phenomenon in premature infants, with no clearly identifiable cause.

The consequence of untreated apnea in infancy is exposure to recurrent episodes of hypoxia, with possible damage to the immature brain.[5] Without intervention, primary apnea may progress to secondary apnea, responsive only to vigorous assisted ventilation. Indeed, infants who require theophylline therapy, continuous positive airway pressure (CPAP), or intubation for prolonged apnea may be at higher risk for development of cerebral palsy,[6] although a simple cause-and-effect relationship has *not* been established.

The exact nature of the central neurologic mechanisms that predispose premature infants to apnea is unclear. What has emerged from research in this area is a better definition of those elements of respiratory function that distinguish the newborn or premature infant from the adult. No single component, such as immaturity of mechanoreceptor reflex input or chemical control, is adequate to explain all the facets of this disorder. Nevertheless, a consideration of each of these factors clearly gives a better understanding of the overall problem of apnea, and those modes of therapy currently available for its treatment.

DETECTION AND CLASSIFICATION OF APNEA

The definition of apnea itself varies among investigators, leading to some difficulty in comparison of observations. An apnea may be defined as a pause in breathing of variable duration (5 seconds or greater), often associated with cyanosis and/or bradycardia. Apnea has been distinguished from periodic breathing, in which the infant exhibits regular cycles of respiration of approximately 10 to 18 seconds interrupted by pauses of at least 3 seconds in duration, this pattern recurring for at least 2 minutes.[7] Episodes of apnea may, however, occur in clusters and their exact relationshps to the cyclic respiratory pattern seen in periodic breathing has yet to be elucidated. The short respiratory pauses that occur during periodic breathing are not associated with significant bradycardia and are thought to be of no pathologic significance.

In the premature infant, respiratory patterns may be monitored by several quantitative or semiquantitative techniques. Among the latter is the impedance pneumogram,[8] commonly used in conjunction with continuous recording of heart rate for clinical apnea monitoring in neonates. This technique measures respiratory patterns by means of changes in electrical resistance across the chest wall during breathing. Rib cage and diaphragmatic movements coincident with breathing may also be assessed in a semiquantitative manner via mercury-filled thoracic and abdominal strain gauges or magnetometers.[9,10] Respiratory inductance plethysmography gives semiquantitative information on tidal volume changes from rib cage and abdominal motion, although calibration can be time-consuming and measurements can only be made in one position.[11]

A widely utilized but largely research technique for monitoring neonatal ventilation employs a nasal mask or nasal prongs modified as a pneumotachograph.[12,13] A fine mesh screen of known resistance may be mounted across

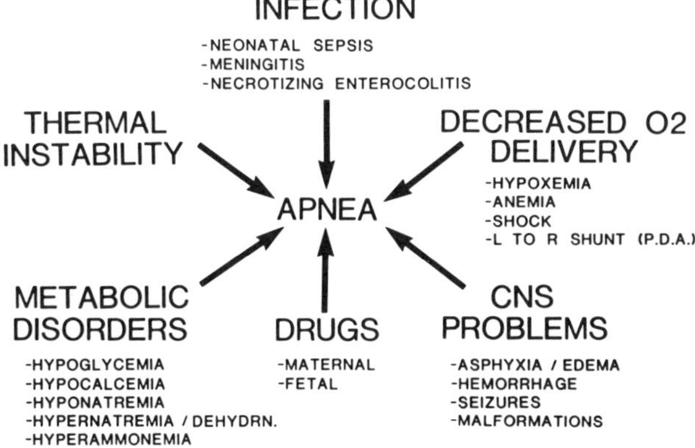

Fig. 8-1 Specific causes of apnea.

the path of airflow; continuous recording of pressure changes across the screen may be converted to units of airflow, which may be electronically integrated to give tidal volume. Unfortunately addition of any kind of mask arrangement probably modifies an infant's respiratory patterns.

Body plethysmography has also been utilized in the laboratory investigation of respiratory function. In this methodology, an infant is placed in a box with his head or face outside. An airtight seal is formed around the face, and volume changes in the box converted via a spirometer or pressure transducer into respiratory volumes.[14,15]

Neonatal apneas were initially believed to involve both cessation of chest wall movement and airflow, signalling a failure of "central" respiratory drive. Recently, Thach and coworkers, utilizing simultaneous measurement of airflow and chest wall movements, have found that upper airway obstruction may occur in premature infants during apnea. Flexion of the neck, whether spontaneous[16] or induced[17] led to airway occlusion, although apneas with an obstructive component have been observed *without* head flexion. In apnea with an obstructive component nasal airflow may entirely cease, although chest wall movements continue. Obstructive apneas would, therefore, be misinterpreted as isolated bradycardia by standard impedance monitoring techniques.

The most common type of apnea observed in premature infants is termed *mixed* apnea, in which a central respiratory pause of $\geq$2 seconds is either preceded or followed by obstructed breaths (see Fig. 8-2). Mixed apneas account for between 53 and 71 percent of all apneic episodes in preterm infants.[18,19] In purely *obstructive* apnea (12 to 20 percent of episodes) obstructed breaths continue throughout the entire apnea, although airflow has ceased (Fig. 8-3). Isolated *central* apneas may also occur during which both airflow and chest wall movement cease simultaneously (Fig. 8-4). The predominant type of apnea varies somewhat between infants and depends on precise diagnostic

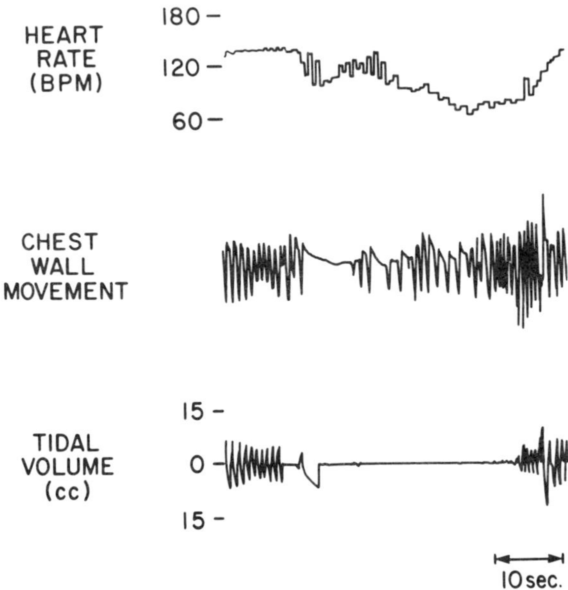

Fig. 8-2 Mixed apnea. Obstructed breaths precede and follow a central respiratory pause.

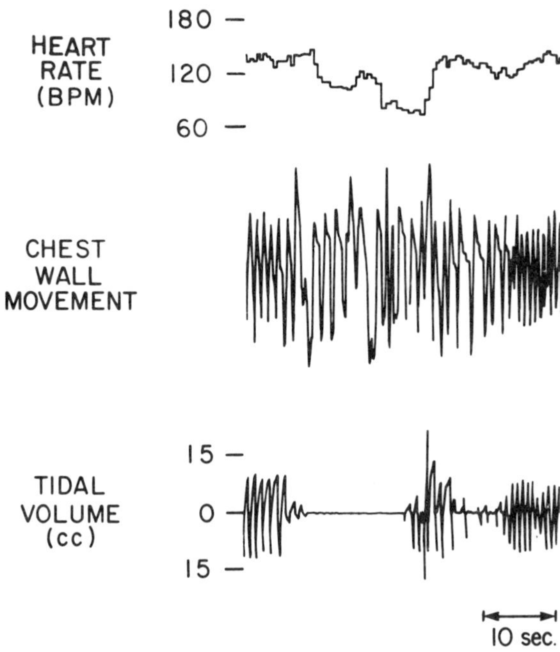

Fig. 8-3 Obstructive apnea. Breathing efforts continue, although no nasal airflow occurs.

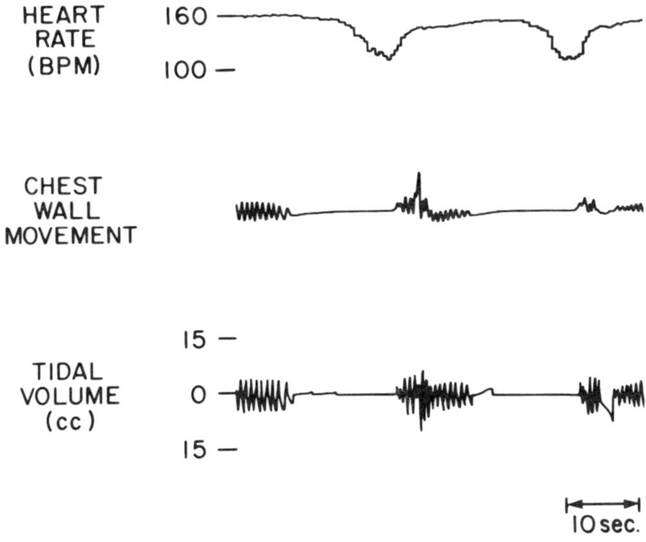

Fig. 8-4 Central apnea. Both nasal airflow and breathing efforts cease simultaneously.

criteria. In any one infant either central apneas or apneas with an obstructive component tend to predominate at any given time.

The airway obstruction that occurs in apneic infants appears to arise at the level of the pharynx.[20] It has been proposed that negative pharyngeal pressure, normally generated during inspiration, may produce pharyngeal collapse particularly in the presence of decreased tone in the pharyngeal dilator muscles (geniohyoid, genioglossus), as has been observed in infants with mandibular hypoplasia.[21] In order for the collapsed airway to open, the infant may need to overcome surface adhesive forces in the pharynx and activate the pharyngeal dilator muscles. Swallows have been noted during obstructive apnea,[20] the etiology of which is unclear. Swallowing may be part of a lower pharyngeal reflex response to collapse of the airway during obstruction.

Bradycardia may accompany all three types of apnea, generally occurring between 10 and 15 seconds after onset of the apnea. This fall in heart rate has been attributed to hypoxia.[22] Bradycardia may, however, occur within 2 seconds of the onset of obstructed breaths,[23] too soon to be due to a peripheral chemoreceptor response. The early onset of bradycardia suggests the presence of a cardiorespiratory reflex that may be triggered during apnea, the physiologic details of which are entirely unknown at this time.

Respiratory pauses may also occur in awake premature infants during autonomic functions, such as defecation or urination, or during crying, yawning, or vigorous spontaneous movement.[24] These pauses can be associated with bradycardia, possibly on a reflex basis, and must be distinguished from true apnea of prematurity, which occurs in sleeping infants.

On the basis of current knowledge of upper airway physiology, a hypo-

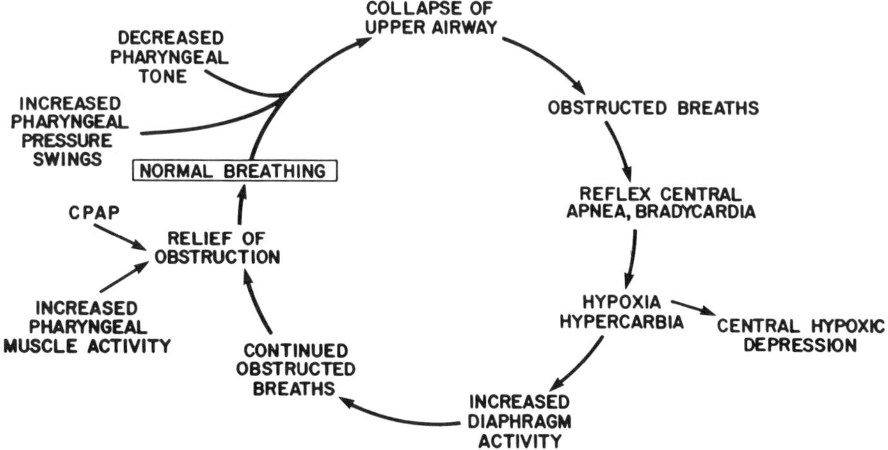

Fig. 8-5 Hypothetical scheme for origin of apnea with an obstructive component.

thetical sequence for the events leading to mixed and obstructive apnea may be constructed (Fig. 8-5), although many details need to be confirmed. Initially, the sleeping premature infant may exhibit a transient decrease in dilator tone of the pharyngeal airway, possibly associated with periodic or oscillatory cycles of respiration, or change in sleep state. In this setting, inspiratory efforts and the resultant negative pressure in the pharyngeal airway may collapse the pharynx completely. This collapse, in turn, may trigger reflex swallowing movements and/or reflex central apnea. Recovery from this airway obstruction could depend on several responses. As the apnea continues, respiratory drive may increase due to chemoreceptor responses to hypoxia and hypercapnia. Diaphragmatic activation may actually precede that of the upper airway, increasing the likelihood of obstructed breaths in the latter portion of an apnea. Finally, increase in tone of pharyngeal dilator muscles would open the airway and terminate the apnea. The influence of sleep state on this sequence of events is discussed later.

MECHANORECEPTOR REFLEXES

The pattern of normal breathing is constantly modified by afferent input to the respiratory control center from a great variety of senosry end organs. These are present in the trachea and bronchi, throughout the smooth muscle of the respiratory tract, in the respiratory bronchioles, alveoli, pleura, the pulmonary vascular bed, and the intercostal muscles. Many respiratory reflexes appear to be prominent in premature or term infants, and may exert a proportionally greater influence over respiratory patterns during the neonatal period. Several reflexes, namely the Hering-Breuer reflex, Head's paradoxical reflex, and the intercostal inhibitory reflex have generated interest in studies of respiration in human infants.

Hering-Breuer Reflex

In 1868 Hering and Breuer[25] reported that distension of the lungs of anesthetized animals decreased respiratory frequency. This reflex response could be abolished by section of the vagus nerve. Man appears to have a generally weaker reflex than experimental animals such as cats, guinea pigs, or rabbits. The afferent limb of the reflex arc originates in slowly adapting pulmonary stretch receptors such as those within the smooth muscle of the tracheobronchial tree.[26] Fibers in the vagus nerve carry stretch receptor input to the medulla, with caudal connections to the nucleus tractus solitarius. The efferent limb of the reflex arc travels within the phrenic nerve to the diaphragm. In anesthetized animals a nearly linear relationship is found between inspiratory inflation volume, and the logarithm of the length of apnea (the larger the inflation volume, the longer the apnea).

The activity of the Hering-Breuer reflex may be elicited in newborn infants by altering lung volume in several ways. Abrupt lung inflation results in an initial gasp (see Head's reflex) followed by an apnea of variable duration. This apnea is thought to result from vagal inhibition of inspiration and/or prolongation of expiration due to the Hering-Breuer inflation reflex. Termination of the apnea will depend on other factors such as rapidly increasing chemical drive. Occlusion of the airway at end-expiration generally results in prolongation of the subsequent inspiratory effort due to a decrease in inspiratory inhibition. This prolongation of inspiratory time has been used as a quantifiable measure of the Hering-Breuer reflex. An alternate approach is to produce a small but sustained lung inflation, as with the administration of CPAP.[27] This has the effect of prolonging expiration (without much effect on inspiratory time) thereby decreasing the respiratory rate. Studies such as these indicate that the Hering-Breuer inspiratory reflex is weak at 32 weeks, increases in strength in infants up to 38 weeks postmenstrual age, and then declines in strength thereafter.[28] The physiologic significance of this change in reflex strength is unknown, but may relate to an early insufficiency of afferent input, and later dominance of other competing reflexes. The influence of the Hering-Breuer inspiratory reflex on respiratory rate and depth may be modulated by central input from other respiratory reflexes such as Head's paradoxical reflex.

Hering and Breuer also noted that sudden deflation of the lungs of animals could increase the frequency and force of inspiratory efforts. The afferent limb of this reflex lies in the vagus, although the receptors are unknown. The nature and importance of this reflex in humans is unclear. Hypothetically, it could counteract sudden deflation of the lung, thus preserving functional residual capacity (FRC), although the presence of this reflex in human infants has not been shown.

Head's Paradoxical Reflex

In 1888, Head observed that a large and rapid lung inflation in rabbits produced a transient increase in phrenic motoneuron discharge, and increased inspiratory effort.[29] The stretch receptors for Head's reflex appear to lie in the larger airways, but their exact structure is unknown. Like the Hering-Breuer reflex, the afferent limb lies in the vagus, and the efferent limb in the phrenic nerve. The presence of this reflex in the newborn human infant is suggested by the observation of Cross et al.[30] that rapid lung inflation in the first few days of life produced an abrupt gasp. The physiologic role of this reflex is unclear, although it has been suggested that the reflex may produce the occasional deep breath seen during resting breathing or immediately after birth.

Intercostal Inhibitory Reflex

Chest wall reflexes originating in the intercostal muscles may be important in the newborn infant. Ordinarily, activity of the intercostal muscles should stabilize the neonatal chest wall against increasing respiratory loads. During rapid eye movement (REM) sleep, significant distortion of the chest wall may occur, particularly in premature infants, manifested by paradoxical inward motion of the rib cage during inspiration (see below). In preterm infants, active distortion of the chest wall may trigger an inspiratory *inhibitory* reflex, originating in the intercostal muscle spindles. Knill and coworkers demonstrated that increased chest wall distortion produced by vibratory stimuli during active sleep was associated with a shortened inspiratory time. Conversely, stabilization of the chest wall with either continuous negative pressure (CNEG) or CPAP reduced chest wall distortion and lenghtened inspiratory time (T_i).[31,32] It was thus postulated that during active sleep, paradoxical inward inspiratory motion of the rib cage may activate intercostal muscle spindles, shortening inspiration. An alternative possibility is that compression or distortion of underlying lung may trigger vagally mediated irritant or deflation reflexes that could also shorten inspiration.

In summary, reflexes from the larger airways, bronchioles, alveoli, and intercostal muscles may regulate the length and depth of inspiration and expiration during normal breathing. In newborns the activity of these reflexes may be relatively enhanced, possibly due to immature chemical control mechanisms or paucity of inhibitory central dendritic interconnections. Direct evidence that these mechanoreceptor reflexes initiate central or obstructive apnea is lacking, although such afferent input could modify the infant's respiratory response to cessation of airflow during apnea, whether central or obstructive. Knowledge of the exact contribution from each class of receptor, and the central organization of this information in the newborn would add greatly to our understanding of respiratory regulation in both apneic and healthy infants.

CHEMICAL CONTROL

The change in ventilation that occurs in response to increased levels of inspired carbon dioxide or to alterations in inspired oxygen traditionally has been used to test the chemical responsiveness of respiratory control mechanisms. The response of the respiratory muscles to a chemical stimulus is initiated by afferent information derived from peripheral or central chemoreceptors, or both. The peripheral receptors are situated in the carotid and aortic bodies, while the central receptors are assumed to be located on the ventrolateral surface of the medulla. The latter is thought to be the primary site at which a hypercapnic stimulus is sensed at steady state. On the other hand, transient and more rapid changes in $PaCO_2$ will largely be sensed peripherally.

As early as 1953, Cross et al.[33] administered up to 2 percent carbon dioxide to premature and term infants and found an increase in minute ventilation mediated primarily by changes in tidal volume and a substantial decrease in periodic breathing. Their observations have been confirmed by several other investigators.[34–37] More recent studies have quantitated the influence of maturation on "carbon dioxide sensitivity," which is defined as the slope of the line describing ventilation (corrected for body weight) versus alveolar PCO_2, usually obtained from at least two steady state levels. The preterm infant's CO_2 sensitivity has been shown to be decreased in comparison with that of the term infant.[35–38]. It remains unclear whether this is the result of an immaturity in some component of the chemical control mechanism, or a mechanical inability on the part of the respiratory muscles to generate an appropriate ventilatory response. Nonetheless, the premature infant's response does increase with either greater gestational age at birth or advancing postnatal age. It has been proposed that CO_2 sensitivity is decreased in apneic preterm infants, but a clear cause-and-effect relationship has never been established.

When challenged with a hypoxic stimulus, both term and neonates respond with a brief increase in minute ventilation over the first minute.[39,40] This response occurs in preterm infants as young as 28 weeks' gestation.[41] While this initial ventilatory response echoes that of the adult, the similarity ends there, because within 2 to 3 minutes the infant's minute ventilation falls, sometimes to less than the resting level. This biphasic response contrasts with that in the hypoxic adult, in whom hyperventilation is maintained. Once the neonate has reached a postnatal age of approximately 7 to 18 days, hyperventilation can be sustained, and this change appears to be independent of gestational age.[41,42] It has been proposed that the characteristic neonatal response to low oxygen is due to initial peripheral chemoreceptor stimulation followed by an overriding depression of the respiratory center as a result of hypoxemia. Postulated mechanisms for this ventilatory depression include release of endorphins (see below), or a hypoxia-induced increase in cerebral blood flow resulting in alkalosis (due to CO_2 washout), which is sensed centrally. Finally, a vagally mediated mechanism cannot be excluded for the decrease in ventilation is primarily the result of a fall in respiratory rate secondary to a prolonged expiratory time. It is

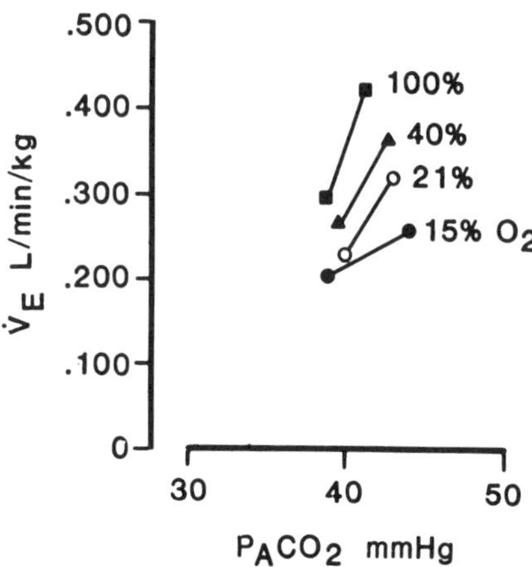

Fig. 8-6 Effect of varying inhaled oxygen concentration on ventilatory response ($\dot{V}_E$) to alveolar PCO_2 (P_ACO_2). (Rigatto H, de la Torre Verduzco P, Cates DB: Effects of O_2 on the ventilatory response to CO_2 in preterm infants. J Appl Physiol 39:896, 1975.)

tempting to speculate that the failure of preterm infants to maintain hyperventilation in response to sustained hypoxemia might destabilize respiratory control and aggravate apneic episodes.

In response to 100 percent F_IO_2 there is a diminution in the incidence of periodic breathing[40] consistent with the observed increase in periodic breathing in the face of hypoxia.[43] Also, there is a potentiation of the response to carbon dioxide, that is, the higher the inspired oxygen, the greater is the infant's carbon dioxide sensitivity (Fig. 8-6).[44] This effect is the reverse of that observed in adults, in whom increasing oxygen depresses carbon dioxide sensitivity. Premature and term infants demonstrate a consistent respiratory response to 100 percent oxygen alone: in the first minute, ventilation acutely falls, then it returns to a level generally higher than baseline.[39–41] This response also is found in newborn lambs but is lost after bilateral carotid sinus denervation.s;4[5]

CENTRAL MATURATION

The area of the brain that both generates rhythmic respiratory activity and integrates input from peripheral receptors lies in the brainstem. Microelectrode studies, largely performed in cats, have demonstrated respiratory neurons in two areas of the medulla; the dorsal respiratory group (DRG), present bilaterally in the area of the nucleus tractus solitarius, and the ventral respiratory group (VRG), located bilaterally in the region of the nucleus ambiguous and nucleus retroambigualis. Respiratory neurons are also found in the dorsolateral rostral pons, associated with the nucleus parabrachialis (NPMB) and the Kolliker-Fuse nucleus. Neurons of the DRG are most active during inspiration, and two types of neurons here are of particular interest. R alpha-neurons exite phrenic motoneurons, and R beta-neurons may include the inhibitory interneurons of the Hering-Breuer inspiratory reflex. In addition, inspiratory and expiratory neurons are also found in the VRG, as well as important motor nuclei for the glossopharyngeal and vagus nerves. At the level of the medulla, there are axonal interconnections between a wide variety of contralateral and ipsilateral respiratory neurons, allowing for complex integration of sensory input and respiratory motor output. In the area of the pons (NPBM) all the respiratory neurons are under strong inhibition by afferent input from pulmonary stretch receptors.

Despite many years of investigation, the exact area of the brain that is necessary for generation of rhythmic respirations is not fully clarified. Recently, a model for organization of medullary respiratory activity has been proposed.[46–48] In this model, a central generator of inspiratory activity continually integrates input from chemoreceptors, other central neurons, and mechanoreceptors. Inspiratory activity increases slowly, until it reaches a firing threshold, the "off-switch" mechanism. The off-switch threshold may be itself modulated by inputs from other areas of the central nervous system (CNS), chemoreceptors, and peripheral reflexes. An example of the latter would be the vagal input from the Hering-Breuer inspiratory reflex, which facilitates inspiratory termination.

From studies in fetal sheep, it appears that central respiratory neurons are active by at least the latter half of the second trimester.[49,50] However, knowledge of the anatomic details of the respiratory control center in the fetal animal or human is incomplete. Chernick et al. have mapped the activity of respiratory neurons in exteriorized fetal sheep, and noted that the respiratory center was more diffuse in the fetus, than in the newborn or adult animal.[51]

Fetal breathing movements have been studied in human newborns prior to term, by the technique of real time ultrasound. Fetal breathing could be defined as inward movement of the rib cage in association with outward movement of the abdomen.[52] Breathing was present 31 percent of the time during the last 10 weeks of pregnancy, being interrupted by periods of fetal apnea. Less mature fetuses had a breathing rate of 58/minutes, which decreased to 47/minutes as term approached, the breathing rates being influenced by fetal sleep state, maternal meals, alcohol ingestion, and cigarette smoking. In the stressed fetus, a regular pattern of respiration may be replaced by gasping prior to fetal death.

From these few studies, a picture emerges of the antenatal development of respiratory control. Respiratory activity can be documented in the second trimester, and is responsive to both central neural input (sleep state) and external influences (glucose, smoking). As the infant approaches term, central respiratory drive as well as peripheral reflex input must develop for the baby to initiate and sustain regular respiration after birth. Clearly the process of respiratory maturation is not complete in the human infant born prematurely. Indeed, in the immature vertebrate brain dendritic synapses are not completely developed.[53] This may explain the observation that breathing patterns in premature infants are very sensitive to external stimuli and change in sleep state. An example of the importance of peripheral input is seen in the bewildering variety of stimuli that may trigger apnea in premature infants (Fig. 8-1). Apnea appears to be a final common response of the immature respiratory control center to stimuli that are considerably less potent in an older child or adult. Presumably, as the preterm brain matures, increasing numbers of interconnections develop between various respiratory regulating areas in the brain, leading to more stability in central respiratory drive, and proportionally less influence from various peripheral sites.

Henderson-Smart et al. have recently described a significant association between brain stem conduction times for auditory evoked responses and clinical apnea in preterm infants.[54] With increasing postconceptional age, apneas decrease in frequency, and auditory brain stem conduction times shorten. Presumably this reflects improved synaptic efficiency, and greater myelination of pathways within the brain.

Sleeping infants show periodic oscillations in breathing pattern, possibly related to apnea and periodic breathing.[55] Frequency analysis has allowed identification of multiple simultaneous frequencies of ventilatory oscillation, with apneas produced when two oscillations are in phase.[56] Periodic breathing has been interpreted by Waggener et al.[56] as an oscillation in the peripheral chemoreceptor control loop (higher frequency 16 to 20 breaths/cycle) or the central medullary chemoreceptor control loop (50 to 60 breaths/cycle), present in the normal infant. The influence of gestational or postnatal age on these periodic oscillations in breathing pattern is not yet known. Similarly, their exact relationship to central and obstructive apnea remains to be clarified.

Much attention has recently been focused on the role of endorphins in respiration. The sites for production of these endogenous opiates in the brain are present as early as embryonic day 16 in the rat.[57] Similarly, in the experimental animal, the level of opiate binding increases with gestational age, due to an increasing number of receptors. In the human fetus, opiate receptors have also been found, and β-endorphin is present in the human placenta.[58] Indeed, the β-endorphin like *activity* in plasma from the newborn is three to four times that in the mother. Fetal hypoxia and stress of delivery are both postulated triggers for the release of fetal endorphins.[59] However, the suggestion that endogenous opiates may regulate breathing in the newborn is controversial.

Administration of FK-33-824, a potent enkephalin, produced a significant reduction in rate of breathing in rabbit pups.[60] In addition, the opiate antagonist, naloxone, has been found to initiate breathing movements in apneic fetal lambs.[61] Hypoxic fetuses may be particularly prone to respiratory depression due to endogenous opiates. Chernick et al.[62] have found that the duration of primary apnea in asphyxiated rabbit fetuses was reduced by pretreatment of the mother with naloxone. In contrast, however, naloxone could not abolish apnea in preterm infants.[63] The studies to date suggest that endogenous opiates may modulate respiratory control, particularly in the asphyxiated neonate. There is no clear evidence, however, for a role of endorphins or enkephalins in apnea of prematurity.

Table 8-1. A Schematic Organization of the Usefulness of Measures in Defining State in the Premature and Young Infant

	Conceptional age (weeks)				
	24	28	32	36	40
Body movements	±	+	+ +	+ + +	+ + + +
Eye movements		+	+ +	+ + +	+ + + +
Respiration pattern			±	+ +	+ + +
EEG			−		+ + +
Chin EMG				+	+ + +

(Parmelee AH, Stern E: Development of states in infants. p. 199. In Clement CD (ed): Sleep and the Maturing Nervous System, Academic Press, New York, 1972)

INFLUENCE OF SLEEP STATE ON NEONATAL RESPIRATION

It is only over the last decade that the profound influence of sleep state on regulation of breathing in newborn infants has become readily apparent. As a result many of the earlier classic studies of neonatal respiration are being reevaluated. There is clear agreement that studies of respiratory control in infants beyond about 34 weeks gestational age can no longer be interpreted if there has been no control of the infant's behavioral state. Nonetheless, differences of opinion remain regarding the criteria for precise definition of the various states, and the clinical significance of sleep state related influences on neonatal respiration.

Phillipson has proposed that during quiet sleep (QS) respiration is largely under metabolic (or autonomic) control, whereas during active sleep (AS), behavioral (or voluntary) influences predominate.[64] The relevance of this approach to the newborn is not entirely clear. The traditional developmental approach is to look on AS as a more primitive state and QS as a more mature, highly controlled state, possibly arising from greater cortical influences.[65] Advancing fetal development is associated with greater organization of states, both prenatally and postnatally. This parallels the rapidly increasing complexity of dendritic interactions at all levels of the maturing central nervous system. Parmelee and Stern defined the two major sleep states in infancy as follows: (1) quiet sleep (QS), characterized by closed eyes with no eye movements, no body movements, and regular respiration and (2) active sleep (AS), characterized by closed eyes with eye movements, frequent body, limb or face movements, and irregular respiration.[65] A schematic organization of the usefulness of measures employed in the definition of neonatal state is shown in Table 8-1. In studying respiration, some investigators have elected to exclude respiratory regularity as a criterion of sleep state, and focused greater attention on the electroencephalogram (EEG). This is a possible reason for some of the disparate results obtained from different centers. Nonetheless, whatever set of parameters is employed, characterization of sleep state is difficult prior to

32 weeks postmenstrual age, and extensive periods will be classified as indeterminate (or transitional) even beyond that time.

In both preterm and term infants apnea occurs predominantly during AS and indeterminate sleep.[66] It is less common for apnea to be observed during QS, when respiration is characteristically regular with little breath-by-breath change in tidal volume or respiratory frequency. Nonetheless, periodic breathing is seen in QS and may even occur predominantly during that state. While the reason for the higher incidence of apnea in AS is unclear, and may be centrally mediated (via the reticular activating system, etc.), many of the physiologic changes noted below may be relevant. It is widely accepted that the three major ventilatory parameters (minute ventilation, tidal volume, and frequency) all show twofold to threefold greater variability during AS versus QS. Minute ventilation and frequency both tend to be higher during AS while tidal volume is not significantly different between sleep states.[67,68]

More recently, Hathorn has shown term infants to have oscillations in tidal volume and frequency with mean periods of 6 to 12 seconds.[55] The oscillations had higher amplitudes during AS and were predominantly out of phase, in contrast to preterm infants exhibiting periodic breathing, in whom tidal volume and frequency oscillations were in phase. This change in the phase relationship between tidal volume and frequency with increasing neonatal maturity and the influence of sleep state on this relationship, raises the question of whether there may be somewhat differing controls for the rate and depth of breathing. During periodic breathing, the two central controllers may operate in phase with each other, while in the more mature baby, they become more closely "locked" out of phase with each other, leading to more efficient, stable ventilation.

The increase in minute ventilation during AS is probably associated with a higher alveolar ventilation, as recent studies indicate both transcutaneous and alveolar PCO_2 to be lower in AS.[69,70] In addition, an increase in O_2 consumption of up to 10 percent has been reported in healthy neonates during AS.[71] Despite alveolar hyperventilation, transcutaneous PO_2 averages 5 to 10 mmHg lower in AS than in QS in both preterm and term neonates, raising the possibility of ventilation/perfusion imbalance in these infants during AS.[72] This observation is consistent with recent data in which the patterns of respiratory muscle behavior have been examined in infants during the various stages of sleep.

Chest wall movements are predominantly out of phase (or paradoxical) during AS, in contrast to QS when paradoxical movements are almost never observed in term infants (although they may persist in preterm infants during QS).[70,72,73] Thus, abdominal expansion during inspiration is frequently accompanied by inward movement of the rib cage during AS, whereas during QS rib cage and abdomen often expand together. These paradoxical chest wall movements during AS appear to be the result of decreased intercostal muscle activity and are clearly more common in preterm than term infants. A fall in FRC also has been observed in term infants during AS, and this, together with the paradoxical chest wall motion, might well impair ventilation/perfusion relation-

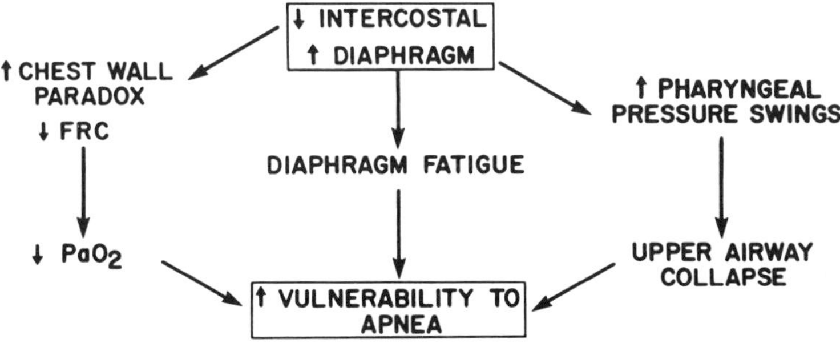

Fig. 8-7 Mechanisms that may lead to apnea during active sleep.

ships throughout the lung as proposed earlier.[74] Bryan reported that these events are accompanied by greater abdominal respiratory excursions and greater diaphragmatic activity during AS.[75] This group of investigators has further proposed that electromyographic changes suggestive of diaphragmatic fatigue accompany these paradoxical chest wall movements in normal preterm and term infants.[76] It is thus tempting to speculate that decreased intercostal muscle and enhanced diaphragmatic activity during AS enhance the vulnerability to apnea by decreasing FRC, lowering PaO_2 and possibly precipitating diaphragmatic fatigue (Fig. 8-7).

As noted earlier, there has recently been increased interest in the role of upper airway obstruction during apneic episodes in human infants.[17] Activation of upper airway muscles may be an important protective mechanism, preventing upper airway collapse due to high negative pharyngeal pressure during inspiration. Activity of pharyngeal muscles, negative pharyngeal pressure, and neck positioning are all thought to interact in the maintenance of airway patency, and small changes in pharyngeal pressure may be critical to the development of upper airway obstruction.[77] In human neonates the greater diaphragmatic activity during AS coincides with the development of larger swings in transdiaphragmatic pressure. These in turn might result in more negative pharyngeal pressure swings and increased vulnerability to obstructive apnea. We have documented a significant increase in alae nasi activity during AS as compared to QS in healthy preterm infants.[78] By lowering transnasal resistance, dilatation of the alae nasi may help to maintain a patent upper airway during AS.[79] There are no current data on the effect of sleep state on other upper airway muscles in neonates.

The influence of sleep state on both mechanoreceptor and chemoreceptor mediated control mechanisms has been less well-defined. Only one study in infants has addressed the influence of sleep state on respiratory timing as mediated via the Hering-Breuer reflex. The data of Finer et al. suggested that this reflex is weaker in AS as determined by less prolongation of inspiratory effort following end expiratory airway occlusions.[67]

The ventilatory effect of inhaled CO_2 has been measured under *steady-*

state conditions as the change in magnitude of ventilation, or as the slope of the relationship between ventilation and arterial PCO_2. Bryan et al. reported a decreased response to CO_2 during AS in seven infants up to 6 months of age.[80] In contrast, Davi et al.[36] and Haddad et al.[70] have subsequently found no difference in the steady-state sensitivity and response to CO_2 between AS and QS in a group of preterm and full-term neonates. Anderson et al.[81] have examined the effect of sleep state on the initial transient portion of the ventilatory response to CO_2 inhalation, that is the first 60 seconds of CO_2 inhalation, in a group of healthy full-term neonates. Our data indicate that, although minute ventilation significantly increased during the first 60 seconds of CO_2 inhalation, there was again no effect of sleep state on the average time course of the total ventilatory response. However, the large variability in ventilation during the control period of AS persisted throughout the transient response. Furthermore, there was a greater increase in end-tidal PCO_2 during the first minute of CO_2 inhalation during AS compared with QS, suggesting a smaller initial increase in alveolar ventilation relative to CO_2 delivery to the lungs. These data suggest that if sleep state alters the ventilatory response to CO_2, the effect is not a profound one. Finally, a possible influence of sleep state on the hypoxic ventilatory response was noted by Rigatto et al., who observed that 1- to 4-week-old premature infants were able to maintain a hyperventilatory response while in QS, in contrast to the biphasic response during AS when hyperventilation could not be sustained.[82] Previous studies describing the characteristic biphasic ventilatory response to hypoxia were not controlled for sleep state, and this area also clearly requires further study.

DIAGNOSIS AND TREATMENT

As discussed above, apnea in the neonatal period may be associated with a specific precipitating factor, although frequently no cause can be identified. An overview of the variety of pathophysiologic disorders that may trigger apnea in infants is depicted in Figure 8-1. This differential diagnosis must be considered before appropriate treatment is commenced. Table 8-2 summarizes the clinical and laboratory evaluation of the infant with apnea. Most frequently, only a few diagnostic studies are required and most of the precipitating disorders can be discarded with a thorough review of the history and physical examination. Treatment of all the contributory causes of apnea is beyond the scope of this chapter and the approach to be presented should only be used for those infants in whom the diagnosis of idiopathic apnea of prematurity is entertained.

Apneic episodes vary widely in severity. The occasionally apneic, otherwise healthy infant may respond well to minimal sensory stimulation while the infant with recurrent and prolonged apneic spells may require more aggressive treatment such as assisted ventilation. It should be noted that none of the

Table 8-2. Evaluation of the Apneic Infant

History
Perinatal complications and Apgar scores
Gestational and postnatal age
Drugs given to mother or infant
Preceding infant and environmental temperatures
Risk factors for infection
Feeding tolerance
Physical examination
Complete examination, emphasizing cardiorespiratory and neurologic status
Laboratory
Consider the following studies when clinically indicated:
Hematocrit
Blood sugar
WBC and differential
Blood culture
Spinal tap
Arterial blood gas
Head ultrasound
Serum electrolytes and calcium
X-Ray (chest, abdomen)

alternative therapeutic approaches is without potential problems in this high risk population.

Probably the most innocuous treatment for apnea comprises various modes of sensory stimulation. Prophylactic cutaneous stimulation, consisting of rubbing of the extremities 5 out of every 15 minutes has been shown to decrease apneic episodes.[83] Irregularly oscillating water beds, used for prolonged or intermittent periods, also reduce apnea.[84,85] In contrast, regularly oscillating water beds have not been reported to prevent apneic episodes.[86] Previously, maintenance of body temperature at a slightly lower level than that routinely used clinically (36°C vs. 36.8°C) was noted to decrease the number of apneic episodes,[1] however, this approach is currently not utilized. It has been proposed that the afferent input resultant from these cutaneous and vestibuloproprioceptive stimuli nonspecifically enhances respiratory drive.

Another therapy proven effective in the treatment of preterm infants with apnea is nasal CPAP (at 2 to 5 cm H_2O).[83,87] Initial studies suggested that the beneficial effects of CPAP are mediated via alteration of the Hering-Breuer reflex,[88] stabilization of the chest wall with consequent reduction of the intercostal inhibitory reflex,[32] or increase in oxygenation.[89] Recently, we have observed that nasal CPAP only reduces apnea with an obstructive component, with no beneficial effect on central apnea.[19] Resolution of obstructive apnea by CPAP has also been recently reported in adults.[90] Interestingly, in an animal model, genioglossus activity increased with pressure fluctuations in the upper airway, but decreased with CPAP.[91] Furthermore, pressure fluctuations in the upper airway were necessary for maintenance of airway patency. Therefore, it is possible that CPAP exerts its effect by splinting the upper airway with positive pressure throughout inspiration and expiration, rather than by reflex activation of upper airway dilating muscles.

Table 8-3. Treatment of Idiopathic Apnea of Prematurity

Mode	Method	Possible mechanisms of action
Cutaneous stimulation	Intermittent skin rubbing	Increased nonspecific neural afferents
Vestibular and propioceptive stimulation	Irregular oscillations with waterbed	Increased nonspecific neural afferents
CPAP	Nasal, low positive pressure (2–5 cmH_2O)	Splinting of upper airway and maintenance of patency Alteration of Hering-Breuer deflation reflex Increased oxygenation Irritant receptor stimulation
Pharmacologic stimulation	Theophylline Loading 5–6 mg/kg Maintenance 1–2 mg/kg, q8h Caffeine Loading 10 mg/kg Maintenance 2.5 mg/kg per day	Central respiratory effect (increased CO_2 sensitivity) Increased diaphragmatic contraction Decreased muscle fatigue Increased metabolic rate Increased catecholamine activity

Multiple studies have now conclusively shown that methylxanthines (theophylline and caffeine) are very effective in treatment of apnea of prematurity.[92–94] Roberts et al. have recently demonstrated that theophylline reduces obstructive as well as central apneas.[95] Furthermore, studies by Kelly and Shannon[96] and Hunt et al.[97] support the use of theophylline in full term infants and infants beyond the neonatal period who are at high risk for apnea. A wide range of dosage regimens has been used and proven to be effective. Serum levels of theophylline of 5 to 10 μg/ml and of caffeine of 8 to 20 μg/ml are usually therapeutic and free of toxicity,[98] although some authors report beneficial effects even at lower levels. Furthermore there is interconversion of theophylline to caffeine in preterm infants. While it is now clear that methylxanthines are effective in the treatment of neonatal apnea, the mechanism whereby respiratory regularity is established is still a subject of controversy. Increased diaphragmatic contraction, decreased muscle fatigue, increased metabolic rate, and increased catecholamine activity may contribute to the respiratory actions of methylxanthines. However, it is possible that the mechanism of action of theophylline may differ somewhat from that of caffeine.[98] Neonatal studies have shown that CO_2 response curves have an increased slope, or are shifted to the left with both caffeine and theophylline treatment.[98–100] This is in agreement with the central respirogenic effect reported in animals and human adults. In newborn rabbits caffeine had no effect on vagal afferent activity,[101] and block of carotid and aortic chemoreceptors in adult animals did not eliminate the effects of caffeine,[102] implying a central site of action of methylxanthines. Additional support for a central site of action upon respiratory activity is provided by Eldridge et al.,[103] who observed that decerebration or transection of the spinal cord did not interfere with the action of theophylline. However, inhibition of the synthesis of dopamine and block of dopamine receptors reduced the respiratory effect of intravenous aminophylline, implicating dopaminergic neurons in the medullary response to methylxanthines.

Most infants respond to one or more of the above mentioned modes of treatment (Table 8-3), but if apnea persists despite these measures, tracheal intubation and intermittent positive-pressure ventilation may be necessary. Such severe apnea is frequently the result of an underlying specific pathologic process, such as sepsis or intraventricular hemorrhage, in which case management efforts are directed accordingly. The overall prognosis is then clearly dependent on the underlying disease. Nonetheless, every effort must be undertaken to minimize the complications of prolonged endotracheal intubation and assisted ventilation in the newborn infant.

SUMMARY AND FUTURE DIRECTIONS

In this chapter, we have discussed the most common disorder of respiratory control in neonates, apnea of prematurity, which is primarily a problem of respiratory regulation during sleep. Our understanding of respiration in the neonate is far from complete. The development of respiratory control may be seen as a continuum from the fetus in utero to the adult. Apnea in the premature infant may then represent exposure of the immature respiratory control system to physiologic demands that it is not equipped to handle. The resolution of apnea with time is, in this context, due to normal development and differentiation within the brain stem. Alternatively, we know little of the possible micropathology that may occur in the immature brain stem due to hypoxic and/or ischemic insult. Small areas of damage in the respiratory control center could lead to ventilatory instability, and to apnea. Resolution of apnea with time could occur if other spared and possibly multipotential areas of the brainstem assume the function of respiratory control.

The events that initiate, terminate, or regulate the duration of an apnea are currently unknown. Central apnea itself appears to represent cessation of firing of inspiratory neurons in the medulla. These neurons are subject to afferent input from mechanoreceptors, chemoreceptors, and other brain stem and cortical centers, any or all of which could theoretically initiate an apnea. The realization that not all apneas are similar, that is, some are accompanied by obstruction of the upper airway, raises the possibility that they are not identical in pathophysiology. Obstructive apnea may involve complex developmental changes in and reflex input from the pharynx, while central apneas may be less dependent on peripheral input. Recent interest in the anatomy, neurophysiology, and function of the upper airway promises greater understanding of this somewhat neglected area of the respiratory tract in newborn infants. Hopefully, a multidisciplinary approach to the control of respiration in premature and full-term neonates will unravel the sequence of events that produces apnea, and may lead to better modes of therapy for this common disorder.

ACKNOWLEDGMENT

This work was supported by grants HL-25830 and HL-31173 from the National Heart, Lung, and Blood Institute and a research award from Radiometer Corporation, Copenhagen.

REFERENCES

1. Daily WJR, Klaus M, Meyer HBP: Apnea in premature infants: Monitoring, incidence, heart rate changes, and an effect of environmental temperature. Pediatrics 43:510, 1969
2. Alden ER, Mandelhorn T, woodrum DE et al: Morbidity and mortality of infants weighing less than 1000 grams in an intensive care nursery. Pediatrics 50:40, 1982
3. Carlo WA, Martin RJ, Versteegh FGA et al: The effect of respiratory distress syndrome on chest wall movements and respiratory pauses in preterm infants. Am Rev Respir Dis 126:103, 1982
4. Henderson-Smart DJ: The effect of gestational age on the incidence and duration of recurrent apnoea in newborn babies. Aust Pediatr J 17:273, 1981
5. Peabody JL, Neese AL, Philip AG et al: Transcutaneous oxygen monitoring in aminophylline-treated apneic infants. Pediatrics 62:698, 1978
6. Kitchen WH, Yu VHY, Orgill AA et al: Collaborative study of very low birth weight infants. Am J Dis Child 137:555, 1983
7. Rigatto H, Brady JP: Periodic breathing and apnea in preterm infants; evidence for hypoventilation possibly due to central respiratory depression. Pediatrics 50;202, 1972
8. Pacela AF, Miller CE, Daily WJR et al: Impedance technique for monitoring the newborn infant. Digest of the seventh international conference on medical and biological engineering, Stockholm, Sweden, Aug. 16, 1967.
9. Konno K, Mead J: Static volume-pressure characteristics of the rib cage and abdomen. J Appl Physiol 24:544, 1968
10. Stark AR, Goldman MD, Frantz ID: Lung volume changes, occulsion pressure and chest wall configuration in human infants. Pediatr Res 13:250, 1979
11. Duffty P, Spriet L, Bryan MH et al: Respiratory induction plethysmography (Respitrace^{TM}): An evaluation of its use in the infant. Am Rev Respir Dis 123:542, 1981
12. Swyer PR, Reiman RC, Wright JJ: Ventilation and ventilatory mechanics in the newborn infant. J Pediatr 56:612, 1960
13. Anderson JV, Martin RJ, Lough MD et al: An improved nasal mask pneumotachometer for measuring ventilation in neonates. J Appl Physiol 53:1307, 1982
14. Drorbaugh JE, Fenn WO: A barometric method for measuring ventilation in infants. Pediatrics 16:81, 1955
15. Polgar G, Lacourt G: A method for measuring respiratory mechanisms in small newborn (premature) infants. J Appl Physiol 32:555, 1972

16. Thach BT, Stark AR: Spontaneous neck flexion and airway obstruction during apneic spells in preterm infants. J Pediatr 94:275, 1979
17. Stark AR, Thach BT: Mechanisms of airway obstruction leading to apnea in newborn infants. J Pediatr 89:982, 1976
18. Dransfield DA, Spitzer AR, Fox WM: Episodic airway obstruction in premature infants. Am J Dis Child 137:441, 1983
19. Miller MJ, Carlo WA, Martin RJ: Continuous positive airway pressure selectively reduces obstructive apnea in preterm infants. J Pediatr 106:91, 1985
20. Mathew OP, Roberts JL, Thach BT: Pharyngeal airway obstruction in preterm infants during mixed and obstructive apnea. J Pediatr 100:964, 1982
21. Roberts JL, Mathew OP, Reed WR et al: A clinical test of pharyngeal airway (PAQ) stability. (Abstract) Pediatr Res 16:1692, 1982
22. Guilleminault C, Peraita R, Sonquist M et al: Apnoea during sleep in infants. Possible relationship with sudden infant death syndrome. Science 190:677, 1975
23. Vyas H, Milner AD, Hopkin IE: Relationship between apnea and bradycardia in preterm infants. Acta Pediatr Scand 70:785, 1981
24. van Someren V, Stothers JK: A critical dissection of obstructive apnea in the human infant. Pediatrics 71:721, 1983
25. Hering E, Breuer J: Die selbsteurung der athmung durch den nervus vagus. Sitzberg Akad Wiss wien 57 (II):672, 1868
26. Widdicombe JG: Receptors in the trachea and bronchi of the cat. J Physiol (Lond) 123:71, 1954
27. Martin RJ, Okken A, Katona PG et al: Effect of lung volume on expiratory time in the newborn infant. J Appl Physiol 45:18, 1978
28. Bodegard G, Schweiler GH, Skoglund S et al: Acta Pediatr Scand 58:567, 1969
29. Head H: On the regulation of respiration. J Physiol (Lond) 10:179, 1889
30. Cross KW, Klaus M, Tooley WH et al: The response of the new-born baby to inflation of the lungs. J Physiol (Lond) 151:551, 1960
31. Knill R, Bryan AC: An intercostal-phrenic inhibitory reflex in human infants. J Appl Physiol 40:352, 1976
32. Hagan R, Bryan AC, Bryan MH et al: Neonatal chest wall afferents and regulation of respiration. J Appl Physiol 42:362, 1977
33. Cross KW, Hooper JMD, Oppe TE: The effect of inhalation of carbon dioxide in air on the respiration of the full-term and premature infant. J Physiol (Lond) 122:264, 1953
34. Avery ME, Chernick V, Dutton RE et al: Ventilatory response to inspired carbon dioxide in infants and adults. J Apply Physiol 18:895, 1963
35. Frantz ID, Adler SM, Thach BT et al: Maturational effects on respiratory responses to carbon dioxide in premature infants. J Appl Physiol 41:41, 1976
36. Haddad GG, Lestner HL, Epstein RA et al: CO_2 induced changes in ventilation and ventilatory pattern in normal sleeping infants. J Appl Physiol 48:684, 1980
37. Rigatto H, Brady JP, de la Torre Verduzco R: Chemoreceptor reflexes in preterm infants. II. The effect of gestational and postnatal age on the ventilatory response to inhaled carbon dioxide. Pediatrics 55:614, 1975
38. Krauss AN, Klain DB, Waldman S et al: Ventilatory response to carbon dioxide in newborn infants. Pediatr Res 9:46, 1975
39. Cross KW, Warner P: The effect of inhalation of high and low oxygen concentrations on the respiration of the newborn infant. J Physiol (Lond) 114:283, 1951

40. Cross KW, Oppe TE: The effect of inhalation of high and low concentrations of oxygen on the respiration of the premature infant. J Physiol (Lond) 117:38, 1952
41. Rigatto H, Brady JP, de la Torre Verduzco R: Chemoreceptor reflexes in preterm infants. I. The effect of gestational and postnatal age on the ventilatory response to inhalation of 100% and 15% oxygen. Pediatrics 55:604, 1975
42. Brady JP, Ceruti E: Chemoreceptor reflexes in the newborn infant: Effects of varying degrees of hypoxia on heart rate and ventilation in a warm environment. J Physiol (Lond) 184:631, 1966
43. Rigatto H, Brady JP: Periodic breathing and apnea in preterm infants. II. Hypoxia as a primary event. Pediatrics 50:219, 1972
44. Rigatto H, de la Torre Verduzco R, Cates DB: Effects of O_2 on the ventilatory response to CO_2 in preterm infants. J Appl Physiol 39:896, 1975
45. Purves MJ: Respiratory and circulatory effects of breathing 100% oxygen in the newborn lamb before and after denervation of the carotid chemoreceptors. J Physiol (Lond) 185:42, 1966
46. Bradley GW, von Euler C, Marttila J, Roos B: A model of the central and reflex inhibition in the cat. Biol Cybernetics 19:105, 1975
47. von Euler C, Trippenbach T: Excitability changes of the inspiratory "off-switch" mechanism tested by electrical stimulation in nucleus parabrachialis in the cat. Acta Physiol Scand 97:75, 1976
48. Cohen MJ: Neurogenesis of respiratory rhythm in the mammal. Physiol Rev 54:91, 1979
49. Bowes G, Adamson TM, Ritchie BC et al: Development of respiratory activity in unanesthetized fetal sheep in utero. J Appl Physiol 50:693, 1981
50. Maloney JE, Bowes G, Wilkinson M: Fetal breathing and the development of patterns of respiration before birth. Sleep 3:299, 1980
51. Chernick V, Havlicek V, Pagtakhan RD, Skelenovsky A: Respiratory response to electrical stimulation of the brain stem of fetal and neonatal sheep. Pediatr Res 7:20, 1973
52. Patrick JK, Campbell K, Carmichael L et al: A definition of human fetal apnea and the distribution of apneic intervals during the last 10 weeks of pregnancy. Am J Obstet Gynec 56:24, 1980
53. Changeux JP, Danchin A: Selective stabilization of developing synapses as mechanism for the specification of neuronal networks. Nature 264:705, 1976
54. Henderson-Smart DJ, Pettigrew AG, Campbell DJ: Clinical apnea and brain stem neural function in preterm infants. N Engl J Med 308:353, 1983
55. Hathorn MKS: Analysis of periodic changes in ventilation in newborn infants. J Physiol (Lond) 285:85, 1978
56. Waggener TB, Frantz ID, Stark AR et al: Oscillatory breathing patterns leading to apneic spells in infants. J Appl Physiol 52:1288, 1982
57. Bayon A, Shoemaker DJ, Bloom FE et al: Perinatal development of the endorphin- and enkephalin-containing systems in the rat brain. Brain Res 179:93, 1979
58. Nahai Y, Nahao K, Oki S et al: Presence of immunoreactive β-lipotropin and β-endorphin in human placenta. Life Sci 23:2013, 1978
59. Wardlaw SL, Stark R, Barc L et al: Plasma β-endorphin and β-lipotropin in human fetus at delivery: Correlation with arterial pH and PO_2. J Clin Endocrin Metab 49:888, 1979
60. Hedner T, Hedner G, Bergman B et al: Transient apnea after the enkephalin analog in the preterm rabbit. Biol Neonate 39:290, 1981

61. Moss JR, Scarpelli EM: Generation and regulation of fetal breathing in utero: Fetal CO_2 response test. J Appl Physiol 47:527, 1979
62. Chernick V, Mandansky DL, Lawson EJ: Naloxone decreases the duration of primary apnea with neonatal asphyxia. Pediatr Res 14:357, 1980
63. Jansen AH, Chernick V: Development of respiratory control. Physiol Rev 63:437, 1983
64. Phillipson EA: Control of breathing during sleep. Am Rev Resp Dis 118:909, 1978
65. Parmelee AH, Stern E: Development of states in infants. p. 199. In Clemente CD (ed): Sleep and the Maturing Nervous System. Academic Press, New York, 1972
66. Hoppenbrouwers T, Hodgman JE, Harper RM: Polygraphic studies of normal infants during the first six months of life. III. Incidence of apnea and periodic breathing. Pediatrics 60;418, 1977
67. Finer WW, Abroms IF, Taeusch HW: Ventilation and sleep states in newborn infants. J Pediatr 89:100, 1976
68. Hathorn MKS: The rate and depth of breathing in newborn infants in different sleep states. J Physiol (Lond) 243:101, 1974
69. Martin RJ, Herrell N, Pultusker M: Transcutaneous measurement of carbon dioxide tension: Effect of sleep state in term infants. Pediatrics 67:622, 1981
70. Davi M, Sankaran K, MacCallum M et al: Effect of sleep state on chest wall distortion and on the ventilatory response to CO_2 in neonates. Pediatr Res 13:982, 1979
71. Stothers JK, Warner RM: Oxygen consumption and neonatal sleep states. J Physiol (Lond) 278:435, 1978
72. Martin RJ, Okken A, and Rubin D: Arterial oxygen tension during active and quiet sleep in the normal neonate. J Pediatr 94:271, 1979
73. Curzi-Dascalova L: Thoracicoabdominal respiratory correlations in infants: Constancy and variability in different sleep states. Early Hum Dev 2:25, 1978
74. Henderson-Smart DJ, Read DJC: Reduced lung volume during behavioral active sleep in the newborn. J Appl Physiol 46:1081, 1979
75. Bryan MH: The work of breathing during sleep in newborns. Am Rev Respir Dis 119:137, 1979
76. Muller N, Gulston G, Cade D et al: Diaphragmatic muscle fatigue in the newborn. J Appl Physiol 46:688, 1979
77. Wilson SL, Thach BT, Brouillette RT et al: Upper airway patency in the human infant: Influence of airway pressure and posture. J Appl Physiol 48:500, 1980
78. Carlo WA, Martin RJ, Abboud EF et al: Effect of sleep state and hypercapnia on alae nasi and diaphragm EMGs in preterm infants. J Appl Physiol 54:1590, 1983
79. Carlo WA, Martin RJ, Bruce EN et al: Alae nasi activation (nasal flaring) decreases nasal resistance in preterm infants. Pediatrics 72:338, 1983
80. Bryan MH, Hagan R, Gulston G et al: CO_2 response and sleep state in infants. (Abstract) Clin Res 24:689, 1976
81. Anderson JV, Martin RJ, Abboud EF et al: Transient ventilatory response to CO_2 as a function of sleep state in full-term infants. J Appl Physiol 54:1482, 1983
82. Rigatto H, Kalapesi Z, Leahy FN et al: Ventilatory response to 100% and 15% O_2 during wakefulness and sleep in preterm infants. Early Hum Dev 7:1, 1982
83. Kattwinkel J, Nearman HS, Fanaroff AA et al: Apnea of prematurity 86:588, 1975
84. Korner AF, Kraemer HC, Haffner ME et al: Effects of waterbed flotation on premature infants: A pilot study. Pediatrics 56:361, 1975
85. Korner AF, Guilleminault C, Van den Hoed J et al: Reduction of sleep apnea and

bradycardia in preterm infants on oscillating waterbeds: A controlled polygraphic study. Pediatrics 61:528, 1978

86. Jones RAK: A controlled trial of regularly cycled oscillating waterbed and a non-oscillating waterbed in the prevention of aponea in the preterm infant. Arch Dis Child 56:889, 1981
87. Speidel BD, Dunn PM: Use of nasal continuous positive airway pressure to treat severe recurrent apnoea in very preterm infants. Lancet 2:658, 1976
88. Martin RJ, Nearman HS, Katona PG et al: The effect of a low continuous positive airway pressure on the reflex control of respiration in the preterm infants. J Pediatr 90:976, 1977
89. Durand M, McCann E, Brady JP: Effect of continuous positive airway pressure on the ventilatory response to CO_2 in preterm infants. Pediatrics 71:634, 1983
90. Sullivan CE, Issa FG, Berthon-Jones M et al: Reversal of obstructive sleep apnea by continuous positive airway pressure applied through the nares. Lancet 1:862, 1981
91. Mathew OP, Abu-Osba YK, Thach BT: Influence of upper airway pressure changes on genioglossus muscle respiratory activity. J Appl Physiol 52:438, 1982
92. Kuzemko JA, Paala J: Apnoeic attacks in the newborn treated with aminophylline. Arch Dis Child 48:404, 1973
93. Shannon DC, Gotay F, Stein IM et al: Prevention of apnea and bradycardia in low birthweight infants. Pediatrics 55:589, 1975
94. Uauy R, Shapiro DL, Smith B et al: Treatment of severe apnea in prematures with orally administered theophylline. Pediatrics 55:595, 1975
95. Roberts JL, Mathew OP, Thach BT: The efficacy of theophylline in premature infants with mixed and obstructive apnea and apnea associated with pulmonary and neurologic disease. J Pediatr 100:968, 1982
96. Kelly DH, Shannon DC: Treatment of apnea and excessive periodic breathing in the full-term infants. Pediatrics 68:183, 1981
97. Hunt CE, Brouillette RT, Hanson D et al: Home pneumograms in normal infants. (Abstract) Am Rev Respir Dis 127:214, 1983
98. Aranda JV, Turmen T: Methylxanthines in apnea of prematurity. Clin Perinatol 6:87, 1979
99. Davi MJ, Sankaran K, Simons KJ et al: Physiologic changes induced by theophylline in the treatment of apnea in preterm infants. J Pediatr 92:91, 1978
100. Gerhardt T, McCarthy J, Bancalari E: Aminophylline therapy for idiopathic apnea in premature infants: Effects on lung function. Pediatrics 62:801, 1978
101. Trippenbach T, Zinman R, Milic-Emili J: Caffeine effect on breathing pattern and vagal reflexes in newborn rabbits. Respir Physiol 40:211, 1980
102. LeMessurier DH: The site of action of caffeine as a respiratory stimulant. J Pharmac Exp Ther 57:458, 1936
103. Eldridge FL, Millhorn DE, Waldrop TG et al: Mechanism of respiratory effects of methylxanthines. Respir Physiol 53:239, 1983

9 Clinical Spectrum of the Sleep Apnea Syndrome

Martin A. Cohn
Marvin A. Sackner

This chapter deals with signs and symptoms of repetitive upper airway obstruction during sleep, a syndrome denoted as obstructive sleep apnea (OSA). The presentations of patients who develop clinical sequelae of inadequate respiratory center drive during sleep (i.e., central apneas and hypoventilation as primary and secondary events) will also be described. The widespread nature of the complaints in such patients and the involvement of multiple organ systems make these syndromes relevant to physicians of diverse specialties. They are not immediately apparent and unless appropriate questions are directed to the patient or bedpartner, diagnostic decision-making procedures will not be ordered. It is important during the taking of the medical history to gather information on sleep-related complaints since many patients with abnormal nocturnal respiration develop their symptoms over many years and may not volunteer such information because they consider their condition to be "normal."

NORMAL BREATHING DURING SLEEP

The control of breathing differs in sleep from wakefulness.[1] Most studies agree that tidal volume is reduced.[2] Bulow,[3] using a noseclip and mouthpiece pneumotachographic system, found that airflow decreased from wakefulness to non-rapid eye movement (NREM) sleep. Duron[4] could not confirm these findings but stressed the difficulty in obtaining true waking measurements in man. Newer noninvasive techniques such as respiratory inductive plethysmography[5,6] permit such measurements without the effects of the mouthpiece-noseclip spirometric or pneumotachographic measurement systems that affect the natural breathing pattern.[7] Using respiratory inductive plethysmography, studies in children[8] and adults[9] demonstrate that respiratory center drive, as reflected by minute ventilation and mean inspiratory flow, is reduced in NREM sleep but similar to wakefulness in rapid eye movement (REM) sleep. Birchfield[10] demonstrated corresponding blood gas changes (small increases in arterial carbon dioxide and decreases in oxygen tension) in NREM sleep. In REM sleep, there is increased variability of tidal volume such that consistent alterations of arterial blood gases are not regularly demonstrated.

In addition to changes in the overall control of breathing, the breathing pattern during sleep in normal subjects may show a few episodes of marked irregularities with central apneas, crescendo-decrescendo tidal volumes (Cheyne-Stokes respiration), and upper airway obstruction. Predisposition to these events is found in males of all ages,[11] postmenopausal women,[12] obese persons,[13,14] and older persons.[15] Although sleep related respiratory disturbances may occur in asymptomatic normals, these are not "healthy events" especially if accompanied by hypoxia and sleep arousals because of the potential for progression and development of secondary symptoms. This situation may be analogous to a slightly elevated fasting blood sugar in an asymptomatic person who may or may not go on to develop complications of diabetes. Medical advice for an asymptomatic diabetic would include attempts to alter those factors that affect blood sugar, including weight reduction and reduced carbohydrate intake in combination with proper exercise and careful follow-up. In a similar way, it may be prudent for an asymptomatic person with nocturnal hypoxemic episodes to alter the contributing factors through weight reduction if obese, avoidance of central nervous system (CNS) depressants (alcohol, tranquilizers, and hypnotics),[16] utilization of nasal decongestants for nasal obstruction should it be present, and avoidance by mechanical means of the supine position during sleep if the events only occur in this posture.

OBSTRUCTIVE SLEEP APNEA SYNDROME

This entity was first described by Gastaut et al.[17] in 1965 in the French literature and in 1972 by Walsh et al.[18] in the American literature. Both groups recognized the role of intermittent upper airway obstruction during sleep as the factor responsible for periodic hypoxia and poor quality sleep. The Pickwickian syndrome,[19] which was described in 1956, may in retrospect, be a subtype of the OSA syndrome associated with congestive heart failure. The

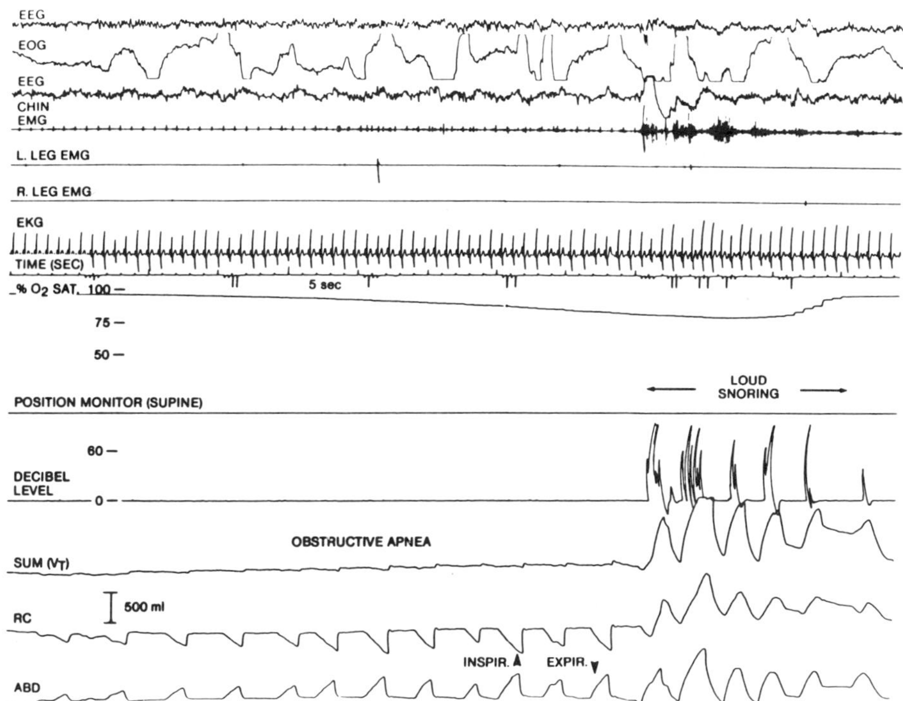

Fig. 9-1 Typical polysomnogram of a 50-year-old obese man with loud nocturnal snoring and excessive daytime sleepiness. Respiration was recorded using respiratory inductive plethysmography (Respitrace). There is absent tidal volume [sum (V_T)] despite persistent paradoxic rib cage and abdominal compartment movements with progressive oxygen desaturation during this REM-sleep-related obstructive apnea. This event is terminated by (1) a sleep arousal as indicated by the altered electroencephalogram, (2) several deep breaths with no paradoxic motion of the rib cage to abdominal compartment, (3) loud snoring sounds greater than 60 decibels in the room as measured with a sound level meter, and (4) improvement of arterial oxygen saturation.

importance of intermittent upper airway obstruction as the basis for this syndrome was not recognized in the original reports.

The diagnosis of OSA syndrome is confirmed with polysomnography. At a minimum, this involves the recording of the electroencephalogram, arterial oxygen saturation, and a measure of breathing pattern. Paradoxic movements of the rib cage and abdominal compartments with little or no deflection of the sum of the two along with a falling arterial oxygen saturation are diagnostic (Fig. 9-1). In about 15 percent of patients with OSA syndrome, little or no respiratory movements of the rib cage and abdominal compartments are detected. Here intrapleural pressure, as reflected by intraesophageal pressure or movement of the suprasternal fossa utilizing surface inductive plethysmography is the standard for respiratory effort.[6] Without these measurements, re-

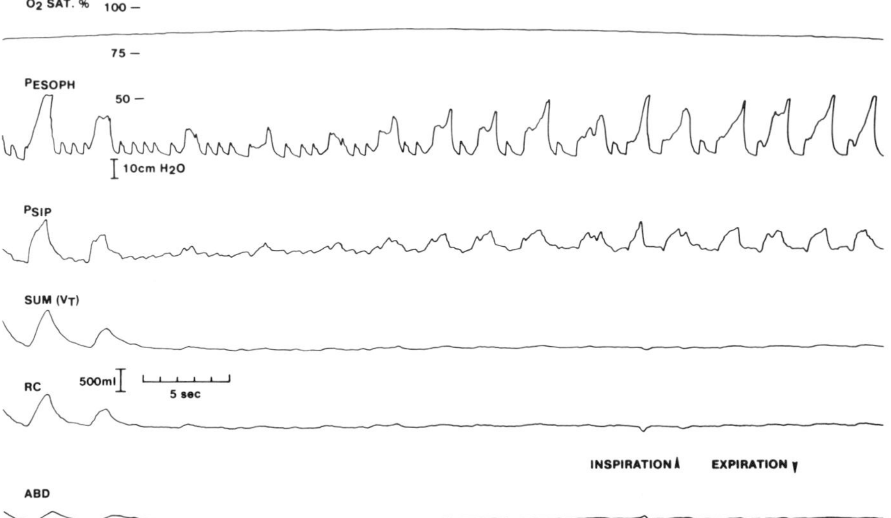

Fig. 9-2 Obstructive sleep apnea. Almost imperceptible movements are seen on sum (V_T), rib cage (RC), and abdominal (ABD) tracings. In this recording, it would be difficult to diagnose obstructive apnea with high degree of confidence but the surface inductive plethysmographic (P_{SIP}) tracing of suprasternal fossa movement clearly indicates regular respiratory efforts during obstruction. Validity of P_{SIP} as qualitative intrapleural pressure indicator can be seen from simultaneous recording of esophageal pressure (P_{ESOPH}). Difference in excursions between these two recordings relates to the fact that P_{SIP} is not calibrated but is displayed as qualitative signal. O_2 SAT% indicates arterial oxygen saturation.

cordings may be falsely diagnosed as central rather than obstructive apneas (Fig. 9-2).

Excessive Daytime Sleepiness

Excessive daytime sleepiness (Table 9-1) refers both to inescapable, inappropriate attacks of sleepiness as well as subtle forms of sleepiness that require the clinician to pose specific questions to the patient or bedpartner. The excessive daytime sleepiness results from the chronic nighttime sleep deprivation due to frequent arousals and/or failure to reach deeper stages of sleep.

Table 9-1. Excessive Daytime Sleepiness

Difficulty achieving full arousal on awakening
Decreased cognitive and motor function
Unavoidable naps—"sleep attack"
Automatic behavior
Fatigue
Depression

Often the patient denies or is unaware of such symptoms, which may be obvious to family members or close friends. Inappropriate daytime sleepiness may be life threatening if it occurs while driving an automobile or operating machinery. Frequent automobile accidents are common in patients with severe OSA syndrome. Patients who have OSA syndrome often describe unusual and often painful methods to prevent attacks of sleepiness including pinching and slapping themselves, sticking pins in the skin, and applying electric shocks to the body.

Sleep attacks may occur while eating, during business negotiations, while conversing on the telephone, and even during sexual intercourse. Patients with OSA syndrome often require frequent daytime naps. Such naps are usually longer than an hour and not as refreshing as the short naps required by patients with narcolepsy, a feature which helps to differentiate the two disorders. Patients with OSA syndrome may complain of excessive fatigue and tiredness as a concomitant or exclusive features of OSA syndrome. Some OSA syndrome patients may not actually fall asleep during the day but require great mental efforts to function in the awake state. Often such patients are unable to completely arouse themselves for several hours upon awakening in the morning.

Automatic behavior without conscious awareness or recollection of having performed an activity may signify another form of daytime sleepiness. Such instances often occur while driving an automobile long distances or instructing a class. For example, patients may miss the correct exits from expressways or complete tasks at work without any recollection of performing them. A teacher or worker who is explaining a lesson or a task may realize that the explanation is nonsensical or that a feeling of being "spaced out" has developed.

Personality changes often occur from the nighttime sleep deprivation in these patients. They are often irritable and tense during the day. Their spouses or friends may recognize that they have become short-tempered. Mental depression, impaired intellectual capacity, and memory impairment may develop gradually and cause failure to hold a job. Successful treatment of OSA syndrome often improves mental depression, but a small fraction of patients become further depressed because removal of the sedating symptoms of OSA syndrome may bring out the inability to cope with ordinary waking mental tasks.

Snoring

The severity of snoring associated with obstructive sleep apnea can be extreme. Following prolonged airway obstruction with progressively increasing respiratory efforts, the patient suddenly arouses (as confirmed by electroencephalographic sleep staging) taking large breaths associated with rapid inspiratory flows often resulting in palatal vibration and extremely loud snoring (Fig. 9-1). The severity may be such that the bedpartner may find it necessary to go to sleep first to avoid hearing such sounds. Some bedpartners choose to sleep in a different room, a situation that may produce considerable interpersonal

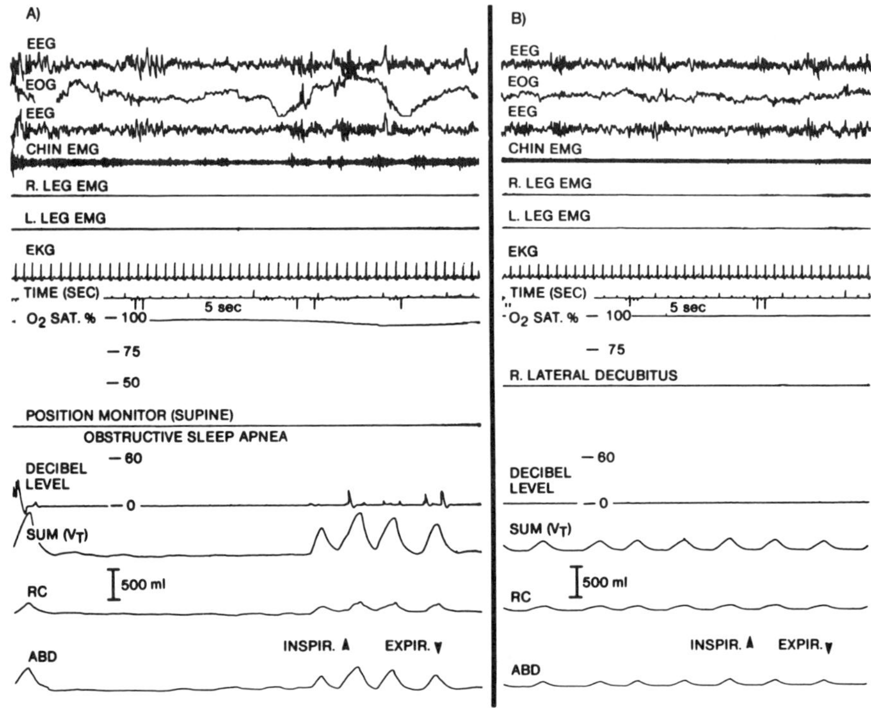

Fig. 9-3 The effect of body position on obstructive sleep apnea is shown on this polysomnogram. (A) While supine (modification of position monitor as described by Schmidt-Nowara: A head position monitor for polysomnography. Sleep 6:384, 1983) in stage 2 NREM sleep, note absent tidal volume [sum (V_T)] despite persistent respiratory effort (paradoxic rib cage and abdominal motion) with slight fall in oxygen saturation during the obstructive apnea episode. (B) However, normal respiration is observed later while patient is in the right lateral decubitus position and the same sleep stage. The obstructive apneas in this patient occurred exclusively in the supine position.

stress. When this occurs, any preexisting humorous attitude toward snoring disappears. The patient is usually unaware of snoring regardless of severity. Family members occasionally record the patient's snoring to prove its existence. Often snoring is increased in intensity and duration following ingestion of alcohol or other CNS depressants, when the patient is overfatigued, or when sleeping in the supine position (Fig. 9-3). The latter may occur as a result of the jaw falling open allowing the tongue to move posteriorly (Fig. 9-4). Snoring may occur during daytime sleep periods and prove a source of embarrassment especially if it occurs during sermons, conferences, or lectures. The patient may develop severe dryness in the mouth or throat during the night, need to sip water frequently during the night, or awaken with a dry mouth or sore throat.

The failure to elicit a history of snoring does not exclude the diagnosis of the OSA syndrome. Patients may terminate apneic periods with less dramatic

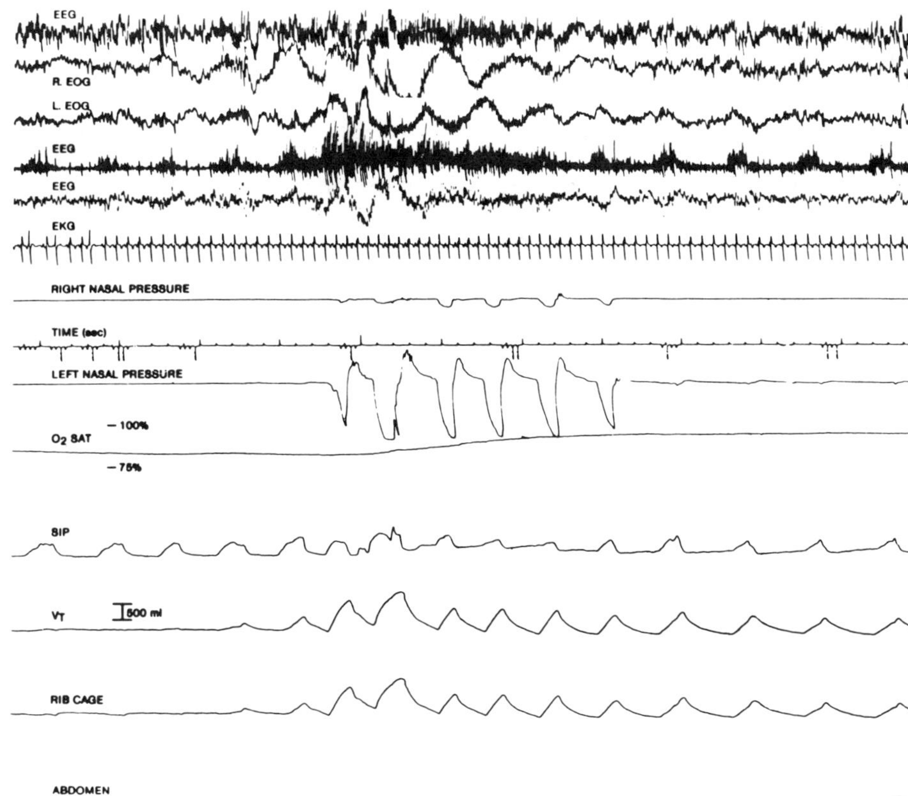

Fig. 9-4 Polysomnogram illustrating the relationship of the jaw to obstructive events. On video recording, the patient's mouth was open with jaw drooping during the obstructive apnea. However, mouth closure with nasal breathing was observed following the apnea. Note the obstructive apnea with absent tidal volume [sum (V_T)] and nasal pressure [(using modified nasal oxygen cannula) despite persistent respiratory effort (paradoxic rib cage and abdominal movements as well as intrapleural pressure swings via surface inductive plethysmography(SIP)]. With arousal and mouth closure, nasal breathing resumes (large nasal pressure swings) and oxygen saturation (O_2 SAT) rises. Toward the end of the record, nasal pressure falls toward zero as the patient breathes almost exclusively through the mouth.

clicking noises preceding the deep breaths. Patients with underlying diaphragmatic weakness secondary to neuromuscular disease or kyphoscoliosis may not generate sufficiently great inspiratory efforts to produce loud sounds. Snoring may occur only during the initial part of the first post-apnea breath. Conversely, loud nocturnal snoring may not be diagnostic of obstructive sleep apnea. Lugaresi[20] has shown that nocturnal snoring occurs in half the population over the age of 40 years. Although the prevalence of hypertension and cardiac disturbances is significantly greater in snorers than in nonsnorers in this age group, many snorers apparently suffer no ill effects.

Family members usually are not able to accurately and sufficiently describe important features of the snoring such as its intermittency and whether or not it is accompanied by chest or abdominal respiratory movements. In addition, loud snoring may occur during the first few breaths following a central apnea. Thus, a subjective description of snoring may be highly suggestive of obstructive sleep apnea but the diagnosis must be confirmed by clinical polysomnography.

Abnormal Motor Behavior During Sleep

The neuromuscular effort associated with arousal at the end of an obstructive apneic episode may be so great as to cause the patient to sit up with a sudden motion in bed. The abruptness of this shift of body posture may frighten the patient. More often, lesser movements of the arms or shift of body position terminates an apneic episode. Uncommon, more coordinated movements may occur. The patient may punch or kick the bedpartner during these events. After a prolonged obstructive apnea, the patient may sit up at the side of the bed or crawl to the floor and then sleep in this position the rest of the night.

Enuresis

Enuresis is more common in children with sleep apnea than adults. When this occurs, it probably results from incomplete arousal with a full bladder. Occasionally, it is seen in association with a cardiac arrhythmia (including asystole) with secondary bladder sphincter relaxation.

Morning Headaches

Patients may awaken with a dull generalized headache that gradually subsides over a few hours. This may be due to increased cerebral blood flow during sleep as a result of frequent apneas and associated hypercapnias.

Hypertension

Systemic and pulmonary arterial hypertension have been shown to accompany repetitive hypoxemic apneic episodes.[21] Sustained systemic hypertension may occur that is refractory to usual antihypertensive medications. Following successful treatment of OSA syndrome, patients may become normotensive or be more responsive to dietary control and drugs.

Cor Pulmonale

Sustained pulmonary hypertension may produce right ventricular failure and its sequelae including severe peripheral edema. In those patients with cor pulmonale, immediately following the establishment of upper airway patency during sleep with surgery or endotracheal intubation, massive diuresis occurs.

Effect of Body Weight

The typical patient with OSA syndrome is usually a middle aged man with gradual or accelerated weight gain associated with an increase in neck collar size. This may be accompanied by description of uncontrollable appetite and increases of food intake with a decrease in physical exertion. However, OSA syndrome may be present in children and adults of normal body weight.

HIGH RISK GROUPS

Obese Adults

Nocturnal hypoxemia related to upper airway obstruction, alveolar hypoventilation, and breathing at low lung volume occur in the overweight OSA syndrome patient.[14] Nocturnal hypoxemia is often greater than that which can be ascribed to hypoventilation alone and is thought to be related to breathing at low lung volume such that the end-expiratory lung volume is below the closing capacity of lung. Thus, closure of small airways of the dependent zone of the lung is present. Since perfusion of this zone still takes place, intrapulmonary right to left shunting of blood causes hypoxemia. Breathing at low lung volume relates to reduced diaphragmatic and other respiratory muscle efficiency in the supine position and/or the relaxation of skeletal muscle tone, which is especially prominent in REM sleep. Those obese patients with alveolar hypoventilation and chronic hypercapnia during the waking state may be at greater risk during sleep due to blunted responses of the respiratory center to carbon dioxide.

The physician treating obesity must consider symptoms and signs of nocturnal breathing abnormalities as part of an overall evaluation. If such events are suspected, a polysomnogram should be performed to identify the type and severity of events so that corrective measures can be planned. Without specific treatment of hypoxemia and the disturbed sleep, weight loss through dietary modification and augmentation of physical activity may not be readily achieved.

Children

Enlargement of tonsils and adenoids are predisposing factors to obstructive sleep apnea and all its features including pulmonary hypertension and cor pulmonale.[22–24] As in adults, other contributing factors include cranial facial deformities (mid-facial hyperplasia and micrognathia), chronic nasal congestion, nasal obstruction and allergies, and obesity. Parents may describe typical loud snoring in a child who may appear to be restless while sleeping or assume unusual sleep positions. The child may be difficult to arouse in the morning and be disoriented, confused, and irritable. Excessive sleepiness may be manifested by falling asleep in class or lapses of attention that often produce a reprimand from the teacher. Enuresis may be causally related to the breathing events and disappear after treatment. Sleep deprivation may also produce developmental delays and impaired intellectual functioning. Children may show mood and personality abnormalities such as being "flat" or emotionless. Indeed, Sir William Osler[25] in 1895 used the term "aprosexia" (slow to respond) to describe mouth-breathing children who did poorly in school and recommended removal of the tonsils and adenoids as a cure.

Old Age

Sleep-related breathing disorders are commonly observed in the elderly. In one series of asymptomatic volunteers over age 60, frequent central sleep apneas often occurred.[26] In another series of insomniac patients over age 60, obstructive apneas were common.[15] The prevalence of habitual snoring increases with age and may reflect an age related decrease in time of activation of upper airway pharyngeal dilator muscles.[20] Hypoxemia attendant with intermittent upper airway obstruction may then contribute to deterioration of brain function and other changes ascribed to senility.[27]

Patients with Pulmonary Disease

Severe nocturnal oxygen desaturation with or without sleep apneas may be associated with chronic obstructive lung disease,[28–32] cystic fibrosis,[33] asthma,[34,35] kyphoscoliosis,[36–38] and diaphragmatic paralysis.[39] Hypoxia may occur exclusively during REM sleep as a result of the decrease of end expiratory lung volume with closure of small airways with attendant right to left intrapulmonary shunting of blood. Hypoxemia is exacerbated if hypopneas or apneas due to upper airway obstruction take place.

Clinical clues that raise the suspicion of nocturnal hypoxemia include insomnia, erythrocytosis, and cor pulmonale. Polysomnography may be necessary to identify the events leading to hypoxia when it is not apparent during wakefulness. Further, polysomnography is useful in ascertaining the proper amount of supplemental oxygen to prescribe. Supplemental nocturnal oxygen can usually be given without fear of worsening the hypercapnia[30,40] but may prolong duration of upper airway obstruction by delaying hypoxic arousal response leading to cardiac disturbances.[41] Polysomnography can be carried out to assure the safety and proper dosing of nocturnal oxygen in patients with pulmonary disease.

Patients with Upper Airway Disease

Obstructive sleep apnea has been reported in "mouth breathers" associated with nasal obstruction due to allergies,[42] postoperative nasal packing,[43] nasal polyps, enlarged adenoid tissue, and nasal septal deviation.[44] Nasal obstruction augments the inspiratory collapsing forces in the pharynx and enhances the potential for obstructive sleep apneas. With unilateral nasal obstruction as in septal deviation, body position is crucial. If the patient assumes a posture such that the unobstructed nostril is placed in the dependent lateral position,[45] the nasal mucosa of this nostril becomes congested and bilateral nasal obstruction occurs. In this circumstance, upper airway obstruction develops since adults are preferential nasal breathers. These patients respond to control of body position during sleep by mechanical means or surgical correction of nasal obstruction.

The decision to remove enlarged tonsils or adenoids in children with repeated bouts of upper respiratory tract infections can often be made on clinical grounds. However, in children with borderline enlargement of these tissues who may have loud nocturnal breathing sounds or symptoms suggestive of obstructive sleep apnea, polysomnography helps to decide if surgery is indicated.[23]

Snoring is common after the age of 40 and may be the major clue to the presence of obstructive sleep apnea. When snoring is loud enough to disturb family members, it is likely to be associated with significant upper airway obstruction. Therefore, polysomnography is recommended to evaluate the severity of the obstruction and associated hypoxemia and cardiac arrhythmias. Uvulopalatopharyngoplasty[46,47] is a recently described corrective operation with morbidity similar to tonsillectomy. It is highly effective in diminishing snoring and in many patients eliminates the obstructive events.[48] In some patients, snoring is improved but apneas persist. Thus, follow-up polysomnography is important to establish the effectiveness of this treatment. Uvulopalatopharyngoplasty should not be performed without an evaluation for the presence and severity of obstructive sleep apnea. Tracheotomy is a curative procedure to eliminate the upper airway obstruction but carries significant morbidity. A new surgical approach currently undergoing evaluation is splitting of the hyoid bone.[49]

Patients with facial deformities such as acquired micrognathia[50] and Treacher-Collins syndrome[51] may develop obstructive sleep apnea. Cephalometric assessment[52] and appropriate surgery such as mandibular advancement[53] eliminate upper airway obstruction by improving the anatomical relationships.

Patients with Heart Disease

In addition to congestive heart failure and cor pulmonale, patients with obstructive sleep apnea may present with other cardiac symptoms such as sleep-related angina and palpitations. Ambulatory electrocardigraphic recordings may reveal nocturnal arrhythmias[54] including apnea related bradytachycardia, various degrees of heart block,[55] and ventricular tachycardia.[56] Such sleep-related events dictate further evaluation for sleep apnea including polysomnography since treatment of the apneas may eliminate need for antiarrhythmic drugs or pacemaker implantation.

Patients with Neurologic Disease

The differential diagnosis of hypersomnolence includes obstructive sleep apnea, narcolepsy, depression, drug abuse, nocturnal myoclonus (repetitive leg jerks), and other neurologic diseases.[57] The naps of patients with narcolepsy are typically shorter in duration and often more refreshing than the naps in obstructive sleep apnea.[58] Appropriate evaluation for mental depression along with a thorough drug history is also important. All night polysomnography is necessary to evaluate the quality of sleep, and the degree of sleep disturbance by sleep apneas or nocturnal myoclonus. The electroencephalogram should be examined for shortened REM latency, which supports the diagnosis of depression[59] or rapid onset into stage REM sleep, which is observed almost exclusively in narcolepsy.[60]

Obstructive sleep apnea has been reported with other neurological diseases including postpoliomyelitis,[61] Shy-Drager syndrome,[62] muscular dystrophy,[39] cerebral infarct,[63] brain stem infarct,[64] and syringobulbiamyelia.[65]

Patients with Endocrinologic Disorders

Endocrine function may play a role in predisposition to upper airway obstruction during sleep. OSA syndrome may occur in patients with acromegaly who have enlarged tongues and soft tissues of the upper airway.[66] In myxedema OSA syndrome is common; both macroglossia and blunted response of the respiratory center to carbon dioxide have been suggested to contribute to the upper airway obstruction.[67]

The male predominance of obstructive sleep apnea has prompted speculation regarding the modulating role of male and female hormones in this disorder.[11] Postmenopausal women with evidence of disordered nocturnal breathing are not protected by administration of female hormone[68] yet others have suggested that medroxyprogesterone may be an effective treatment in obstructive sleep apnea.[69] Conversely, upper airway obstruction may be induced by testosterone administration.[70]

Miscellaneous Diseases

In addition to the diseases described above, obstructive sleep apnea has been reported to contribute to the morbidity of sickle cell disease,[71] the development of pectus excavatum,[72] paranoid psychosis,[73,74] endocardial fibroelastosis,[75] and pulmonary hypertension in Down's syndrome.[76,77] In addition, obstructive sleep apnea has been reported as a complication of lymphocytic lymphoma,[78] irradiation-induced fibrosis of the neck,[79] the mucopolysaccharidosis of Scheie's symptom,[80] and western equine encephalitis.[81]

REFERENCES

1. Phillipson EA: Respiratory adaptations in sleep. Ann Rev Physiol 40:133, 1978
2. Magnussen G: Studies on the respiratory during sleep. H.K. Lewis, London 1944
3. Bulow K: Respiration and wakefulness in man. Acta Physiol Scand 59 (Suppl. 209):1, 1963
4. Duron B: La fonction respiratoire pendant le commeil physiologique. Bull Physiolpath Respir 8:1031, 1972
5. Cohn M, Rao ASV, Broudy M et al: The respiratory inductive plethysmograph: A new noninvasive monitor of respiration. Bull Eur Physiopathol Respir 18:643, 1982
6. Tobin MJ, Cohn MA, Sackner MA: Breathing abnormalities during sleep. Arch Intern Med 143:1221, 1983
7. Gilbert R, Auchincloss JH, Brodsky J, Boden W: Changes in tidal volume, frequency, and ventilation induced by their measurement. J Appl Physiol 133:252, 1972
8. Tabachnik E, Muller NL, Bryan AC, Levison H: Changes in ventilation and chest wall mechanics during sleep in normal adolescents. J Appl Physiol 51:557, 1981
9. Cohn MA: Pattern of breathing during sleep in insomniac adults. Sleep Res, 12:232, 1983
10. Birchfield RI, Sieker HO, Heyman A: Alterations in blood gases during natural sleep and narcolepsy. Neurology 8:107, 1959
11. Block AJ, Boysen PG, Wynne JW, Hunt LA: Sleep apnea, hypopnea and oxygen desaturation in normal subjects. N Engl J Med 300:513, 1979
12. Block AJ, Wynne JW, Boysen PG: Sleep-disordered breathing and nocturnal oxygen desaturation in postmenopausal women. Am J Med 69:75, 1980
13. Orr WC, Martin RJ, Imes NK et al: Hypersomnolent and nonhypersomnolent patients with upper airway obstruction during sleep. Chest 75:418, 1979
14. Harman E, Wynne JW, Block AJ, Malloy-Fisher L: Sleep-disordered breathing and oxygen desaturation in obese patients. Chest 79:256, 1981
15. Ancoli-Israel S, Kripke DF, Mason W, Messin S: Sleep apnea and nocturnal myoclonus in a senior population. Sleep 4:349, 1981
16. Scrima L, Broudy M, Nay KN, Cohn MA: Increased severity of obstructive sleep apnea after bedtime alcohol ingestion: Diagnostic potential and proposed mechanism of action. Sleep 5:318, 1982
17. Gastaut H, Tassinair C, Duron B: Etude polygraphique des manifestations episodiques (hypniques et respiratoires) diurnes et nocturnes du syndrome de Pickwick. Rev Neurol 112:573, 1965
18. Walsh RE, Michaelson ED, Harklerood LE et al: Upper airway obstruction in obese patients with sleep disturbance and somnolence. Ann Intern Med 76:185, 1972
19. Burwell CS, Robin ED, Whaley RD et al: Extreme obesity associated with alveolar hypoventilation: A Pickwickian syndrome. Am J Med 21:811, 1956
20. Lugaresi E, Coccagna G, Cirignotta F: Snoring and its clinical implications. p. 13. In Guilleminault C, Dement WC (eds): Sleep Apnea Syndromes. Alan R. Liss, New York, 1978
21. Tilkian AG, Guilleminault C, Schroeder JS et al: Hemodynamics in sleep-induced apnea: Studies during wakefulness and sleep. Ann Intern Med 85:714, 1976
22. Loughlin GM: Obstructive sleep apnea in older children. J Respir Dis 3:10, 1982

23. Eliaschar I, Lavie P, Halperin E et al: Sleep apneic episodes as indications for adenotonsillectomy. Arch Otolaryngol 106:492, 1980
24. Guilleminault C, Eldridge FL, Simmons FB, Dement WC: Sleep apnea in eight children. Pediatrics 58:23, 1976
25. Osler W: Principles and Practice of Medicine. D. Appleton and Co., New York, 1895
26. Carskadon MA, Dement WC: Respiration during sleep in the aged human. J Gerontol 4:420, 1981
27. Smallwood RG, Vitiello MV, Giblin EC, Prinz PN: Sleep apnea: Relationship to age, sex, and Alzheimer's dementia. Sleep 6:16, 1983
28. Flick MR, Block AJ: Continuous in vivo monitoring of arterial oxygenation in chronic obstructive lung disease. Ann Intern Med 86:725, 1977
29. Wynne JW, Block AJ, Hemenway J et al: Disordered breathing and oxygen desaturation during sleep in patients with chronic obstructive lung disease (COLD). Am J Med 66:573, 1979
30. Kearley R, Wynne JW, Block AJ et al: The effect of low flow oxygen on sleep-disordered breathing and oxygen desaturation. Chest 78:682, 1980
31. Calverley PMA, Brezinova V, Douglas NJ et al: The effect of oxygenation on sleep quality in chronic bronchitis and emphysema. Am Rev Respir Dis 126:206, 1982
32. Fleetham J, West P, Mezon B et al: Sleep, arousals, and oxygen desaturation in chronic obstructive pulmonary disease. Am Rev Respir Dis 126:429, 1982
33. Muller NL, Francis PW, Gurwitz D et al: Mechanism of hemoglobin desaturation during rapid-eye-movement sleep in normal subjects and in patients with cystic fibrosis. Am Rev Respir Dis 121:463, 1980
34. Barnes P, Fitzgerald G, Brown M, Dollery C: Nocturnal asthma and changes in circulating epinephrine, histamine, and cortisol. N Engl J Med 303:263, 1980
35. Montplaisir J, Walsh J, Malo JL: Nocturnal asthma: Features of attacks, sleep and breathing patterns. Am Rev Respir Dis 125:18, 1982
36. Guilleminault C, Kurland G, Winkle R, Miles LE: Severe kyphoscoliosis, breathing, and sleep. Chest 79:626, 1981
37. Mezon BL, West P, Israels J, Kryger M: Sleep breathing abnormalities in kyphoscoliosis. Am Rev Respir Dis 122:617, 1980
38. Hoeppner VH, Cockcroft DW, Dosman JA, Cotton DJ: Nighttime ventilation improves respiratory failure in secondary kyphoscoliosis. Am Rev Respir Dis 129:240, 1984
39. Skatrud J, Iber C, McHugh W et al: Determinants of hypoventilation during wakefulness and sleep in diaphragmatic paralysis. Am Rev Respir Dis 121:587, 1980
40. Nocturnal Oxygen Therapy Trial Group: Continuous or nocturnal oxygen therapy in hypoxemic chronic obstructive lung disease. A clinical trial. Ann Intern Med 93:391, 1980
41. Guilleminault C, Cummiskey J, Motta J: Chronic obstructive airflow disease and sleep studies. Am Rev Respir Dis 122:397, 1980
42. Lavie P, Gertner R, Zomer J, Podoshin L: Breathing disorders in sleep associated with "microarousals" in patients with allergic rhinitis. Acta Otolaryngol 92:529, 1981
43. Taasan V, Wynne JW, Cassisi N, Block JA: The effect of nasal packing on sleep-disordered breathing and nocturnal oxygen desaturation. Laryngoscope XCI:1163, 1981

44. Heimer D, Scharf SM, Lieberman A, Lavie P: Sleep apnea syndrome treated by repair of deviated nasal septum. Chest 84:184, 1983
45. Hasegawa M: Nasal cycle and postural variations in nasal resistance. Ann Otol Rhinol Laryngol 91:112, 1982
46. Fujita S, Conway W, Zorick F et al: Surgical correction of anatomic abnormalities in obstructive sleep apnea syndrome: Uvulo-palato-pharyngoplasty. Otolaryngol Head Neck Surg 39:923, 1981
47. Hernandez SF: Palatopharyngoplasty for the obstructive sleep apnea syndrome: Technique and preliminary report of results in ten patients. Am J Otolaryngol 3:229, 1982
48. Cohn MA, Hernandez S, Foster AC et al: Uvulo-palato-pharyngoplasty (UPP) in obstructive sleep apnea: Clinical evaluation in 92 consecutive patients. Chest 84:336, 1982
49. Kaya N: Sectioning the hyoid bone as a therapeutic approach for obstructive sleep. Sleep 7:77, 1984
50. Coccagna G, di Donato G, Verucchi P et al: Hypersomnia with periodic apneas in acquired micrognathia. Arch Neurol 33:769, 1976
51. Roa NL, Moss KS: Treacher-Collins Syndrome with sleep apnea: Anesthetic considerations. Anesthesiology 60:71, 1984
52. Riley R, Guilleminault C, Herran J, Powell N: Cephalometric analyses and flow-volume loops in obstructive sleep apnea patients. Sleep 6:303, 1983
53. Kuo PC, West RA, Bloomquist DS, McNeil RW: The effect of madibular osteotomy in three patients with hypersomnia sleep apnea. Oral Surg 48:385, 1979
54. Guilleminault C, Connolly SJ, Winkle RA: Cardiac arrhythmia and conduction disturbances during sleep in 400 patients with sleep apnea syndrome. Am J Cardiol 52:490, 1983
55. Deedwania PC, Swiryn S, Dhingra RC, Rosen KM: Nocturnal atrioventricular block as a manifestation of sleep apnea syndrome. Chest 76:319, 1979
56. Imaizumi T: Arrhythmias in sleep. Am Heart J 100:513, 1980
57. Roffwarg HP: Diagnostic classification of sleep and arousal disorders. Sleep 2:1, 1979
58. Zarcone V: Narcolepsy. N Engl J Med 288:1156, 1973
59. Coble PA, Foster FG, Kupfer DJ: Electroencephalographic sleep diagnosis of primary depression. Arch Gen Psych 33:1124, 1976
60. Guilleminault C, Dement WC: 235 cases of excessive daytime sleepiness. J Neurol Sci 31:13, 1977
61. Hill R, Robbins AW, Messing R, Arora N: Sleep apnea syndrome after poliomyelitis. Am Rev Respir Dis 127:129, 1983
62. Chokroverty S, Sharp JT, Barron KD: Periodic respiration in erect posture in Shy-Drager Syndrome. J Neurol Neurosurg Psych 41:980, 1978
63. Power WR, Mosko SS, Sassin JF: Sleep-stage-dependent Cheyne-Stokes respiration after cerebral infarct: A case study. Neurology 32:763, 1982
64. Levin BE, Margolis G: Acute failure of automatic respirations secondary to a unilateral brain stem infarct. Ann Neurol 1:583, 1977
65. Haponik EF, Givens D, Angelo J: Syringobulbia-myelia with obstructive sleep apnea. Neurology 33:1046, 1983
66. Perks WH, Horrocks PM, Cooper RA et al: Sleep apnoea in acromegaly. Br Med J 280:894, 1980

67. Orr WC, Males JL, Imes NK: Myxedema and obstructive sleep apnea. Am J Med 70:1061, 1981
68. Block AJ, Wynne JW, Boysen PG et al: Menopause, medroxyprogesterone and breathing during sleep. Am J Med 70:506, 1981
69. Strohl KP, Hensley MJ, Saunders NA et al: Progesterone administration and progressive sleep apneas. JAMA 245:1230, 1981
70. Sandblom RE, Matsumoto AM, Schoene RB et al: Obstructive sleep apnea syndrome induced by testosterone administration. N Engl J Med 308:508, 1983
71. Scharf MB, Lobel JS, Caldwell E: Nocturnal oxygen desaturation in patients with sickle cell anemia. JAMA 249:1753, 1983
72. Olsen KD, Kern EB, O'Connell EJ: Pectus excavatum: Resolution after surgical removal of upper airway obstruction. Laryngoscope XC:832, 1980
73. Martin PR, Lefebvre AM: Surgical treatment of sleep-apnea-associated psychosis. Can Med Assoc J 124:978, 1981
74. Berrettini WH: Paranoid psychosis and sleep apnea syndrome. Am J Psychiatry 137:493, 1980
75. Suzuki M: Pickwickian syndrome and endocardial fibroelastosis. Am J Med 53:123, 1972
76. Loughlin G, Wynne J, Victorica B, Cassisi N: Intermittent upper airway obstruction during sleep causing accelerated pulmonary hypertension in Down's Syndrome. Chest 78:529, 1980
77. Clark RW, Schmidt HS, Schuller DE: Sleep-induced ventilatory dysfunction in Down's Syndrome. Arch Intern Med 140:45, 1980
78. Zorick F, Roth T, Kramer M, Flessa H: Exacerbation of upper airway sleep apnea by lymphocytic lymphoma. Chest 77:689, 1981
79. Polnitsky CA, Sherter CB, Sugar JO: Irradiation-induced fibrosis of the neck and sleep apnea. Arch Otolaryngol 107:629, 1981
80. Perks WH, Cooper RA, Bradbury S et al: Sleep apnoea in Scheie's syndrome. Thorax 35:85, 1980
81. White DP, Miller F, Erickson RW: Sleep apnea and nocturnal hypoventilation after Western Equine Encephalitis. Am Rev Respir Dis 127:132, 1983

10 Therapy of Sleep Apnea Syndromes

Teodoro V. Santiago
Marie C. Trontell

As is evident in earlier discussions, the pathogenesis of sleep-disordered breathing has not been fully elucidated. In certain cases where a clear-cut underlying etiology is present (e.g., hypothyroidism) therapy directed against the underlying etiology will be effective in resolving the sleep-related respiratory irregularities. However, therapy of most cases of sleep-disordered breathing continues to remain difficult since mechanisms of their genesis remain obscure. Nonetheless, important and impressive advances have been made in the past few years and a better understanding of these disorders has evolved. In this chapter, therapy will be divided into general measures that are recommended for the management of all cases of sleep-disordered breathing and specific measures that are recommended for particular disorders.

GENERAL MEASURES

Weight Loss for Obese Patients

The increased frequency of sleep-disordered breathing and nocturnal oxygen desaturation in obese patients has been well documented.[1] These abnormalities included a higher incidence of both apneas and hypopneas when compared to nonobese, sex and age-matched subjects. Symptomatic sleep apnea is also frequently associated with obesity. Weight reduction is therefore strongly recommended for the obese patient with sleep-disordered breathing.

Surprisingly there are only a few studies that have examined the effects of weight reduction on the incidence of sleep-related breathing abnormalities. One study reported that a small number of patients with sleep apnea continued to have significant episodes of obstructive apnea after moderate weight loss.[2] However, several studies have noted improvement in nocturnal oxygenation,[3] resolution of upper airway obstruction and of daytime hypersomnolence.[4,5] While it appears clear that there is some controversy regarding the effect of weight reduction on the incidence of upper airway obstruction during sleep, there is general agreement that nocturnal oxygenation improves after weight loss, perhaps to a great degree, secondary to an increase in awake arterial oxygen tensions. The latter would allow a greater reduction in PO_2 before significant arterial oxygen desaturation is induced by respiratory irregularities during sleep.

Oxygen Inhalation

It has been suggested that the use of supplemental oxygen in patients with sleep apnea may be deleterious since oxygen may prolong the apneas by preventing arousal, thus potentiating the associated cardiovascular risks of arrhythmias and decreased myocardial contractility.[6] However, there is evidence indicating that hypoxia is a poor arousal stimulant[7] and hypoxemia remains a significant source of morbidity in these patients because it may induce bradycardia, pulmonary hypertension and cor pulmonale. The ease of inducing hypoxemia in sleep apnea is supported by data in healthy subjects demonstrating that a period of apnea that increases alveolar PCO_2 by less than 12 mmHg will decrease alveolar PO_2 by 50 mmHg. This is presumably because of the low respiratory exchange ratio that develops during apnea.[8] Martin et al.[9] followed five eucapnic patients with obstructive sleep apnea for 30 to 90 days while on low flow oxygen and reported an improvement (i.e., a decrease) both in total apnea time and in the degree of oxygen desaturation. These findings have been recently confirmed.[10] In addition, the apnea-associated bradycardia was prevented by oxygen, confirming an earlier report by Zwillich et al.[11] that this phenomenon is mediated by the carotid bodies. It is apparent from the above studies that the use of oxygen can be recommended in the management of sleep-disordered breathing including sleep apnea and would be especially helpful if additional steps are being taken to treat the underlying disorder.

Avoidance of Alcohol and Depressant Drugs

Previous studies have indicated that ingestion of alcohol increases the frequency and duration of apneic events during sleep in asymptomatic men[12] as well as in patients with sleep apnea.[13,14] Similar findings have been reported with sedative or hypnotic drugs such as flurazepam.[15] The exact mechanisms of action of these agents in inducing these effects are still unclear; however, evidence has been presented recently that they may do so by selectively depressing genioglossal muscle activity.[16,17] Strict proscription of alcohol and sedative drugs in patients with sleep apnea as well as asymptomatic snorers is therefore strongly recommended.

SPECIFIC MEASURES

Obstructive Sleep Apnea

The pathogenesis of obstructive sleep apnea has remained obscure. There are several existing theories of its generation, however, and several approaches to therapy have evolved based, at least in part, on these theories.

Mechanical Narrowing of the Upper Airway. Mechanical narrowing of the upper airway accompanied by the normal reduction of upper airway muscle tone during sleep was initially believed to be the main mechanism leading to obstructive sleep apnea. This theory accounts for the frequency of obesity in patients with this disorder as well as the development of sleep-disordered breathing in some patients with hypertrophied tonsils and/or adenoids. Careful examination of the upper airway should always be the first step in the management of obstructive sleep apnea. Two surgical approaches, tracheostomy and uvulopalatopharyngoplasty have been recommended as therapy, based at least in part on the above theory unless hypertrophied tonsils and/or adenoids are present. In the latter instance, tonsillectomy with or without adenoidectomy has resulted in dramatic improvement of symptoms and resolution of obstructive sleep apnea.[18,19]

Tracheostomy. Tracheostomy bypasses the site of upper airway obstruction during sleep, and therefore should be effective in obstructive sleep apnea, regardless of its pathogenesis. This procedure has been technically more difficult to perform in sleep apneic patients because they are frequently obese and have large but short necks. The procedure is poorly accepted by patients because of its interference with their day-to-day activities and carries its own morbidity.[20] Furthermore, it is difficult to wean a patient from a tracheostomy once performed, since plugging the tracheostomy site usually leads to reappearance of the apneas. At the present time, it is best to think of doing this procedure as a temporizing measure in very symptomatic patients or when no other form of therapy is successful in alleviating the sleep-disordered breathing.

Uvulopalatopharyngoplasty. Because of poor patient acceptance of tracheostomy, other surgical procedures on the upper airway have been introduced. One such procedure is uvulopalatopharyngoplasty (UPP). UPP consists of resection of excess or redundant tissue from the lateral pharynx along with the uvula, the entire posterior border of the soft palate and one-half of the anterior tonsillar pillar.[21] The goal is the removal of as much soft palate as possible without causing permanent nasal regurgitation. Despite impressive results that accompanied the initial report,[21] no systematic follow-up of patients treated with this procedure has been reported until recently.[22,23] In the first report, 14

Table 10-1. Effect of Nasal CPAP on Obstructive Sleep Apnea

	Without Nasal CPAP			With Nasal CPAP		
No. of patients	Apnea index	Lowest SaO_2(%)	Mean SaO_2 (%)	Apnea index	Lowest SaO_2 (%)	Mean SaO_2 (%)
12	43.2 ± 14.3	77.4 ± 11.1	86.4 ± 4.0	1.06 ± 1.0	93.2 ± 1.6	94.7 ± 1.3

patients were studied before and 8 weeks after the procedure. They reported that 12 of 14 patients had improvement of daytime hypersomnolence. However, no significant improvement in apnca and hypopnea index, longest apnea duration, or lowest O_2 saturation occurred. Significantly better nocturnal oxygenation resulted however and, if individual subjects are examined, 10 of the 14 showed a reduction in apnea and hypopnea index and 12 of 14 exhibited a reduction in total number of apneas. The second study[23] reported on 66 consecutive patients who underwent UPP and who were restudied a year later. Thirty-three of the 66 showed a reduction of apnea index by at least 50 percent 6 weeks after surgery and 20 of the 33 who were studied a year later showed persistence of the improvement. These data suggest that UPP may have a place in the management of obstructive sleep apnea, especially in those patients who fail to respond to nonsurgical therapy (see below). These data also indicate that while anatomic factors are undoubtedly important in the genesis of obstructive sleep apnea, they are not the sole determinant of the generation of these respiratory irregularities.

Increased Suction Pressures. When mechanical narrowing of the upper airway requires increased suction pressures to maintain inspiratory airflow, the suction pressures per se may cause closure when upper airway muscle tone is reduced. In order to minimize excessive negative pressures in the airway that may promote or perpetuate upper airway occlusion during sleep, continuous positive airway pressure (CPAP) applied to the nose via a mask (i.e., nasal CPAP) was introduced by Sullivan et al. in 1981 and found to cause dramatic reversal of obstructive sleep apnea.[24] A similar experience in a majority of patients suffering from obstructive sleep apnea was reported by others.[25,26] Our experience with this device is just as favorable (Table 10-1) in terms of improvement of apnea index, oxygen saturation, and sleep quality. Some patients cannot tolerate (i.e., sleep with) the device although they are in the minority. Those who tolerate nasal CPAP adapt quite well to chronic usage at home. The obvious advantage of nasal CPAP is that it represents the only form of therapy that can be evaluated directly as part of the diagnostic sleep study, thus assuring a careful selection of responding patients. This form of therapy also appears to be remarkably free of side effects despite theoretical disadvantages of CPAP such as impedance of expiration or reduction of cardiac output and renal function. Use of the lowest effective pressures would help avoid the development of these problems. Nasal CPAP in patients showing a beneficial response must be considered the initial therapy of choice for moderate-to-severe obstructive sleep apnea.

Normal Airway Geometry with Loss of Muscle Tone. Normal airway geometry with excessive loss of muscle tone during sleep leading to airway narrowing and obstruction has prompted the search for selective stimulants of upper airway muscles, especially the genioglossus. Although no such selective agent has been found, a drug, protriptyline, which has been used effectively in the treatment of obstructive sleep apnea may work, at least in part, by this mechanism. Protriptyline is a nonsedating, tricyclic antidepressant drug that was found to reduce daytime hypersomnolence initially in the narcolepsy-cataplexy syndrome[27] and later in obstructive sleep apnea.[28] Other studies[29,30] have since confirmed the drug's efficacy in reducing hypersomnolence and improving oxygenation in obstructive sleep apnea. In reporting the drug's efficacy, both groups of investigators noted that the percentage of rapid eye movement (REM) sleep declined in their subjects after administration of protriptyline. Since REM-sleep-associated apneas were usually associated with greater oxygen desaturation, they speculated that the drug may act by changing the patient's sleep profile to one with less REM sleep. However, recent reports in animals indicate that protriptyline may selectively stimulate the upper airway muscles.[31] This action, if exhibited during sleep, would of course help prevent upper airway occlusion. At the present time, it is unclear what the exact mechanism of action of the drug is in obstructive sleep apnea.

Central Sleep Apnea

Central sleep apnea, which is characterized by generally periodic loss of rhythmic breathing movements, is encountered much less frequently than obstructive apnea. There are some reports, however, that suggest that it may be present but unrecognized much more frequently in the elderly.[32] The exact pathogenesis is also uncertain but is believed to involve either an unstable respiratory control mechanism similar to Cheyne-Stokes respiration[33] or an accentuation of changes in CO_2 chemoreception during sleep. The former mechanism would account for the frequent occurrence of central apneas in newcomers to high altitude while the latter would explain its occurrence in patients with impairment of CO_2 chemoreception, for example the obesity-hypoventilation (Pickwickian) syndrome.

Agents that have been found useful in central sleep apnea appear to act by enhancing CO_2 chemoreception and may produce their beneficial effects by minimizing respiratory oscillations during sleep. These agents include acetazolamide and medroxyprogesterone acetate. Acetazolamide has been used successfully to treat periodic breathing during sleep at high altitude.[34] White et al.[35] administered the drug to six patients with central sleep apnea (250 mg four times daily) and reported a 69 percent reduction in total apneas, improvement in sleep quality and decreased daytime hypersomnolence. Medroxyprogesterone acetate (Provera) was first proposed as treatment for the obesity-hypoventilation syndrome in 1968[36] and was successfully administered on an outpatient basis in this condition in 1975.[37] Patients with the obesity-hypoventilation syndrome frequently exhibit both obstructive and central apneas. The pathophysiologic hallmark of this condition is waking hypercapnia occurring on a background of normal or near normal lung function. Conditions such as hypothyroidism and ingestion of depressant drugs must be excluded. In view of the efficacy of progesterone in the Pickwickian syndrome, hypercapnic patients with sleep apnea should have a trial of progesterone treatment before other therapeutic modalities are explored. It is important to note that the drug takes several days to manifest its effect.[38] There is some disagreement regarding the effectiveness of progesterone in sleep-disordered breathing[39,40] but it is very likely that these differences merely indicate that the drug's usefulness is limited to the sub-group of patients with sleep-disordered breathing secondary to the Pickwickian syndrome.

In summary, the specific therapy of sleep-disordered breathing has seen significant advances but, with a few exceptions, data are still lacking, especially with regards to long-term efficacy of therapy. At the present time, obstructive sleep apnea is best handled by first making sure that no obstructing lesion or abnormality is present in the upper airway. If this is ruled out, protriptyline (10 to 20 mg at bedtime) is recommended for the mild disorder (apnea index $<$15 events/hour). For the moderate and severe disorder, nasal CPAP should be tried if a second polygraphic study documents its effectiveness. If nasal CPAP is not tolerated or is ineffective in reducing the apneic events significantly, surgical procedures (uvulopalatopharyngoplasty or tracheostomy) are recommended. In the patient with central sleep apnea, acetazolamide is the recommended therapy. In the obese-hypercapnic (i.e., Pickwickian) patient with no underlying lung disease who is suffering from sleep-disordered breathing of whatever nature, progresterone should be initially tried because of its proven effectiveness in many patients with this disorder. If progesterone causes no improvement, therapy should be directed against the predominant sleep-related breathing abnormality.

REFERENCES

1. Harman EM, Wynne JW, Block AJ, Malloy-Fisher L: Sleep-disordered breathing and oxygen desaturation in obese patients. Chest 79:256, 1981
2. Guilleminault C, van den Hoed J, Mitler MM: Clinical overview of apnea syndromes. In Guilleminault C, Dement W (eds): Sleep apnea syndromes. Kroc Foundation Series. Vol II. Alan R. Liss, New York, 1978
3. Harman EM, Wynne JW, Block AJ: The effect of weight loss on sleep-disordered breathing and oxygen desaturation in morbidly obese men. Chest 82:291, 1982
4. Remmers JE, de Groot WJ, Sauerland EK: Neural and mechanical factors controlling pharyngeal occlusion during sleep. In Guilleminault C, Dement W (eds): Sleep apnea syndromes. Kroc Foundation Series. Vol II. Alan R. Liss, New York, 1978
5. Sharp JT, Barrocas M, Chokroverty S: The cardiorespiratory effects of obesity. Clin Chest Med 1:103, 1980

6. Motta J, Guilleminault C. Effects of oxygen administration in sleep-induced apneas. In Guilleminault C, Dement W (eds): Sleep apnea syndromes. Kroc Foundation Series. Vol II. Alan R. Liss, New York, 1978
7. Neubauer JA, Santiago TV, Edelman NH: Hypoxic arousal in intact and carotid chemodenervated sleeping cats. J Appl Physiol 51:1294, 1981
8. Otis AB, Rahn H, Fenn WO: Alveolar gas changes during breath holding. Am J Physiol 152:674, 1948
9. Martin RJ, Sanders MH, Gray BA, Pennock BE: Acute and long-term ventilatory effects of hyperoxia in the Adult Sleep Apnea Syndrome. Am Rev Respir Dis 125:175, 1982
10. Gold AR, Bleecker ER, Smith PL: A shift from central and mixed sleep apnea to obstructive sleep apnea resulting from low flow oxygen. Am Rev Respir Dis 132:220, 1985
11. Zwillich C, Devlin T, White D et al: Bradycardia during sleep apnea. J Clin Invest 69:1286, 1982
12. Taasan VC, Block AJ, Boysen PG, Wynne JW: Alcohol increases sleep apnea and oxygen desaturation in asymptomatic men. Am J Med 71:240, 1981
13. Issa FG, Sullivan CE: Alcohol, snoring and sleep apnoea. J Neurol Neurosurg Psychiat 45:353, 1982
14. Scrima L, Broudy M, Nay KN, Cohn MA: Increased severity of obstructive sleep apnea after bedtime alcohol ingestion: Diagnostic potential and proposed mechanism of action. Sleep 5:318, 1982
15. Dolly FR, Block AJ: Effect of flurazepam on sleep-disordered breathing and nocturnal oxygen desaturation in asymptomatic subjects. Am J Med 73:239, 1982
16. Krol RC, Knuth SL, Bartlett, Jr D: Selective reduction of genioglossal muscle activity by alcohol in normal human subjects. Am Rev Respir Dis 129:247, 1984
17. Leiter JC, Knuth SL, Krol RC, Bartlett, Jr D: The effect of diazepam on genioglossal muscle activity in normal human subjects. Am Rev Respir Dis 132:216, 1985
18. Orr WC, Martin RJ: Obstructive sleep apnea associated with tonsillar hypertrophy in adults. Arch Intern Med 141:990, 1981
19. Kravath RE, Pollak CP, Borowiecki B: Hypoventilation during sleep in children who have lymphoid airway obstruction treated by nasopharyngeal tube and T and A. Pediatrics 59:865, 1977
20. Conway WA, Victor LD, Magilligan, Jr DJ et al: Adverse effects of tracheostomy for sleep apnea. JAMA 246:347, 1981
21. Fujita S, Conway W, Zorick F, Roth T: Surgical correction of anatomic abnormalities in obstructive sleep apnea syndrome: Uvulopalatopharyngoplasty. Otolaryngol Head Neck Surg 89:923, 1981
22. Silvestri R, Guilleminault C, Simmons FB: Palatopharyngoplasty in the treatment of obstructive sleep apneic patients. p. 163. In Guilleminault C, Lugaresi E (eds): Sleep/wake disorders: Natural history, epidemiology and long-term evolution. Raven Press, New York; 1983
23. Conway W, Fujita S, Zorick F et al: Uvulopalatopharyngoplasty: One year followup. Chest 88:385, 1985
24. Sullivan CE, Issa FG, Berthon-Jones M, Eves L: Reversal of obstructive sleep apnoea by continuous positive airway pressure applied through the nares. Lancet 1:862, 1981
25. Rapoport D, Sorkin B, Garay SM, Goldring RM: Reversal of the "Pickwickian

syndrome" by long-term use of nocturnal nasal-airway pressure. N Engl J Med 307:931, 1982
26. Sanders MH: Nasal CPAP effect on patterns of sleep apnea. Chest 86:839, 1984
27. Schmidt HS, Clark RW, Hyman PR: Protriptyline: An effective agent in the treatment of the narcolepsy-cataplexy syndrome and hypersomnia. Am J Psychiat 134:183, 1977
28. Clark RW, Schmidt HS, Schaal SF: Sleep apnea: Treatment with protriptyline. Neurology (NY) 29:1287, 1975
29. Brownell LG, Perez-Padilla R, West P, Kryger MH: The role of protriptyline in obstructive sleep apnea. Bull Europ Physiopath Resp 19:621, 1983
30. Smith PL, Haponik EF, Allen RP, Bleecker ER: The effects of protriptyline in sleep-disordered breathing. Am Rev Respir Dis 127:8, 1983
31. Bonora M, St John WM, Bledsoe TA: Differential elevation by protriptyline and depression by diazepam of upper airway respiratory motor activity. Am Rev Respir Dis 131:41, 1985
32. Coleman RM, Miles LE, Guilleminault C et al: Sleep-wake disorders in the elderly: A polysomnographic analysis. J Am Geriatr Soc 29:289, 1981
33. Cherniack NS: Respiratory dysrhythmias during sleep. N Engl J Med 305:325, 1981
34. Weil JV, Kryger MH, Scoggin CH: Sleep and breathing at high altitude. In Guilleminault C, Dement W (eds): Sleep apnea syndromes. Kroc Foundation Series. Vol II. Alan R. Liss, New York, 1978
35. White DP, Zwillich CW, Pickett CK et al: Central sleep apnea: Improvement with acetazolamide therapy. Arch Intern Med 142:1816, 1982
36. Lyons HA, Huang CT: Therapeutic use of progesterone in alveolar hypoventilation associated with obesity. Am J Med 44:881, 1968
37. Sutton FD, Zwillich CW, Creagh CE et al: Progesterone for outpatient treatment of Pickwickian syndrome. Ann Intern Med 83:476, 1975
38. Skatrud JB, Dempsey JD, Kaiser DG: Ventilatory response to medroxyprogesterone acetate in normal subjects: Time course and mechanism. J Appl Physiol 44:939, 1978
39. Hensley MJ, Saunders NA, Strohl KP: Medroxyprogesterone treatment of obstructive sleep apnea. Sleep 3:441, 1980
40. Orr WC, Imes NK, Martin RJ: Progesterone therapy in obese patients with sleep apnea. Arch Intern Med 139:109, 1979

11 Sleep and Breathing in Patients with Lung Disease

N. R. Anthonisen
Meir Kryger

RISK FACTORS COMMON TO PATIENTS WITH LUNG DISEASE

Previous chapters have reviewed in detail the respiratory physiology of sleep. When compared to wakefulness, physiological responses that tend to preserve arterial blood gas homeostasis are depressed during sleep, especially in rapid eye movement (REM) stage. We will consider the implications of these findings in patients with lung disease.

Ventilatory responses to hypoxia and hypercapnia are attenuated but not obliterated during sleep in normals.[1-3] Patients with severe lung disease often have very blunted chemical ventilatory responses while awake.[4] If the sleep state further attenuated these responses, then in such patients hypoxemic or hypercapnic episodes during sleep would tend to be more severe and prolonged than in normals. Arousing or awakening in response to a physiological stimulus is another potentially useful protective mechanism. For example, if hypoxemia were present in a patient whose hypoxic ventilatory response was obliterated by the sleep state, than awakening would restore the response to its awake level and arousal would lead to an increase in ventilation. Hypoxia, unfortunately, is an unreliable arousal stimulus in humans—arterial oxygen saturations on the order of 70 percent waken subjects only about half the time.[2,3,5] Thus,

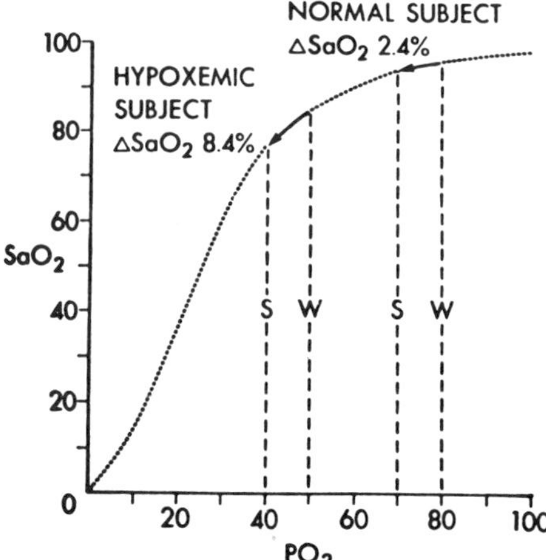

Fig. 11-1 Influence of initial arterial oxygen saturation upon changes in saturation with sleep. Shown is the blood oxygen dissociation curve plotting saturation (ordinate) against PO_2 (abscissa). The effects of a decrease in PO_2 of 10 mmHg going from wakefulness (w) to sleep (s) are much larger in terms of O_2 saturation in a subject with hypoxemia than in a subject without. (Kryger M: Abnormal control of breathing. p. 118. In Kryger MH (ed): Pathophysiology of Respiration. John Wiley and Sons, New York, 1981.)

hypoxic patients may be left without protective arousal or a ventilatory response.

Other normal physiological changes consequent to sleep may be disadvantageous to patients with lung disease. Arousal in response to airway irritation, may be impaired in sleeping patients as it is in experimental animals.[6] Airway resistance increases during sleep in lung disease patients and there are suggestions that during sleep compensatory increases in breathing efforts may be decreased.[7] The sleep state causes a loss of tone of the muscles surrounding the upper airway so that it becomes lax and prone to collapse. This mechanism may contribute to obstructive sleep apnea in patients with lung disease.[8] Finally, mucociliary clearance and the cough reflex may also be impaired.

The breathing pattern may change during sleep in normals, with periods of irregular breathing and reduction in tidal volume. Such patterns do not meet the criteria of Cheynes-Stokes respiration and some investigators use the term hypopnea to describe them. Apneas also occur in normals, but less frequently than irregular breathing. In addition, particularly in REM sleep, discoordination of the respiratory muscles may occur with abolition of intercostal and accessory muscle activity.[9,10] Loss of intercostal accessory muscle activity increases the amount of effort or work that the one remaining inspiratory muscle, the diaphragm, must achieve in order to attain a given level of ventilation. Further, loss of inspiratory muscle activity may produce a decrease in functional residual capacity (FRC), which in turn predisposes the subject to airway closure and hypoxemia.

Probably because of decreases in the chemical drive to breathe, normals hypoventiliate during sleep. This does not result in a significant decrease in arterial O_2 saturation because in normals at sea level, the arterial PO_2 is 80 to 100 mmHg, and substantial decreases in arterial PO_2 are not associated with large decreases in oxygen saturation. In patients with lower arterial PO_2 during wakefulness, hypoventilation can lead to substantial decreases in arterial O_2

saturation. When waking arterial $PO_2 < 60$ mmHg, further decreases of PO_2 are associated with major decreases of oxygen saturation, because in this range of PO_2 the slope of the oxyhemoglobin disassociation curve is relatively steep (Fig. 11-1). Thus, a normal degree of sleep hypoventilation will cause distinct sleep hypoxemia in subjects who have some daytime hypoxemia.

In summary, lung disease patients become hypoxemic during sleep because they have the same kind of sleep-induced abnormalities in the breathing pattern and control as do normals; but they are at increased risk because (1) they are on a steep portion of the oxyhemoglobin dissociation curve and (2) because respiratory drive that may be abnormally reduced during wakefulness are probably further attenuated by the sleep state. This permits hypoxemia to persist.

HYPOXEMIA IN CHRONIC OBSTRUCTIVE PULMONARY DISEASE

Extent of Hypoxemia

Hypoxemia during sleep in chronic obstructive pulmonary disease (COPD) has been documented in a large number of reports. In the earlier reports, hypoxemia was confirmed by intermittent measurement of arterial blood gases,[11,12] and more recently by the continuous measurement of oxygen saturation using ear oximetry.[13,14] Although the spot arterial blood gas measurements gave valuable "snapshots" of oxygenation in sleep, it was not until continuous measurements were made that the dynamic changes of saturation could be appreciated. In spite of these methodologic differences, most studies have qualitatively similar findings: when COPD patients sleep, arterial oxygen saturation falls from awake levels, and saturation is uniformly lowest in REM.[11,15]

Severe sleep hypoxemia in COPD is episodic. The number of episodes reported in various studies differs because of differences in patient selection and how episodes were defined. When hypoxemia episodes are defined as being more than 1 minute duration (i.e., sustained) and the drop in saturation exceeds 10 percent, it was found that patients with severe daytime hypoxemia had a mean of three to four such episodes per night, while those with less had an average of about one such episode per night.[14] In a large group of patients with a mean awake supine saturation of 84.6 ± 1.6 (SEM), 25 percent of sleep time was spent below a saturation of 80 percent, 13 percent of sleep below 75 percent; 5 percent of sleep time below 70 percent and 2 percent sleep time below 65 percent.[16] Thus these patients may spend a great deal of time desaturated. Patients may also have short hypoxemic dips. These are often only 20 to 30 seconds long; their incidence is not clear.

Three reports have found significant relationships between awake oxygenation and the worst oxygenation of the night. In one,[16] describing 24 hypoxemic patients (mean awake saturation 84.6 percent) the average minimum

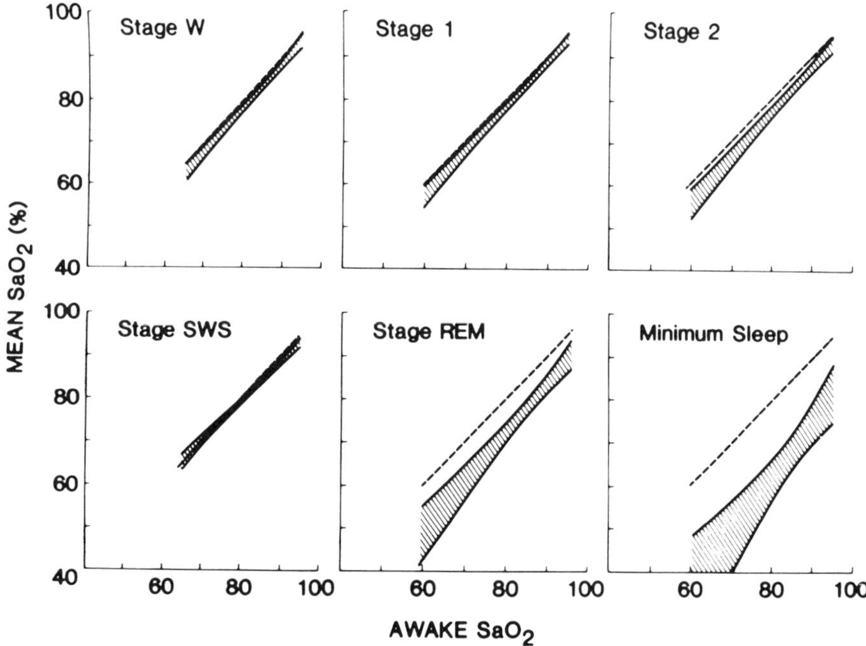

Fig. 11-2 Correlation of waking with nocturnal hypoxemia in patients with COPD. Abscissae: waking arterial oxygen saturation. Ordinates: sleep arterial oxygen saturation. Each panel represents data gathered during a specific sleep stage except for the lower right that shows the minimum value attained during sleep. Dashed lines are lines of identity and shaded areas enclose the 95 percent confidence limit for the results gathered (Fleetham J, West P, Mezon B et al: Sleep arousals and oxygen desaturation in chronic obstructive pulmonary disease. Am Rev Resp Dis 126:429, 1982.)

saturation was 17.5 percent less than the waking value (Fig. 11-2). Other studies[17–19] are in general agreement with the data of Figure 11-2. In one,[19] normals and a variety of patients with COPD were compared in terms of the maximum decrease of arterial PO_2 that was obtained from direct blood samples. A decrease of arterial PO_2 of approximately 24 mmHg was observed in all groups but this decrease was associated with a large decrease in arterial O_2 saturation in patients who were initially hypoxemic, a smaller fall in patients who were not and only a minor decrease in saturation in normals. Thus, the minimum saturation observed was very strongly related to oxygenation during wakefulness and was explicable on the basis of a similar decline in arterial PO_2 occurring in subjects with different values of the initial waking PO_2.

Though the degree of nocturnal hypoxemia is related to daytime oxygenation, there is substantial variability, especially when the maximum decrease in arterial O_2 saturation is considered. The maximal change in saturation—that is the size of the large decreases in O_2 saturation—appear to be related to CO_2, in that they are uncommon in patients without CO_2 retention,[20] or in those showing a vigorous ventilatory response to CO_2.[17] These results are congruent since CO_2 retention is associated with decreased CO_2 response in COPD, and suggest that CO_2 sensitivity may be an important protective mechanism against severe sleep hypoxemia in COPD.

Hypoxemia and Sleep Stage

More than 80 percent of hypoxemic episodes occur during REM sleep even though REM usually accounts for less than 20 percent of sleep time. Thus, it is not surprising that the mean arterial oxygen saturation in REM is much lower than it is in wakefulness or the other sleep stages. In a report based on spot blood gases in patients with a mean awake arterial PO_2 of 62 mmHg, arterial PO_2 was about 57 mmHg in non-rapid eye movement (NREM) sleep and about 50 mmHg in REM sleep.[12] These results were qualitatively quite similar to those obtained with continuous measurements of arterial oxygenation;[16] in more hypoxic patients with mean awake saturation of 84.6 percent the drop from awake in stage 1 was 1.7 percent, in stage 2, 3.1 percent, in slow-wave sleep (SWS) 1.4 percent and in REM stage 7.7 percent. In another report[21] that also documented the most severe hypoxemia in REM, hypoxemia in SWS was slightly more severe than in stages 1 and 2. The common thread of all these reports is that in patients with awake hypoxemia there occurs a small drop (in the range of about 1 to 4 percent) when the patient goes into NREM sleep, and a large drop in SaO_2 when the patient is in REM sleep.

Mechanisms Causing Sleep Hypoxemia in COPD

There are several areas of controversy concerning the mechanisms causing hypoxemia in COPD. We will try to deal with the two we believe are the most pertinent: (1) the relative contributions of hypoventilation and ventilation-perfusion mismatching, and (2) the importance of breathing pattern dysrhythmias.

There is no question that arterial PCO_2 increases during sleep in COPD. Pierce et al.[11] found that COPD patients had a 6.6 mmHg rise in PCO_2 with sleep, not different from normal subjects in a group of patients (mean forced expiratory volume (FEV_1) = 0.96 L) studied with spot blood gases. Koo et al.[12] reported the highest PCO_2 of the night was 8.3 ± 4.4 mmHg higher than during wakefulness. PCO_2 went up about 5 mmHg during NREM sleep and about another 5 mmHg during REM sleep. In a similar group of patients, Cocagna and Lugaresi[22] also found a 3 to 5 mmHg increase in arterial PCO_2 in NREM sleep and about a 8 mmHg increase REM. Catteral et al.[19] found only a 4.2 mmHg rise in PCO_2 in patients who were hypoxemic while awake. Though the increase in arterial PCO_2 was greater than normal in some studies of COPD patients, this was not always the case, and further measurements are needed before firm conclusions can be reached concerning degrees of hypoventilation in normals versus COPD patients.

All of the above studies showed a larger fall in arterial PO_2 than rise in arterial PCO_2. It has been suggested that this shows that the worsening gas exchange is due to worsening ventilation-perfusion matching; that is, the addition of units with low ventilation-perfusion ratios.[12] Such suggestions are based on assumptions that are probably not valid. In the steady state, that is when O_2 uptake, CO_2 output, ventilation, cardiac output, and gas concentrations in mixed venous blood and inspired gas are all constant, decreases in ventilation are associated with increases in arterial and alveolar PCO_2 that are nearly as large as the decreases in arterial PO_2. It is most unlikely, however, that all requirements for steady state analysis are met during the episodes of severe sleep hypoxemia to which this kind of analysis has been applied. Indeed, during nonsteady state decreases in ventilation, best exemplified by breath-holding, decreases in arterial PO_2 are much larger than associated increases in arterial PCO_2. Because the body stores of CO_2 are relatively large, a sudden decrease in ventilation produces a slow rise in arterial PCO_2 with an apparent decrease in CO_2 output that lasts minutes before a steady state is reestablished. Thus, episodes of hypoxemia without comparable CO_2 retention are as explicable on the basis of transient hypoventilation as they are on the basis of changes in the distribution of ventilation and perfusion within the lung, a point usefully emphasized by Catterall et al.[19]

Other workers have drawn inferences regarding the mechanism of sleep hypoxemia by measuring the rate of decline of arterial O_2 saturation. If the decline were faster during sleep than during breath-hold while awake, then the decline during sleep must have been related at least in part to mechanisms other than hypoventilation. This reasoning is correct if lung volumes, cardiac output, and alveolar and mixed venous gas tensions are the same in the two situations. These criteria have not been fulfilled in studies of COPD patients.

There are suggestions that distributions of ventilation and perfusion may change during sleep,[9,23] especially during REM stage when loss of intercostal and accessory muscle activity may result in decreased lung volumes. Decreases in lung volume are likely to be associated with airway closure, so that loss of intercostal-accessory muscle activity in REM sleep may well be associated with the development of units with little ventilation in relation to their perfusion.

In summary, there is evidence that hypoventilation contributes to sleep hypoxemia in COPD and this may be accentuated by changes in the distribution of ventilation and perfusion in the lung, but this has neither been proven nor excluded.

The types of breathing pattern dysrhythmias associated with hypoxemia have been a major source of controversy. The controversy stems from two factors—patient selection and imprecise terminology. Guilleminault et al.[24] found that 21 of 26 patients with chronic obstructive pulmonary disease demonstrated the sleep apnea syndrome as defined by more than five apneas per hour of sleep. The vast majority of abnormal respiratory events of the night were due to upper airway obstruction or occlusion during NREM sleep. This group of patients had been referred to a sleep disorders clinic because of suspected sleep apnea; 23 of 26 complained of excessive daytime sleepiness and weighed more than 90 kg. None of these patients had an FEV_1 of less than 1.0 L, and 11 had an FEV_1 of more than 2.5 L. It is likely that the obesity of the patients had a greater influence on their sleep quality than the very mild to moderate obstruction documented in most of them. The patients studied by Guilleminault et al.[24] probably were an atypical group: patients referred to exclude sleep apnea are likely to have sleep apnea, whether or not they have COPD, the degree of gross obesity reported is not common in COPD patients, and most other workers have studied patients with much more severe obstruction. Nevertheless, other investigators have noted obstruction of the upper airway in sleeping COPD patients. Douglas et al.[14] report this in one of their 10 patients with severe COPD. At least one of the patients reported by Wynne et al.[25] had episodes of obstructive apnea. One of the 10 patients reported by Arand[26] clearly had obstructive sleep apnea, while 3 had evidence of partial upper airway obstruction. These latter patients snored, demonstrated increased respiratory effort (swings in intrathoracic pressure) and changes in sleep state, arterial saturation, and heart rate that were similar to those seen in patients with obstructive sleep apnea. Episodes of desaturation were short and repetitive and were seen in all sleep stages. The fact that the episodes were in all sleep stages clearly separates this group of patients from most COPD patients, in whom prolonged severe desaturation occurs almost exclusively in REM stage.

It is not known whether the incidence of obstructive sleep apnea is increased in patients with COPD, but since both syndromes are common and largely occur in older men, their chance coincidence should be expected. Should this occur, the impact of the combined disorders on sleep quality might be greater than either alone. It is clear, however, that the severe nocturnal hypoxemia that occurs in some COPD patients is usually not attributable to obstructive sleep apnea.

Most investigators have noted changes in breathing pattern in COPD patients during REM associated hypoxemia. These changes, usually termed "hypopnea" most often involved a decrease in oronasal gas flow or chest wall motion, indicating a decrease in tidal volume. Unfortunately, some workers included the presence of hypoxemia in their definition of hypopnea. This definition biased their results toward an association between hypoxemia and changes in breathing pattern and further implies that because hypoxemia, here defined as decreases in arterial O_2 saturation, did not occur in normals, neither did hypopnea. It is clearly preferable, therefore, to define hypopnea solely in terms of changes in the volume and timing of ventilation. Quantitative measurements of ventilation during sleep are extremely difficult to make and are not available in a representative series of COPD patients. However, semiquantitative data are available in small numbers of patients who developed sleep hypoxemia.

Skatrud et al.[27] reported hypopnea in three patients who demonstrated one to four episodes/hour of REM. Though their definition of hypopnea included O_2 desaturation, they also found a substantial decrease in the fractional contribution of the rib cage to tidal volume. The rib cage contribution was 48 percent while awake and fell to 34 percent and 19 percent respectively during the tonic and phasic manifestations of REM. These changes probably reflect loss of tone of intercostal and accessory respiratory muscles as part of the general loss of muscle tone in REM. Arand et al.[26] found that the prolonged oxygen desaturation in REM sleep in COPD was related to decreased respiratory effort, quantified by reduced swings in intrathoracic pressure measurements. Catterall et al.[19] who defined hypopnea as a 50 percent reduction in rib cage motion for more than 10 seconds, found that hypopnea was repetitive over a period of several minutes and occurred primarily in REM sleep. About 75 percent of all the hypoxemic episodes occurred during hypopnea; in the remainder, breathing pattern remained regular. Since this group was examining rib cage motion alone, it is possible that abnormalities in abdominal motion may have been associated with the unexplained hypoxemic episodes. The results of Catteral et al.[19] are consistent with the finding of reduced rib cage contribution in REM by Skatrud et al.[27] A potentially important contribution by the former group was the finding that the incidence of abnormal breathing patterns in COPD was not different from the incidence in healthy subjects. These results were quite similar to those reported in chronic mountain sickness patients,[28] of whom 25 percent had a detectable breathing pattern abnormality as compared to 22.6 percent in controls. Yet only the chronic mountain sickness patients had severe O_2 desaturation in sleep. Thus some patients become hypoxemic when they develop the normal breathing pattern dysrhythmias of sleep.

In summary, COPD patients develop normal irregularities in the breathing pattern during sleep. If, before sleep, they are hypoxemic so that arterial PO_2 lies on a steep part of the oxyhemoglobin dissocilation curve, these irregularities will result in decreases in arterial O_2 saturation. Because chemical drives to breath are blunted by the lung disease and further by the sleep state, the hypoxemia persists. Such patients become hypoxemic primarily in REM when breathing pattern abnormalities are most common. In a minority of COPD patients, the above explanation is inadequate and the hypoxemia may be due to obstruction that may represent simple snoring in a patient who is already hypoxemic. In these patients, decreases in O_2 saturation are short, frequent, and occur in all sleep stages. Hypoxemic episodes occasionally are not associated with breathing pattern abnormalities. The importance of changes in the distribution of ventilation and perfusion in contribution to hypoxemia are unclear at present.

COMPLICATIONS AND SEQUELA OF SLEEP HYPOXEMIA IN COPD

Sleep Quality

There is no single series comparing sleep quality in well selected COPD patients with that in similarly instrumented age and sex-matched normals. Therefore, comparisons of sleep quality must be made among data acquired by different laboratories under somewhat different conditions, and results of such comparisons must be regarded as provisional. Nevertheless, available data indicate that in patients with severe COPD sleep quality is abnormal.

Time spent actually sleeping is reduced in COPD patients being only 4 to 5 hours per night; about one-third of the night in bed is spent awake. The distribution of sleep stages expressed as a fraction of actual sleep time appears to be not statistically different from normals.[16] This "nondifference" stems from the huge scatter of findings in the normal sleeping population. Larger, better controlled studies may find significant differences. When examining data from several centers, several findings are consistent. Very light sleep is increased, and REM sleep reduced. The patients have many arousals (about 10/hour) and therefore have a shortened duration of uninterrupted sleep episodes. There are also very frequent sleep stage changes—15 to 20/hour or about three times the normal rate. The cause of the disturbed sleep is not clear. Fleetham et al.[16] found that 40 percent of arousals occurred during decreases in arterial O_2 saturation. However, O_2 administration, though increasing oxygenation, did not improve sleep or change arousal frequency. Arousals were still associated with decreases in saturation, but these decreases were relatively minor so that arousals occurred at much higher levels of O_2 saturation. These results suggest that arousals were not caused by hypoxemia but were due to associated phenomena such as hypercapnia or acidemia. This is consistent with the recent finding that hypoxemia in humans is an unreliable arousal stimulus. In a group of patients with severe waking hypoxemia, Calverly et al.[21] showed that the greater the number of hypoxemic episodes, the less disturbed the sleep. In this study, an episode was defined as being more than a minute with at least 10 percent drop in arterial saturation; arousal frequency was not reported. These investigators suggested that unstable sleep may, in fact, have been protective, preventing prolonged episodes of hypoxemia. In the same report, O_2 therapy improved some measures of sleep quality in five of six very hypoxic patients, suggesting that hypoxemia may have disturbed their sleep in the first place. These results appear to contradict those of Fleetham et al.,[16] but may relate to the more severe hypoxemia exhibited by the patients of Calverly et al.[21] Sleep may differ with the degree of hypoxemia. In patients with moderate hypoxemia, the predominant arousal stimulus or factor disturbing sleep may be CO_2; arousal frequency would thus not decrease with O_2 therapy. On the other hand, in very hypoxic patients with CO_2 retention during wakefulness, hypoxemia may be an important arousal stimulus because it is very severe. Thus O_2 therapy might be expected in improve sleep quality.

There are other factors that are potentially important in disturbing sleep. In our experience, coughing is always associated with the electrophysiological features of arousal. Patients may nap in the daytime and not require as much nocturnal sleep. It is also possible that medications used to treat COPD, such as methylxanthines, may contribute to abnormal sleep.

Cardiac Complications

It is possible that the high incidence of sudden death in COPD patients is caused by cardiac arrhythmias or myocardial ischemia occurring during sleep. The incidence of cardiac arrhythmias is quite high having been reported to involve 30 to 100 percent of hypoxic COPD patients.[29,30] The differences in the various series reflect patient selection—in some series patients were not as stable as in others—and methods of data collection.

The most commonly reported arrhythmias are premature contractions of atrial, junctional and ventricular origin. Premature ventricular contractions were twice as common at night as during the daytime.[29] Episodes of ventricular tachycardia have also been noted. It is still unclear whether the ectopic activity occurs primarily during the hypoxemic dips or simply occurs at random in patients whose baseline arterial O_2 saturations are low. Some well oxygenated COPD patients may have premature ventricular contractions indicating perhaps that coincidental coronary artery disease in this elderly population contributes to the arrhythmias. Other contributors to arrhythmias could be the medications used in treatment (methylxanthines, beta-adrenergic agents) and the sleep state itself. It is not known whether arrhythmias are related to sleep stage in these patients.

In general, COPD patients have a rapid heart rate, which is inversely related to the arterial PO_2 and this tachycardia tends to be maintained during sleep. Sustained hypoxemia seems to play a role in the tachycardia since nocturnal O_2 therapy systematically reduces heart rate.[30] It is unclear whether heart rate in COPD is related to sleep stage per se or whether heart rate changes consistently with hypoxemic episodes. Arand et al.[26] reported a slight decrease in heart rate during desaturation in sleeping COPD patients including those without any evidence of upper airway obstruction. More data on the interrelationship of heart rate respiratory rate, arterial oxygenation and sleep stage are required.

Besides premature contractions, ECG evidence of myocardial ischemia has been observed in COPD patients, including S-T segment depression, lengthening of the Q-T interval, and development of partial right bundle branch block.[30] Again, these abnormalities were probably related to oxygen saturation level since O_2 therapy improved several of the ischemic markers. In general, severely hypoxemic patients had much more improvement with O_2 than did less hypoxemic ones. Thus, evidence suggests that sustained sleep hypoxemia has a deleterious effect on the myocardium and conducting system.

Pulmonary Hypertension

Alveolar hypoxia causes pulmonary vascular constriction and chronic hypoxia causes structural changes in pulmonary arteries that maintain pulmonary hypertension. Hypoxemia during sleep is associated with increased pulmonary artery pressure.[22,30] Since saturation may differ in the different sleep stages, being lowest in REM, it would be expected that pulmonary artery pressure would be highest during REM. This was shown by Coccagna and Lugaresi.[22] In their series, pulmonary artery pressure rose on the average by 1.29 mmHg for each 1 percent drop in arterial saturation, a value quite similar to that reported by Boysen et al.[30] Pulmonary artery pressure may also increase in response to changes in arterial PCO_2 and pH. The transient changes in oxygen saturation and pulmonary artery pressure documented by Boysen et al.[30] were probably too short in duration—about 30 seconds—to have been accomplanied by significant elevations in PCO_2. In addition, Coccagna and Lugaresi[22] reported that pulmonary artery pressure changes in specific sleep stages correlated with arterial PO_2 much better than with PCO_2 or pH. In further support of the primary importance of oxygenation in influencing pulmonary artery pressure, is the finding that O_2 therapy markedly reduced episodic pulmonary hypertension during sleep.

Although it has been suggested[31] that repetitive episodes of pulmonary hypertension during sleep may produce continuous pulmonary hypertension, there is no direct evidence for this in humans. It is thus not clear that abolishing episodic sleep hypoxemia will ameliorate or prevent pulmonary hypertension.

Chronic O_2 therapy may attenuate the pulmonary vascular response to hypoxia.[32] Patients taken off O_2 after 8 weeks of treatment showed degrees of sleep hypoxemia similar to those noted before therapy, but the associated increases in pulmonary artery pressure were smaller. These changes were not due to changes in cardiac output and are compatible with the hypothesis that O_2 therapy had caused regression of hypoxia associated increase in vascular smooth muscle that had rendered the pulmonary artery pressure very sensitive to further hypoxia.

Neuropsychiatric Impairment

Because the central nervous system (CNS) is very sensitive to oxygen lack, it would not be surprising if neuropsychiatric impairment resulted from the very severe nocturnal hypoxemia frequently observed in patients with COPD. There is, however, little clinical evidence to support this hypothesis, though there is ample evidence that patients with severe COPD demonstrate neuropsychiatric abnormalities and that the degree of impairment is inversely related to *waking* arterial oxygenation.[33] It may be that neuropsychiatric abnormalities are related more to sustained than to episodic hypoxemia, an hypothesis supported by the finding that they tended to improve more with continuous than with nocturnal O_2 therapy.[34]

Chronic hypoxemia and hypercapnia may be associated with EEG abnormalities, with a slowing of the dominant wave frequently similar to that observed with agents known to impair cerebral function. Similar abnormalities are common in patients with elevated hematocrits, another consequence of chronic hypoxemia. In hypoxemic COPD patients, acute O_2 administration does not reverse EEG abnormalities, but there is evidence that this does occur in patients on long term O_2 therapy.[35] Since the treatment was 15 to 20 hr/day, it is not clear whether the EEG effects were due to relief of daytime or nocturnal hypoxemia, or even whether they were related to an associated reduction in hematocrit.

With the exception of patients with coincident obstructive sleep apnea, daytime somnolence is not a prominent feature of stable COPD patients. It may be in COPD patients who are acutely ill, but these patients usually have iatrogenically induced sleep disorders.

TREATMENT OF SLEEP HYPOXEMIA IN COPD

Oxygen Therapy

It is clear that sleep hypoxemia in COPD can be prevented by nocturnal O_2 therapy. Tirlapur and Mir[29] administered 24 percent O_2 to 12 COPD patients. This dose increased saturation to normal and virtually abolished hypoxemic dips in patients with little daytime hypoxemia. In patients with moderate to severe waking hypoxemia this O_2 dose was probably too low—five of seven patients had mean arterial saturations less than 85 percent with hypoxemic episodes. Douglas et al.[14] administered 2 L/minute O_2 using nasal prongs to hypoxemic COPD patients. Although mean sleep saturation was not reported, the lowest saturations of the night were greatly increased. The same group[21] later administered O_2 at 2 L/minute to six very hypoxic patients (mean awake saturation = 81 percent). Mean sleep saturation was increased from 53 to 90 percent, the lowest from 33 to 76 percent. The number of sustained hypoxemic episodes was reduced by more than half. When O_2 dosage is individualized, better results can be obtained. One major trial utilized a dose of 1 L greater than the lowest O_2 flow rate (in whole L/min) that demonstrably increased resting semirecumbant arterial PO_2 to 65 mmHg.[33] Using this guideline in 15 patients, mean sleep saturation was increased to over 90 percent and average lowest saturation of the night exceeded 85 percent.

Nocturnal O_2 therapy is well tolerated by COPD patients. Initial fears that it might induce severe CO_2 retention have proven groundless, at least in stable patients. Of a total of 12 patients who underwent careful measurement of arterial PCO_2 by a variety of investigators,[14,15,36] only one showed a substantial increase with nocturnal O_2 therapy, and this one may not have been stable. Though these numbers were small, they accord with the lack of clinical evidence of CO_2 narcosis in much larger groups of patients receiving nocturnal O_2.

The effect of nocturnal O_2 administration on sleep quality has been systematically examined by two groups. Calverly et al.[21] examined six severely hypoxemic patients (mean awake saturation = 81 percent); some measures of sleep quality were improved with O_2 therapy in five of six patients. Fleetham et al.[16] examined less severely hypoxemic patients (mean awake saturation = 85 percent) and found no systematic improvement in sleep quality with O_2 administration—sleep was unstable with many arousals and stage changes, and time actually asleep was small. Differences in results are probably related to the types of patients—the British patients were all hypercapnic, the Canadian patients were not. In addition, the former group were apparently treated with only inhaled beta$_2$-sympathomimetic agents while the latter group was treated in addition with methyxanthines, which may themselves worsen sleep quality.

Just as it is difficult to separate the consequences of nocturnal hypoxemia from those of associated daytime hypoxemia, it is at present impossible to assess the therapeutic value of oxygen therapy administered exclusively during sleep. Recent multicenter trials[37] have firmly established that in patients with daytime hypoxemia due to COPD, O_2 administration for at least 15 hours/day, including the hours of sleep, is associated with better survival than no O_2 therapy. In similar patients it has been shown that mortality is lower when O_2 is administered approximately 20 hours/day than when nocturnal oxygen therapy is given for 12 hours/day.[33] In these patients sleep oxygenation was worse than that during the daytime, but correction of only sleep hypoxemia produced less benefit than continuous O_2 therapy. Thus patients with COPD who are hypoxemic while awake—arterial PO_2 <60 mmHg—should be treated with O_2 as continuously as possible, the dose being increased with sleep as noted above. Specific sleep studies are not needed to make this decision. Since more severe nocturnal hypoxemia in COPD patients occurs in those who are also hypoxemic while awake, acting on this recommendation will probably deal with most sleep hypoxemia problems in these patients. However, there may be patients who are not hypoxemic while awake but who demonstrate significant sleep hypoxemia. The physician who deals with such patients should be careful to rule out obstructive sleep apnea as a cause of the hypoxemia. Severe episodic nocturnal hypoxemia in the absence of upper airway obstruction or daytime hypoxemia should probably be treated with nocturnal O_2 therapy, but the value of this treatment has not been established.

Drug Therapy of Sleep Hypoxemia

There are few published reports of the effect of respiratory stimulant agents on sleep hypoxemia in COPD and no long term clinical trials, so the use of these agents at present must be considered experimental.

Medroxyprogesterone (MPA) has been evaluated in five sleeping hypercapnic COPD patients.[38] With MPA there was an increase in nocturnal ventilation and a reduction in arterial PCO_2. Sleep oxygenation also improved, the changes being largest during REM stage, though this sleep stage was studied in only three patients. These patients were selected for sleep studies because they had previously been shown to increase their ventilation in response to MPA while awake. In chronic mountain sickness, a disorder afflicting high altitude residents who demonstrate waking hypoxemia and hypoventilation with worsening hypoxemia during sleep, MPA has been shown to increase ventilation and to improve sleep oxygenation and has been an effective form of chronic therapy.[28]

Acetazolamide, a carbonic anhydrase inhibitor, has been evaluated in five sleeping hypercapnic COPD patients.[27] In three, sleep arterial PCO_2 became normal, but arterial PO_2 increased in all five, the mean increase being 9 mmHg. In both the MPA and acetazolamide trials patients were carefully selected. Patients with very severe disease or who are unable to lower arterial PCO_2 by more than 5 mmHg with voluntary hypoventilation were excluded.

Almitrine, an agent that stimulates the carotid body without causing widespread nervous system excitation has been shown to increase ventilation in COPD patients.[39,40] In addition, the arterial PO_2 may increase out of proportion to the reduction in arterial PCO_2, indicating that the matching of the distributions of ventilation and perfusion may be improved. Preliminary investigation of this agent in sleeping COPD patients are promising.

CYSTIC FIBROSIS

Though relatively few studies have been published[9,41] it appears that patients with cystic fibrosis behave like COPD patients during sleep. When the disease is severe enough to be associated with decreased waking arterial O_2 saturation, further decreases in saturation are the rule with sleep and some patients have episodes of severe hypoxemia associated with REM. Apneic episodes are not common. The decreases in saturation during both REM and NREM sleep are correlated with lung function and waking arterial oxygenation;[38] the sicker the patient the more likely he or she is to demonstrate sleep hypoxemia. We are aware of no studies that systematically examined associations between sleep hypoxemia in cystic fibrosis and either waking CO_2 retention or the chemical control of ventilation.

The mechanism of sleep hypoxemia in cystic fibrosis has been studied in some detail.[9] The shift from NREM and REM sleep is probably accompanied by a decrease in ventilation. Further, there is evidence favoring a decrease in tonic, continuous activity of the inspiratory muscles, which would favor a decrease in FRC, and independent measurements of rib cage and abdominal diameters indicate that FRC may indeed be decreased in REM sleep. Such a decrease would favor airway closure and decreased ventilation of closed units would accentuate hypoxemia. However, the relative contributions to sleep hypoxemia of hypoventilation and airway closure induced changes in the distribution of ventilation-perfusion ratios remains obscure in cystic fibrosis, as in COPD.

The treatment of chronic hypoxemia, either during sleep or wakefulness, has not been systematically studied in cystic fibrosis. Similarities between this disease and COPD, however, suggest that until specific data are available it would be reasonable to employ guidelines derived from experience with COPD to the study and treatment of cystic fibrosis.

KYPHOSCOLIOSIS

We are aware of detailed sleep studies in 10 middle-aged patients with severe kyphoscoliosis, the angle of deformity being greater than 90° in each.[42,43] In one series[42] three of five patients had symptoms of disordered sleep, and all demonstrated abnormally low arterial blood saturation while awake. They all had distinct decreases of saturation during NREM sleep and further, dramatic decreases in REM sleep were evident in four of five. All patients demonstrated apneic episodes, which were predominantly central in some and obstructive in others, though none were obese. During REM sleep, episodes of hypoxemia were not necessarily related to apneic episodes in that severe hypoxemia could occur in the absence of apnea.

In the other series,[43] five patients with severe deformity and grossly abnormal respiratory mechanics were examined. Only two had arterial PO_2 <65 mmHg at rest and it was these two patients who showed the most severe sleep hypoxemia. During REM they demonstrated mean saturations of 71 percent and 79 percent with lows of 45 percent and 48 percent. These patients also had episodes of central apnea that were prominent in REM and associated with severe hypoxemia. In the other three patients no apneas were demonstrated and sleep hypoxemia was less severe, the saturation averaging 79 to 81 percent during REM with the lowest saturation observed being 70 percent.

As in other respiratory diseases it appears that severe sleep hypoxemia is common in kyphoscoliotic patients with hypoxemia during wakefulness. In contrast to patients with COPD, it appears that apneic episodes may be common in such patients, and no clear relationship has been demonstrated between sleep hypoxemia and CO_2 retention or ventilatory response to CO_2. It is possible that some patients with kyphoscoliosis have significant sleep hypoxemia in the absence of treatable hypoxemia during wakefulness.

We routinely employ O_2 therapy guidelines developed for COPD in patients with kyphoscoliosis. However, there is no good evidence that O_2 treatment is of benefit, and when hypoxemia develops in this disease the prognosis is usually poor. Recently a small series of such patients has been reported to show remarkable benefit from nocturnal artificial ventilation.[44] The maneuver apparently rehabilitated patients who were doing very badly on home oxygen therapy. A tracheostomy and positive pressure respirator was employed. This and other forms of nocturnal artificial ventilation should be further examined, though previous studies using cuirass respirators were not encouraging.[42]

ASTHMA

Many asthmatics give a history of symptomatic attacks beginning in early morning hours. Asthmatics have been shown to have consistent diurnal variations in the degree of airways obstruction, peak expiratory flow and FEV_1

reaching nadirs between 2:00 and 6:00 AM.[45,46] This cycle is related to sleep: it is not due to posture or to bed-clothes-associated allergens, and patients who work at night demonstrate increased airways obstruction during daytime sleep hours. It is not clear whether or not all asthmatics demonstrate this kind of cycle, or how it relates to their airways reactivity, but it appears that diurnal changes in airways obstruction are most prominent in asthmatics who during the daytime have intermediate levels of airway obstruction. Patients who are very ill show little diurnal variation and at least some patients with little demonstrable abnormality also may have no diurnal variation.

The cause of diurnal variations in airways obstruction is not clear. Though blood adrenocorticoid concentrations normally have a diurnal cycle with a minimum in the early morning, this can be obliterated by administration of exogenous corticoids without obliterating cyclic changes in airways obstruction.[47] Recently asthmatics have been shown to have diurnal cycles of blood epinephrine, cyclic AMP, and histamine, the last reaching maximum levels in the early morning, when the first two attain their minimum values.[48] Blood levels of all three substances correlated well with changes in peak expiratory flow, which was minimal when histamine was maximal and epinephrine and cyclic AMP were low. Normals showed similar diurnal cycles of these agents though blood histamine levels were lower. The authors postulated that the diurnal changes in histamine and cyclic AMP were secondary to the observed changes in blood epinephrine. Epinephrine by its activation of adenylate cyclase would cause proportional changes in cyclic AMP, and might cause reciprocal changes in blood histamine by inhibiting its release from mast cells. Cyclic inhibition of release of mediators such as histamine might cause cyclic changes in airways obstruction. Low dose infusions of epinephrine during the night decreased blood histamine and increased peak expiratory flow. If this intriguing hypothesis is correct, the blood histamine levels observed must reflect either much higher local airway histamine concentrations, or the release of other mediators of bronchoconstriction, since when similar blood levels are achieved by histamine infusion in asthmatics, notable bronchoconstriction does not result.[49]

In sleeping dogs, airway smooth muscle tone decreases during slow wave sleep and may increase substantially during REM, apparently by vagal mechanisms.[50] One might, therefore, expect human nocturnal asthma attacks to arise chiefly during REM. This is apparently not the case. The probability of nocturnal asthma attacks is as great during stage II sleep as it is during REM.[47,51,52] In some studies there were few attacks—defined as waking with symptoms—during stage III to IV sleep.[51,52] This could have been because these levels of sleep prevented bronchoconstriction, but might have also been because bronchoconstriction was a less effective arousal stimulus in slow wave sleep. Finally, the negative association between attacks and stage III to IV sleep might have simply reflected the fact that this type of sleep tends to occur soon after the onset of sleep, when attacks are relatively few.

Due to the 4 to 6 hour duration of maximum effect of most bronchodilator agents, the prevention of nocturnal asthmatic attacks may pose a difficult therapeutic problem.

Exclusive of attacks, sleep in asthma has been relatively well studied.[53–56] Asthmatics demonstrate larger decreases in mean arterial saturation with sleep than do normals, and have more episodic decreases of saturation. These episodes are more likely to occur during REM according to most but not all workers. However, severe sleep hypoxemia is apparently uncommon in relatively stable asthmatics, probably reflecting the fact that daytime hypoxemia is uncommon. As might be expected nocturnal hypoxemia is more striking in asthmatics at high altitude than it is at sea level. Some investigators have reported that asthmatics have more apneas during sleep than normals,[53] but other[52,54] have found that asthmatics did not have abnormal breathing patterns. Young asthmatics decrease their minute ventilation with NREM sleep and REM sleep may be associated with disproportionate loss of intercostal muscle tone, so that the rib cage actually decreases its volume during inspiration.[54]

Sleep quality is disturbed in patients who have nocturnal asthma attacks, with a greater time spent awake and arousing, and less time in slow wave sleep, though the amount of time spent in REM approximates that of normal subjects.[47,51,52] It seems likely that in these patients the sleep disturbance can be ascribed to attacks of bronchoconstriction.

In summary, asthmatics demonstrate a sleep associated increase in airways obstruction that is frequently manifested by early morning attacks of bronchoconstriction. These attacks may be difficult to manage and may be related to diurnal variations in mediator release that in turn may be dependent in cyclic variations in blood levels of neurohumors such as epinephrine. Nocturnal asthma attacks are relatively uncommon during slow-wave sleep and when present disturb sleep quality. In the absence of attacks, asthmatics tend to have greater nocturnal decreases in arterial oxygen saturation than normals, but at least in ambulatory populations these decreases are seldom severe, probably reflecting the fact that these patients have little hypoxemia during wakefulness.

PULMONARY FIBROSIS

Two studies of sleep in patients with restrictive lung are consistent with findings in patients with obstructive disease.[57,58] These patients show decreases in mean nocturnal arterial O_2 saturation and REM associated episodes of severe hypoxemia, which are related to waking oxygenation: the lower the saturation during the daytime the more striking the hypoxemia during sleep. Of interest is the fact that the abnormally high breathing frequency demonstrated by these patients while awake was maintained during sleep. The presumably neural mechanism that drives breathing frequency in these patients is well preserved during sleep.

REFERENCES

1. Reed DJ, Kellogg RH: Changes in respiratory responses to CO_2 during natural sleep at sea level and at altitude. J Appl Physiol 13:225, 1958
2. Douglas NJ, White DP, Weil JV et al: Hypoxic ventilatory response decreases during sleep in man. Am Rev Resp Dis 125:286, 1982
3. Berthon-Jones M, Sullivan CE: Ventilatory and arousal responses to hypoxia in sleeping humans. Am Rev Resp Dis 125:632, 1982
4. Bradley CA, Fleetham JA, Anthonisen NR: Ventilatory control in patients with hypoxemia due to obstructive lung disease. Am Rev Resp Dis 120:21, 1979
5. Gothe B, Goldman MD, Cherniack NS, Mantey P: Effect of progressive hypoxia on breathing during sleep. Am Rev Resp Dis 126:429, 1982
6. Sullivan CE, Murphy E, Kozar LF et al: Waking and ventilatory responses to laryngeal stimulation in sleeping dogs. J Appl Physiol 45:681, 1978
7. Iber C, Bersenbrugge A, Skatrud J, Dempsey J: Ventilatory adaptations to resistive loading during wakefulness and non REM sleep. J Appl Physiol 52:607, 1982
8. Remmers JE, Anch AM, DeGroot WJ: Respiratory disturbances during sleep. Clin Chest Med 1:57, 1980
9. Muller NL, Francis PW, Gurwitz D: Mechanisms of hemoglobic desaturation during rapid eye movement sleep in normal subjects and in patients with cystic fibrosis. Am Rev Resp Dis 121:463, 1980
10. Tusiewicz K, Moldofsky H, Bryan AC, Bryan MH: Mechanics of the rib cage and diaphragm during sleep. J Appl Physiol 43:600, 1977
11. Pierce AK, Jarrett CE, Werkle G, Miller WF. Respiratory function during sleep in patients with chronic obstructive lung disease. J Clin Invest 45:631, 1966
12. Koo KW, Sax DS, Snider GL: Arterial blood gases and pH during sleep in obstructive lung disease. Am J Med 58:663, 1975
13. Flick MR, Block AJ: Continuous in vivo monitoring of arterial oxygenation during sleep in patients with chronic obstructive lung disease. Am Int Med 86:725, 1977
14. Douglas NJ, Legge RJE, Calverly PA et al: Transient hypoxemia during sleep in chronic bronchitis and emphysema. Lancet 1:1, 1979
15. Leitch AG, Clancy LJ, Leggett RJE et al: Arterial blood gas tensions, hydrogen ions and electroencephalogram during sleep in patients with chronic ventilatory failure. Thorax 31:730, 1976
16. Fleetham J, West P, Mezon B et al: Sleep, arousals and oxygen desaturation in chronic obstructive pulmonary disease. Am Rev Resp Dis 126:429, 1982
17. Fleetham JA, Mezon B, West P et al: Chemical control of ventilation and sleep arterial oxygen desaturation in patients with COPD. Am Rev Resp Dis 122:583, 1980
18. Littner MR, McGinty DT, Arand DL: Determinants of oxygen desaturation in the course of ventilation during sleep in chronic obstructive pulmonary disease. Am Rev Resp Dis 122:849, 1980
19. Catteral JR, Douglas NR, Calverly PMA et al: Transient hypoxemia during sleep in COPD is not a sleep apnea syndrome. Am Rev Resp Dis 128:24, 1983
20. Conway WA, Kryger M, Timms RM, Williams GW: Hypercarbia predicts nocturnal desaturation in COPD. Am Rev Resp Dis 125:100, 1982
21. Calverly PMA, Brezinova V, Douglas NJ et al: The effect of oxygenation on sleep quality in chronic bronchitis and emphysema. Am Rev Resp Dis 126:205, 1982

22. Coccagna G, Lugaresi E: Arterial blood gases and pulmonary and systemic arterial pressure during sleep in chronic obstructive lung disease. Sleep 1:117, 1978
23. Fletcher EC, Gray BA, Levin DC: Nonapneic mechanisms of arterial oxygen desaturation during rapid eye movement sleep. J Appl Physiol 54:632, 1983
24. Guilleminault C, Cammiskey J, Motta J: Chronic obstructive air flow disease and sleep studies. Am Rev Resp Dis 122:397, 1980
25. Wynne JW, Block AJ, Hemenway J et al: Disordered breathing and oxygen desaturation during sleep in patients with chronic obstructive lung disease. Am J Med 66:573, 1979
26. Arand DL, McGinty DJ, Littner MR: Respiratory patterns associated with hemoglobin desaturation during sleep in chronic obstructive pulmonary disease. Chest 80:193, 1981
27. Skatrud JB, Dempsey JA: Relative effectiveness of acetagolamide versus medroxyprogesterone acetate in correction of chronic carbon dioxide retention. Am Rev Resp Dis 27:405, 1983
28. Kryger M, Glas R, Jackson D et al: Impaired oxygenation during sleep in excessive polycythemia of high altitude. Sleep 1:3, 1978
29. Tirlapur VG, Mir MA: Nocturnal hypoxemia and associated electrocardiographic changes in patients with chronic obstructive airways disease. N Engl J Med 306:125, 1982
30. Boysen PG, Block AJ, Wynne JW et al: Nocturnal pulmonary hypertension in patients with chronic obstructive pulmonary disease. Chest 76:536, 1979
31. Block AJ: Dangerous sleep: Oxygen therapy for nocturnal hypoxemia. N Engl J Med 306:166, 1982
32. Fletcher EC, Levin DC: Cardiopulmonary hemodynamics during sleep in subjects with chronic obstructive pulmonary disease. Chest 85:6, 1984
33. Nocturnal Oxygen Therapy Trial Group: Continuous or nocturnal oxygen therapy in hypoxemic obstructive lung disease. Ann Int Med 93:391, 1980
34. Heaton RK, McSweeny AJ, Grant I et al: Psychological effects of continuous and nocturnal oxygen therapy in hypoxemic chronic obstructive pulmonary disease. Arch Int Med 143:1941, 1983
35. Brezinova V, Calverly PMA, Flenley DC, Townsend HRA: The effect of long term oxygen therapy on the EEG in patients with chronic stable ventilatory failure. Bull Euro Physiopath Resp 15:603, 1979
36. Kearly R, Wynne JW, Block AJ et al: The effect of low flow oxygen on sleep disordered breathing and oxygen desaturation. Chest 78:682, 1980
37. Medical Research Council Working Party: Long term domiciliary oxygen therapy in chronic hypoxic cor pulmonale complicating chronic bronchitis and emphysema. Lancet 1:681, 1981
38. Skatrud JB, Dempsey JA, Iber C, Berssenbrugge A: Correction of CO_2 retention during sleep in patients with chronic obstructive pulmonary disease. Am Rev Resp Dis 124:260, 1981
39. Powles ACP, Tuxen DV et al: The effect of intravenously administered almitrine, a peripheral chemoceptor agonist, on patients with chronic air-flow obstruction. Am Rev Resp Dis 127:284, 1983
40. Connaughton JJ, Douglas NJ, Morgan AD et al: Almitrine improves oxygenation when both awake and asleep in patients with hypoxia and carbon dioxide retention caused by chronic bronchitis and emphysema. Am Rev Resp Dis 132:206, 1985

41. Francis PWJ, Muller NL, Gurawitz D et al: Hemoglobin desaturation—its occurrence during sleep in patients with cystic fibrosis. Am J Dis Child 134:734, 1980
42. Guilleminault C, Kurland G, Winkel R, Miles LE: Severe kyphoscoliosis, breathing, and sleep. Chest 79:626, 1981
43. Mezon B, West P, Israels J, Kryger M: Sleep breathing abnormalities in kyphoscoliosis. Am Rev Resp Dis 122:617, 1980
44. Hoeppner VH, Hodgson WC, Graham BL: Night time ventilation in kyphoscoliosis. Chest 80:364, 1981
45. Clark TJH, Hetze MR: Diurnal variation of asthma: Br J Dis Chest 71:87, 1977
46. Turner-Warwick M: On observing patterns of airflow obstruction in chronic asthma. Br J Dis Chest 71:73, 1977
47. Kales A, Beall GN, Bajor GF et al: Sleep studies in asthmatic adults: Relationship of attacks to sleep stage and time of night. J Allergy 41:164, 1968
48. Barnes P, Fitzgerald G, Brown M, Dollery C: Nocturnal asthma and changes in circulating epinephrine, histamine, and cortisol. N Engl J Med 303:263, 1980
49. Drazen J: Histamine and nocturnal wheezing. N Engl J Med 303:278, 1980
50. Sullivan CE, Laurel N, Kozar LF et al: Regulation of airway smooth muscle tone in sleeping dogs. Am Rev Resp Dis 119:87, 1979
51. Kales A, Kales JD, Sly RM et al: Sleep patterns of asthmatic children: All night electroencephalographic studies. J Allergy 46:300, 1970
52. Montplaisir J, Walsh J, Malo JL: Nocturnal asthma: Features of attacks, sleep, and breathing patterns. Am Rev Resp Dis 125:18, 1982
53. Catterall JR, Calverly PMA, Brezinova V et al: Irregular breathing and hypoxemia during sleep in chronic stable asthma. Lancet 1:302, 1982
54. Tabachnik E, Muller NL, Levison H, Bryan AC: Chest wall mechanics and pattern of breathing during sleep in asthmatic adolescents. Am Rev Resp Dis 124:269, 1981
55. Smith TF, Hudgel DW: Arterial oxygen desaturation during sleep in children and its relation to airway obstruction and ventilatory drive. Pediatrics 66:746, 1980
56. Chipps BE, Mak H, Schuberth KC et al: Nocturnal oxygen saturation in normal and asthmatic children. Pediatrics 65:1157, 1980
57. Bye PTP, Issa F, Berthon-Jones M, Sullivan CE: Studies of oxygenation during sleep in patients with interstitial lung disease. Am Rev Resp Dis 129:27, 1984
58. Perez-Padilla R, West P, Lentzman M et al: Breathing during sleep in patients with interstitial lung disease. Am Rev Resp Dis 132:224, 1985

12 Sleep and Breathing in Neurological Disorders

Sudhansu Chokroverty

The effect of neurological lesions on the pattern and control of breathing has been described.[1-11] However, the role of sleep state on the control of breathing in various acute and chronic neurological disorders has received scant attention.[2,12] The long-term effects on breathing of acute neurological lesions has received even less attention.[12]

Many neurological diseases affect central or peripheral respiratory pathways causing acute respiratory failure in wakefulness as well as sleep, while others may affect the control of ventilation only during sleep. Either can eventually lead to undesirable and often catastrophic results including cardiorespiratory failure and even sudden unexplained death. This chapter is concerned with sleep-related respiratory dysrhythmias in central and peripheral neurological disorders. The description follows the anatomical level of the nervous system in a rostrocaudal manner. In addition, sleep-related respiratory dysfunction in autonomic neuropathies and in certain other miscellaneous disorders that cannot be localized to precise anatomical levels will be briefly discussed.

Before discussing disturbances of sleeping and breathing in neurological disorders, a brief description of the physiological changes in the control of breathing that occur in wakefulness and sleep in normal individuals is necessary in order to understand the pathophysiology of sleep-related breathing abnormalities in various neurological disorders. A more comprehensive description of respiratory neural activity in sleep and control of breathing during sleep in adults is given elsewhere in this volume.

PHYSIOLOGY OF SLEEP

Electroencephalographic (EEG) and behavioral observations have led to the recognition of two types of sleep:[13–15] non-rapid eye movement (non-REM) or slow wave sleep; and rapid eye movement (REM) or paradoxical sleep. The non-REM sleep accounts for approximately 75 to 80 percent and REM sleep 20 to 25 percent of sleep time in adults. The percentage of REM sleep is considerably greater in infants. Four stages of non-REM sleep have been identified by EEG criteria. Stage 1 non-REM sleep is characterized by general disorganization of activity, diminution of the alpha rhythm and the appearance of a mixture of theta (4 to 7 Hz) and beta (>13 Hz) rhythms. There are no spindles or K complexes. Occasional slow-rolling eye movement may be seen. Stage II EEG is characterized by K complexes and sleep spindles of 12 to 14 Hz and the record contains less than 20 percent delta (<4 Hz) activity. In stage III EEG there is more (20 to 50 percent) delta activity. In stage IV the EEG contains a large (>50 percent) amount of delta waves. The different stages of sleep are distributed approximately as follows: stage I non-REM 10 percent; stage II non-REM 55 percent; stage III and IV non-REM 15 percent; REM sleep 20 percent.

REM sleep normally begins 60 to 90 minutes after sleep onset and recurs in 90 minute cycles throughout the night. The REM periods are more intense and longer in duration towards the morning. REM sleep consists of tonic and phasic events.[15,16] Tonic events are characterized by desynchronized EEG, hypotonia of the axial muscles (antigravity muscles, neck and orofacial, and posterior neck muscles) and depression of monosynaptic and polysynaptic reflexes. The EEG shows low voltage fast activities mixed with a small amount of theta rhythm and sometimes contains "sawtoothed" waves. The tonic stage lasts throughout REM sleep. Phasic events are discontinuous and superimposed on tonic events. They are characterized by bursts of rapid eye movements (both vertical and horizontal), myoclonic twitchings of the facial and limb muscles, irregular heart rate and respiration with variable blood pressure, spontaneous middle ear muscle activity,[17] and phasic tongue movements.[18]

Two theories of sleep have been proposed: the passive theory of Bremer,[19,20] Moruzzi and Magoun;[21,22] and the active theory of Hess,[23] Von Economo,[24] Batini et al.,[25,26] and Jouvet.[27] In 1935 Bremer[19,20] postulated a passive theory of sleep based on two classical experimental preparations in cats: the "cerveau isole" produced by midcollicular transection of the midbrain below the nucleus of the third nerve that removed all sensory input to the cerebrum except that from cranial nerves I and II; and the "encephale isole" resulting from section at the junction of the medulla and spinal cord. The "cerveau isole" preparation exhibits the EEG pattern and eye signs of sleep, and sensory stimulation fails to cause arousal. The second preparation shows the EEG pattern and eye signs of both wakefulness and sleep but can easily be aroused by sensory stimulation to exhibit a complete sequence of wakefulness and sleep. From these observations Bremer deduced that the afferent inflow via the specific sensory pathways was important for the maintenance of the wakeful state. However, in 1949 Moruzzi and Magoun[21] showed that the maintenance of wakefulness depended mainly on the impulses travelling in the extralemniscal pathways in the center of the brain stem, called the ascending reticular activating systems, which receive collaterals from the main sensory afferent roots. These authors concluded that the loss of alertness and wakefulness resulted from withdrawal of a tonic facilitatory influence of the reticular formation on the cerebral cortex.

The active theory of sleep was first proposed by Von Economo[24] in 1926 who suggested the presence of an active sleep center in the hypothalamic region to account for the somnolence of encephalitis lethargica (Von Economo's encephalitis). Encephalitis lesions located in the posterior hypothalamic region produced hypersomnia while lesions in the preoptic and anterior hypothalamic areas caused insomnia. Experiments in rats by Nauta[28] supported Von Economo's proposal.[24] Hess,[23] based on stimulation experiments in cats, proposed a diencephalic (median thalamic) sleep center.

The midpontine pretrigeminal preparation in cats of Batini et al.[25,26] has revived the question of cerebral hypnogenic centers. Persistent wakefulness in this preparation contrasted with the comatose state of midcollicular section. Stimulation and lesion experiments have suggested that there is a hypnogenic center in the region of the medullary reticular formation near the nucleus of the tractus solitarius. The previously suggested hypnogenic center in the preoptic region of the hypothalamus is supported by stimulation experiments and the effects of lesions on the basal forebrain in cats.

Currently, it is believed that both the active and passive theories for non-REM or synchronized sleep are correct. Two active sleep centers are thought to exist: a diencephalic center in the basal preoptic region of the hypothalamus and a lower brain stem center in the region of the nucleus tractus solitarius. Non-REM sleep results from a combination of two factors: reduced activity of the ascending reticular activating system and increased activity of the two hypnogenic centers.

REM sleep is dependent upon an interaction between the locus ceruleus and the gigantocellular tegmental field located in the pons.[15,16,29,30] The caudal one-third of the locus ceruleus is responsible for muscle hypotonia and the middle one-third triggers the phasic events of REM sleep. The locus ceruleus inhibits the gigantocellular tegmental field during non-REM sleep; during REM sleep this inhibition disappears and the gigantocellular tegmental field triggers the phasic events by generating pontinegeniculateoccipital spikes and desynchronizes the EEG. The neurotransmitter substrates of REM and non-REM sleep are located in the brain stem and comprise cholinergic and aminergic neurotransmitters.[27,31,32] The serotonergic neurons located in the midline raphe nuclei of the brain stem are involved in the production of non-REM sleep. The noradrenergic neurons of the locus ceruleus are associated with the process of REM sleep. In REM sleep there is maximum cholinergic hyperactivity and aminergic hypoactivity. The sertonergic neurons initiate and maintain non-REM sleep by inhibiting the cholinergic ascending reticular activating system; they also trigger REM sleep. The noradrenergic neurons of the locus ceruleus are responsible for inactivation of muscle tone in REM sleep. According to Bremer[20] the brain stem serotonergic neurons should be considered as hypnotonic rather than hypnogenic neurons. Catecholaminergic transmitters (norepinephrine or serontonin or both) inhibit the gigantocellular tegmental field. Therefore, excess medication containing these transmitters would reduce REM. When these drugs are withdrawn abruptly, REM rebound, that is more REM per night is noted and the REM becomes more intense for up to 4 weeks.

CONTROL OF BREATHING AS IT RELATES TO NEURAL LESIONS AND SLEEP

Respiration is thought to be mediated by two separate and independent controlling systems:[4–6,33–36] a metabolic or "automatic" system; and a voluntary or "behavioral" system. During wakefulness both voluntary and metabolic systems operate, but during sleep respiration depends upon the inherent rhythmicity of the metabolic or "automatic" respiratory control system located in the medulla.[37–41] Similarly in coma respiration is wholly dependent upon the metabolic system. A third system, the reticular arousal system exerts a tonic influence on the brain stem respiratory neurons.[41] Reticular inhibition and the loss of wakefulness or arousal stimuli[40,42] on automatic respiration are the two fundamental mechanisms responsible for various changes in respiration occurring in normal sleep.

The respiratory neurons governing the automatic system are located in the medulla. There is ample evidence from animal experiments and human clinical-pathological studies that respiratory neurons are located dorsally in the nucleus tractus solitarius and ventrally in the nucleus ambiguus and retroambigualis.[33,36,43] Axons from these neurons decussate below the obex and descend in the reticulospinal tracts in the ventrolateral spinal cord to synapse with spinal motoneurons innervating respiratory muscles.[6,35,36,44] Respiratory rhythmicity depends on tonic inputs converging on the medullary neurons. The proprioceptive afferents, vagal afferents, the carotid and aortic body chemoreceptors, the central chemoreceptors located on the ventral surface of the medulla, the supramedullary (pontine and cortical), and the reticular activating system (sensitive to the general level of excitation) all influence the medullary respiratory neurons to regulate the rate, rhythm, and amplitude of breathing and acid–base and oxygen homeostasis.[34–36]

The voluntary breathing system controls respiration during wakefulness in addition to participating in nonrespiratory functions,[5,6,34–37] (e.g., coughing,

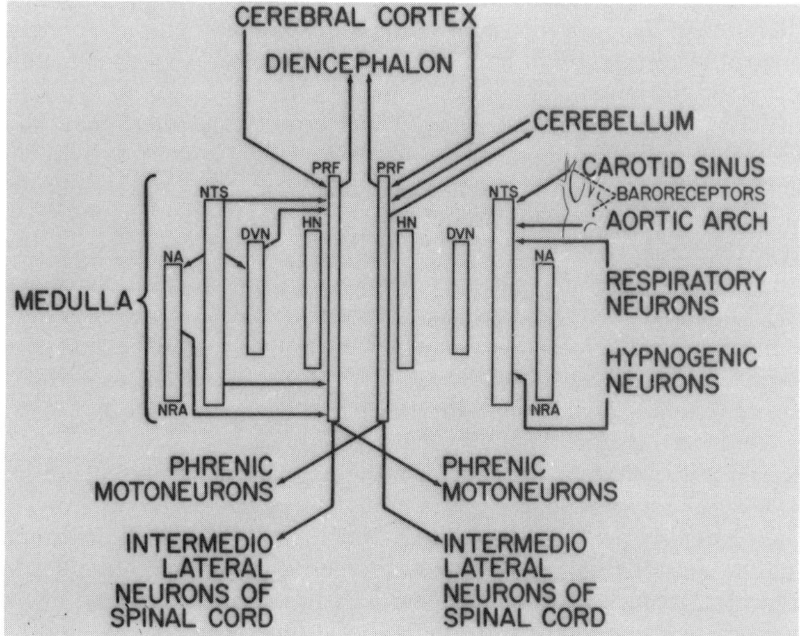

Fig. 12-1 Schematic diagram showing the interrelationship between the baroreceptor afferents, respiratory neurons, and the hypnogenic neurons in the medulla. PRF, paramedian reticular formation; HN, hypoglossal nucleus; DVN, doral vagal nucleus; NTS, nucleus tractus solitarius; NA, nucleus ambiguus; NRA, nucleus retroambigualis.

voice production, breath-holding, sneezing, laughing, etc.). Its exact origin is uncertain but probably originates in the cerebral cortex (forebrain and limbic system)[6] and descends partly to the automatic controlling system in the medulla but largely descends within the corticobulbar and corticospinal tracts to the spinal respiratory motoneurons where this system of fibers integrates with the automatic controlling system.[6,35,36,44] Axons of the spinal respiratory motoneurons innervate the diaphragm, intercostal muscles, upper airways, and the accessory muscles of respiration. Feedback is from the peripheral respiratory muscles to the controlling centers travelling via the sensory afferents and proprioceptive projection.[34–36] The automatic and voluntary respiratory controlling systems can be damaged separately giving rise to two major types of respiratory dysrhythmia.[6,35,36,44] Figure 12-1 schematically shows the close relationship between the respiratory and the hypnogenic neurons.

Respiratory Changes in Sleep in Normal Individuals

In non-REM sleep ventilation, tidal volume and respiratory rate decrease and there may be a few periods of apnea or hypopnea during stages I and II non-REM sleep.[37–40,45–47] Changes may be due to hyposensitivity of the control system to CO_2[45,46] as a result of the inhibition of the reticular activating system and alteration of the metabolic control of the respiratory neurons during sleep. The control of respiration in non-REM sleep in normal persons is mainly dependent upon the automatic control system.[37–39]

In REM sleep respiration is rapid and erratic, and there may be brief periods of apnea or hypopnea.[37,40] There is a decrease of activity in the intercostal and upper airway muscles while activity is maintained in the diaphragm.[37–39,48] There is uncertainty about the ventilatory responses to CO_2 and hypoxia during REM sleep.[37–39] In summary, the REM-related respiratory control system is, at least in part, independent of thc non-REM related system, and the "voluntary" respiratory control system may be active during REM sleep. In normal individuals respiration is vulnerable during sleep, that is, sleeping adversely affects breathing. These respiratory alterations in normal individuals may produce mild respiratory irregularities and pauses, but in disease states these may assume a pathological significance.

Respiratory abnormalities in sleep may arise from neuromuscular disorders in two ways. First, functional or structural deficiencies of the respiratory neurons in the central nervous system (CNS) may impair metabolic or automatic respiratory control resulting in apnea or hypopnea during both non-REM and REM sleep. During REM this problem may be enhanced because of the additional complicating factor of oropharyngeal muscle hypotonia contributing to a possible upper airway obstructive apnea. Second, in patients with weak respiratory muscles (e.g., patients with myopathy and those with lesions in the lower motoneurons to the respiratory muscles) the breathing difficulties occurring during wakefulness may be enhanced during sleep. During wakefulness the central respiratory ncurons may increase the rate of firing or recruit additional respiratory neurons to maintain ventilation at an adequate level to drive weak respiratory musculature in such patients. The normal vulnerability of the respiratory neurons during sleep may thus aggravate the ventilatory problems causing more severe hypoventilation and even apnea during sleep. Also, upper airway muscle weakness (in fact these muscles are respiratory muscles whose function is partially controlled by the respiratory centers of the brain stem) may cause obstructive apnea.

The pattern of breathing in neurological lesions generally depends upon the anatomical location of the lesions. The neurological disorders may affect the breathing by the following mechanisms: (1) direct involvement of the medullary respiratory neurons (automatic controlling system); (2) interference with the voluntary system of respiration; (3) involvement of both 1 and 2; (4) interference with the afferent inputs to the medullary respiratory neurons, [e.g., involvement of peripheral chemoreceptors (vagal and glossopharyngeal nerve endings), supramedullary pathways, and central chemoreceptors in the dorsolateral medulla]; and (5) interference with the efferent mechanism—respiratory muscle weakness may result from direct involvement of the muscles or indirectly through involvement of the lower motoneurons to the respiratory muscles.

The respiratory abnormalities due to the above mechanisms may appear or worsen during sleep because of the normal vulnerability of the central respiratory neurons during sleep. Before ascribing sleep-related alveolar hypoventilation to lesions in the brain stem or high cervical spinal cord, one must exclude other causes of hypoventilation, such as intrinsic bronchopulmonary disease, dysfunction of the thoracic bellows (disease of the chest wall, extreme obesity, and kyphoscoliosis), and neuromuscular defects affecting the respiratory muscles.

TYPES OF SLEEP RELATED RESPIRATORY DYSRHYTHMIAS IN NEUROLOGICAL DISORDERS

Sleep apnea during non-REM and REM sleep is characterized by recurrent episodes of apnea of at least 10 seconds occurring irregularly.[49] To be significant the patient should have at least 30 periods of apnea during 7 hours of all-night sleep or an apnea index (number of apneas per hour of sleep) of at least five.[49,50] Three types of apnea may be recognized from the pattern of breathing: central, upper airway obstructive, and mixed types.

Central apnea is caused by decreased respiratory center output and is characterized by the suppression of diaphragmatic and intercostal muscle activity and absence of air exchange through the nose or mouth. Upper airway obstructive apnea is manifested by an absence of air exchange detected by the oronasal thermistors but persistence of the diaphragmatic and intercostal muscle activities. Mixed apnea is manifested by an initial period of central apnea followed by a period of upper airway obstructive apnea before resumption of regular breathing. Normal men may have an average of 7.0 episodes per night and normal women an average of 2.1 episodes of apneas, usually central in type.

Apneas occurring in sleep in neurological diseases constitute secondary sleep apnea syndromes, in contrast to primary sleep apnea in which no cause is found to account for the appearance of apnea. Secondary sleep apnea may aggravate neurological illness by the adverse effects of sleep-induced hypoxemia and hypercapnia, and in chronic cases by pulmonary hypertension, congestive cardiac failure, sleep deprivation, and sleep fragmentation.

Sleep-related hypopnea is diagnosed when the amplitude of the oronasal thermistor or pneumographic signal is reduced to one-third or less of its value measured during the preceding or following respiratory cycles. These should have the same significance as sleep apneas.[50]

Cheyne-Stokes pattern breathing is characterized by cyclical changes in breathing with a crescendo-decrescendo sequence separated by central apneas. This type of breathing is mostly noted in bilateral cerebral hemispheric lesions[5,6] and worsens during sleep.

Cheyne-Stokes variant pattern of breathing is distinguished by the sub-

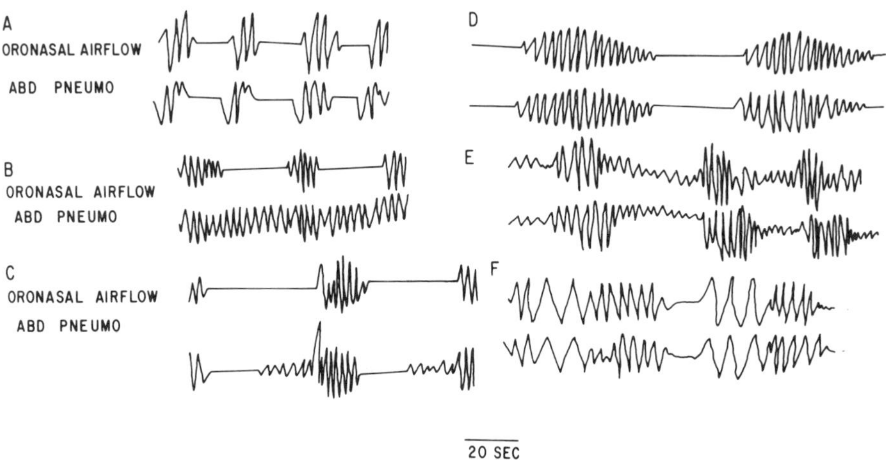

Fig. 12-2 Different sleep-related respiratory patterns in neurological disorders are shown schematically. A: central apnea. B: upper airway obstructive apnea. C: mixed apnea. D: Cheyne-Stokes breathing. E: Cheyne-Stokes variant pattern. F: Dysrhythmic breathing (irregular in rate, rhythm, and amplitude).

stitution of hypopneas for apneas.[8,10] This type of breathing may be seen in bilateral cerebral hemispheric disease or sometimes in brain stem lesions.

Abnormal breathing pattern is characterized by a nonrhythmic irregularity in rate and rhythm of respiration during sleep due to an abnormality in the automatic respiratory pattern generator[41] in the brain stem during sleep.

Figure 12-2 schematically shows different sleep-related breathing patterns observed in neurological disorders.

EVALUATION OF PATIENTS WITH DISORDERS OF SLEEPING AND BREATHING

Clinical Manifestations

In acute neurological disorders the clinical features of neurological dysfunction may overshadow the sleep-related respiratory problems, as many patients with acute neurological disorders that affect sleep are in stupor or coma. The clinical manifestations of disorders of sleeping and breathing consist of general and specific features. The specific features would depend upon the nature of the neurological illness. The general features become relevant and important in the diagnosis of sleep-related hypoventilation in chronic neurological diseases and consist of the following:[49,51,52] (1) breathlessness; (2) hypersomnolence; (3) early morning headache; (4) daytime fatigue; and (5) disturbed nocturnal sleep. Other features that may be present in long-standing cases of sleep deprivation include personality changes, intellectual deterioration, and impotence (in males). Often the patient has abnormal motor activity in the form of excessive body movements during sleep. Examination may reveal respiratory irregularity in rate, rhythm, and depth with asynchrony in wakefulness and sleep. Paradoxical movements of the chest wall and abdomen may suggest diaphragmatic paresis. Most illnesses affecting the lower motoneurons to the respiratory muscles are accompanied by breathlessness. But, breathlessness is not an important symptom in patients with impairment of the voluntary control of breathing nor in patients with medullary lesion causing dysfunction of the automatic respiratory control system.

The general symptoms of excessive daytime somnolence, morning headache and daytime fatigue may be related to two factors:[52] frequent arousals at night due to repeated apnea or hypopnea; and CO_2 retention. It is important to recognize alveolar hypoventilation during sleep because assisted ventilation at night will improve the symptoms, protect the patients from fatal apnea during sleep and may prevent the development of serious complications, such as pulmonary hypertension, cor pulmonale, and congestive cardiac failure to which these patients are susceptible because of episodic or prolonged hypoxemia, hypercapnia, and respiratory acidosis in sleep.

Pulmonary Function Tests

Measurements of spirometry, lung volumes, pulmonary diffusing capacity, and blood gases are obtained to assess respiratory function and to differentiate intrinsic bronchopulmonary disease from the neurological disorders causing respiratory dysfunction. Muscle weakness must be specifically tested. According to Black and Hyatt[53] the values of the maximal static inspiratory and expiratory pressures are more important than the values of the dynamic maneuvers for detection of the respiratory muscle weakness. The measurement of the static pressure, however depends upon the cooperation of patients which may be difficult to obtain in many patients with neurological disorders.

Hypercapnic or hypoxic ventilatory and mouth occlusion pressure ($P_{0.1}$) responses, with or without load, are used to measure the chemical control of breathing.[54] Mouth occlusion pressure reflects CNS respiratory drive and inspiratory muscle strength independent of pulmonary mechanical factors. These measurements may be impaired in patients with dysfunction of the metabolic respiratory control systems.

Impedance Pneumography and Respiratory Magnetometry

Impedance Pneumography[7] and the respiratory magnetometer[55] recording are useful methods for diagnosis and classification of abnormal breathing patterns. Impedance pneumography is used more frequently than the magnetometer.

Neurophysiological Study

Polysomnographic study is an important means of evaluating sleep-related respiratory dysrhythmia. The study should include simultaneous recording of multiple channels of the EEG, electromyograms, electrocardiogram, electro-oculogram, respiration recording by nasal and oral thermistors to detect air-flow, abdominal pneumograph, and continuous oxygen saturation (ear oximeter).[56] It is important to record multiple channels of the EEG to diagnose accurately different sleep stages and their relationship to respiration. Furthermore, EEG is an important test to diagnose focal and diffuse neurological lesions and to diagnose seizure disorders that may sometimes be complicated by sleep apnea. It is also important to record electrooculogram and electromyograms of multiple orofacial muscles in order to recognize REM sleep accurately. For example it is essential for electrophysiological documentation of sleep-onset REM to diagnose narcolepsy. The recording should include REM sleep because the most severe breathing abnormalities are often noted during this sleep stage.

Phrenic nerve conduction study[57] may be necessary to document phrenic nerve abnormalities causing diaphragmatic malfunction.

Brain stem auditory[58] and *somatosensory*[59] *cortical* and *subcortical evoked response studies* may be helpful in many cases. The structures responsible for mediating brain stem auditory and somatosensory impulses are in close proximity to the brain stem respiratory neurons and, therefore, may be affected in neurological diseases causing breathing dysfunction in sleep.

CEREBRAL HEMISPHERIC AND DIENCEPHALIC DISEASES

Neurological disease affecting the cerebral hemispheres and the diencephalon may produce instability of breathing, which increases during sleep. According to Plum and coworkers[3–6,11] the major effects of cerebral hemispheric diseases on respiration in sleep consist of (1) Cheyne-Stokes respiration—long-cycle Cheyne-Stokes breathing associated with hypocapnia is usually found in brain-damage deep in both cerebral hemispheres. In unilateral cerebral infarction this may occur due to the phenomenon of diaschisis. (2) Posthyperventilation apnea—Plum et al.[3] found posthyperventilation apnea in 79 percent of patients with bilateral and 6 percent of patients with unilateral cerebral dysfunction. This becomes more marked in sleep.

Lee et al.[10] found Cheyne-Stokes respiration and Cheyne-Stokes variant pattern in patients with extensive bilateral pontine lesions. These observations are in contrast to those of Plum and coworkers[4–6,11] who found Cheyne-Stokes respiration in bilateral cerebral hemispheric or diencephalic lesions, but rarely in lesions located as low as the upper pons. According to Lee et al.[10] the types of respiratory rate and pattern abnormalities in these patients depend on the size and bilaterality of the lesions. It should be noted that many patients with cerebral hemispheric and diencephalic lesions remain in stupor and coma. Therefore, respiration during sleep in these patients cannot be assessed.

Respiration in Sleep in Alzheimer's Disease

Alzheimer's disease or senile dementia of the Alzheimer type is the most common dementing illness in the elderly population and is characterized by progressive intellectual deterioration associated with a characteristic neuropathological findings including cerebral cortical atrophy and neuronal loss in the nucleus basalis of Meynert. There is also evidence of cholinergic system deficiency.[60] The exact prevalence of sleep-related respiratory dysrhythmia in this condition is not known. Smallwood et al.[61] investigated by polygraphic monitoring 45 elderly subjects, 15 of whom had Alzheimer's disease. They found that the mean apnea-hypopnea index and the percentage of subjects with an index greater than five were not significantly different between the Alzheimer's patient and age- and sex-matched controls. These data failed to confirm the author's hypothesis that primary neuronal degeneration might accentuate sleep apnea by altering neural control of centers regulating sleep-wakefulness and respiration. They concluded that sleep apnea is not significantly increased in Alzheimer's disease. Smirne et al.[62] found that 37.5 percent of men and 33 percent of women with Alzheimer's disease had apnea indices greater than five; these findings are comparable to those of Smallwood et al.[61] Polysomnographic study undertaken by the present writer in a 68-year-old man with advanced Alzheimer's disease revealed central, upper airway obstructive, and mixed apneas associated with oxygen desaturation (Fig. 12-3). However, in view of the recent documentation by Carskadon and associates as summarized by Miles and Dement[63] of a high prevalence of predominantly central sleep apnea in noncomplaining ambulatory elderly volunteers and the findings of Smallwood et al.[61] it is difficult to estimate the true incidence of sleep apnea in Alzheimer's disease patients.

Epilepsy Complicated by Sleep Apnea

The combination of sleep apnea and epilepsy is rare. Wyler and Weymuller[64] reported a 26-year-old man with intractable generalized and focal seizure disorder who also had central sleep apnea. Permanent tracheotomy alleviated the sleep apnea and reduced his generalized seizures. This writer encountered a patient with a posttraumatic generalized seizure disorder and upper airway obstructive and central sleep apneas that necessitated a permanent tracheotomy for relief of sleep apnea but his seizures did not improve following this procedure (Chokroverty, unpublished observations).

Respiratory arrest from seizure discharges in the limbic system has been described by Nelson and Ray.[65] Experimentally Kaada[66] observed apnea after stimulation of the limbic system and related cortical areas. Whether lesion of

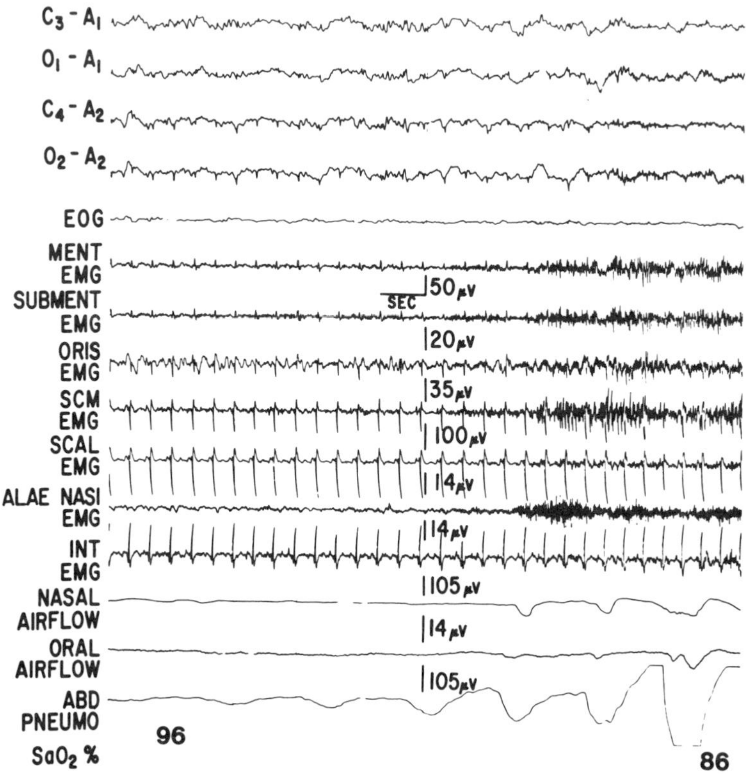

Fig. 12-3 Polygraphic recording in a patient with advanced Alzheimer's disease showing four channels of EEG (C_3-A_1, O_1-A_1, C_4-A_2, O_2-A_2: International Electrode Placement system), vertical electrooculogram (EOG), electromyograms (EMG) of mental (MENT), submental (SUBMENT), orbicularis (ORIS), sternocleidomastoid (SCM), scalenus anticus (SCAL), alae nasi and intercostal (INT) muscles, nasal and oral airflow, abdominal pneumogram (ABD PNEUMO), and oxygen (SaO_2 percent) saturation (ear oximeter). The patient has mixed apnea during stage II non-REM sleep.

the limbic system can be associated with clinical sleep-related respiratory dysrhythmias is not known. However, patients with partial complex and generalized seizures may have sleep apnea.[138]

BASAL GANGLIA

Parkinson's Disease

A systematic study to evaluate sleep-related respiratory dysfunction has not been undertaken in a large number of patients with basal ganglia disease. There have been isolated reports of sleep-related respiratory dysrhythmias, but there are also several reports of pulmonary dysfunction and other respiratory abnormalities in patients with Parkinson's disease.[67–69] In many reports of pulmonary function abnormalities in Parkinson's disease these deficits were thought to be due to restrictive pulmonary disease related to extrapyramidal muscular rigidity. Lilker and Woolf[68] found reduced forced expiratory volume, maximal midexpiratory flow rate and reduced maximal voluntary ventilation in 21 Parkinson's disease patients. They ascribed these abnormalities to several factors: (1) a defective central control of respiration; (2) an impairment of control of respiratory muscles due to extrapyramidal rigidity; (3) a defective autonomic control of tracheobronchial tree; and (4) alterations in respiratory tract secretions. In the absence of a polysomnographic study it is not known whether these patients had sleep apnea. Paulson and Tafrate[70] found in 22 Parkinson's disease patients a problem in repetitive deep breathing that suggested a possible defect in the voluntary respiratory control system. I have observed sleep apnea in some patients with Parkinson's disease (Chokroverty, unpublished observation).

A variety of respiratory disturbances have been described in postencephalitic Parkinson's disease patients[71,72] (e.g., disorder of rate, rhythm, and respiratory tics). Krum[72] described impairment of the voluntary control of respiration in nine postencephalitic patients. Garlind and Linderhold[73] described the syndrome of hypoventilation in cases of postencephalitic Parkinson's disease. Spirometry in their patients was normal but there was hypoventilation associated with hypoxemia and impairment of hypercapnic ventilatory response suggesting a possible decrease in the sensitivity of the central respiratory chemoreceptors.

Purdy et al.[74] described a new syndrome of familial parkinsonism and alveolar hypoventilation. These authors described an illness in identical twins characterized by mild parkinsonism and alveolar hypoventilation due to failure of the automatic respiratory control mechanism. Their patients had ataxic breathing with periods of apnea that worsened during sleep. The defect could be overcome by voluntary breathing necessitating the patient to remain alert most of the day and night. The spirometric tests were normal, but the patients had reduced responses to inspired CO_2. The authors thought that their patients fulfilled the criteria of "Ondine's curse." Postmortem examination in these two patients showed degenerative changes including cell loss and gliosis in the substantia nigra, caudate nucleus, periaqueductal gray area, pontine reticular formation, dorsal motonucleus of the vagus, nucleus tractus solitarius, lateral reticular formation, nucleus ambiguus, and retroambigualis. The authors suggested that in view of the focal gliosis in the areas crucial to respiratory control the patients' respiratory failure may have been related to these lesions. Streider et al.[75] described chronic hypoventilation of central origin in a 62-year-old man in association with Parkinson's syndrome and a past history of encephalitis lethargica. His ventilatory response to CO_2 was impaired suggesting dysfunction of central chemosensory neurons, but hypoxic ventilatory response was unimpaired indicating intact peripheral chemoreceptors.

Tardive Dyskinesia

Weiner and Klawans[69] described respiratory embarassment in tardive dyskinesia patients but did not mention sleep-related respiratory dysrhythmias. Casey and Rabins[76] stated that respiratory distress may be present in tardive dyskinesia and may be due to diaphragmatic dyskinesia causing hypoxemia. Chokroverty et al.[77] studied respiration with multiple electromyograms in tardive dyskinesia in six men. In one patient the respiratory control system was studied by measuring mouth occlusion pressure ($P_{0.1}$) and minute ventilation after hyperoxic hypercapnia. The standard spirometric study in this patient showed evidence of mild obstructive pulmonary disease. Hypercapnic ventilatory and mouth occlusion pressure responses with and without load were subnormal. The authors found that three patients had many periods of central apneas and one of them also had a few periods of upper airway obstructive apnea during light non-REM sleep accompanied by oxygen desaturation and orofacial muscle hypotonia. The authors suggested that sleep apnea in tardive dyskinesia may have resulted from a disturbed balance between central and peripheral dopaminergic opposing actions on breathing. Dopamine-containing neurons are thought to be involved in the respiratory control system in a biphasic manner:[78,79] stimulation of ventilation by its central action, but depression through its effect on peripheral chemoreceptor reflex. The subnormal hypercapnic ventilatory and mouth occlusion pressure response in one patient suggested impaired central chemoreceptor output. The authors concluded that the respiratory control mechanism may become unstable in some patients with tardive dyskinesia. This instability may be related to the presumed dopamine supersensitivity or dopamine receptor blocking effect of neuroleptics.

Cerebellum

Experimental studies in animals have shown distinct cerebellar influence on the sleep-wakefulness mechanism.[80] But the role of the cerebellum on the respiratory control mechanism in sleep is not known. Chokroverty et al.[81] described five patients with olivopontocerebellar atrophy (OPCA) and sleep apnea. OPCA is characterized by a chronic progressive cerebellar-parkinsonian syndrome beginning in middle or later life associated with a specific anatomical pattern of degeneration.[82] Brain stem neurons, which are known to be degenerated in OPCA,[82] are in close proximity to the respiratory[35] and hypnogenic neurons.[20] Therefore, it is plausible to expect dysfunction of respiratory control in parallel fashion along with somatic structural dysfunction in OPCA. Polygraphic study[81] documented repeated episodes of central, upper airway obstructive, and mixed apneas (Fig. 12-4) during sleep ranging from 10 to 62 seconds of apneic periods and with an apnea index of 30 to 55. Three patients had pure central apnea and two had all three types of apneas. Most of the apneic episodes occurred during non-REM sleep stage II. From these observations we concluded that the presence of sleep-related central and upper air-

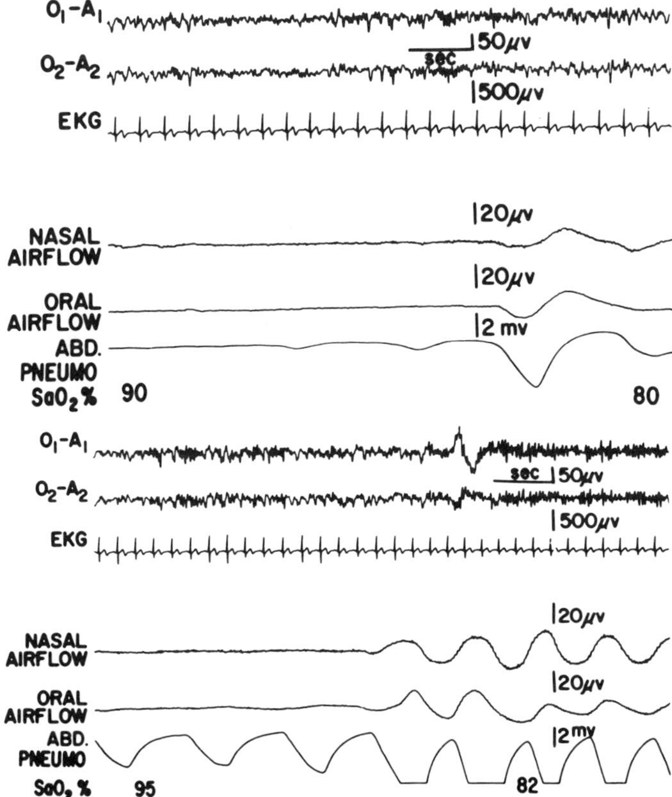

Fig. 12-4 Central (top six channels) and upper airway obstructive (lower six channels) apneas (only a portion is shown) in non-REM sleep stage II in a patient with olivopontocerebellar atrophy.

way obstructive apneas in OPCA suggested a central neuronal dysfunction in an area where respiratory and sleep-waking systems are closely interrelated, such as the nucleus tractus solitarius and the pontomedullary reticular formation. In another subtype of OPCA associated with glutamate dehydrogenase deficiency we[83] observed sleep apnea on polygraphic study in two patients.

BRAIN STEM

Sleep-related respiratory dysrhythmias have been described in neurological lesions of the brain stem, and in particular lesions affecting the medullary respiratory neurons. The lesions have included infarction,[8,10,84,85] tumor,[6] localized ischemic damage,[86] bulbar poliomyelitis,[2,12,87] trauma,[7,9] multiple sclerosis,[88–90] motoneuron disease involving the bulbar nuclei, syringobulbia,[91] and encephalitis.[75,92]

Severinghaus and Mitchell[93] first coined the term "Ondine's curse" to describe three patients who had long periods of apnea even when awake, but breathed on command. They became apneic following surgery involving the brain stem and high cervical spinal cord and required artificial ventilation when asleep. They also became apneic when consciousness was altered with nitrous oxide or thiopental. Their carbon dioxide response curve showed low sensitivity. One patient died in apnea and two improved over a week's time. The authors suggested that the Ondine's curse resulted from damage of the medullary carbon dioxide chemoreceptors. The term Ondine's curse was derived from the sea nymph in German mythology whose curse was supposed to have resulted in the death of her unfaithful lover due to loss of automatic respiratory function. There has been considerable controversy and confusion regarding this eponymic syndrome.

Brain Stem Infarction

Devereaux et al.[84] described two women, ages 36 and 59, with bilateral tegmental medullary infarcts (one autopsy proven) who had apnea necessitating ventilatory support during sleep, but were able to maintain breathing unaided while awake. The CO_2 response, studied in one patient, was markedly depressed. The cases described by Devereaux et al. localized the lesion to the lateral medullary tegmentum emphasizing the importance of this area in the control of automatic respiratory functions. These authors stated that acute automatic failure did not usually evolve into a chronic alveolar hypoventilation syndrome. However, their second patient with brain stem infarction continued to have sleep-induced apnea after many months.

The syndrome of primary failure of automatic respiration or "Ondine's curse" associated with sleep apnea but preservation of voluntary respiratory control is usually caused by bilateral lesions anywhere caudal to the fifth cranial nerve in the pons down to the upper cervical spinal cord in the ventrolateral region. But Levine and Margolis[85] reported a 52-year-old man with unilateral medullary infarction associated with loss of automatic respiratory control. The lesion extended from the left lower pons through the left lateral medullary tegmentum to the upper cervical spinal cord involving the left paramedian reticular formation in the pons. The authors postulated that the observations in their patient suggested that in some patients automatic respiratory control can be represented unilaterally in the pontomedullary tegmentum.

Lee et al.[8] studied respiratory rate and pattern using impedance pneumography in 49 patients with acute brain stem or cerebral infarctions and in a later study[10] reported another 23 patients with acute brain stem infarction. They found a frequent occurrence of respiratory rate and pattern abnormalities and arterial blood gas changes in patients with acute brain stem infarction. These abnormalities were noted more frequently during sleep in patients with depressed sensorium, and in those with severe neurological deficits. The abnormalities included Cheyne-Stokes breathing, Cheyne-Stokes variant pattern, and tachypnea. They also noted cluster breathing in four patients. They found Cheyne-Stokes respiration in patients with extensive bilateral pontine lesions in contrast to Plum and coworkers[4–6,11] who found this pattern of breathing in bilateral cerebral hemispheric or diencephalic lesions, but rarely in lesions located as low as upper pons. Lee et al.[10] stated that the types of respiratory rate and pattern abnormalities in these patients depended on the size and bilaterality of the lesions. The brain stem lesion usually causes central sleep apnea but other types of apneas have been noted occasionally.

Demyelinating Lesion in the Brain Stem

Newsom Davis[88] described a 38-year-old man with an autonomous breathing pattern. The patient could neither take a voluntary breath nor stop breathing, illustrating the apparent independence of the mechanisms controlling metabolic and behavioral respiratory control systems. The patient presented with paralysis of all four limbs and a clinical diagnosis of acute demyelinating lesion at the cervicomedullary junction was made. The patient did not have a sleep-related respiratory problem.

Rizvi et al.[89] reported a 16-year-old woman with brain stem dysfunction that was thought to be consistent with multiple sclerosis. The patient was able to breathe when awake, but became apneic when asleep. However, hypercapnic and hypoxic ventilatory responses did not show significant abnormality.

Boor et al.[90] reported a 40-year-old man with evidence of lower brain stem dysfunction who had simultaneous onset of paralysis of automatic respiration and severe proprioceptive loss. His respiration had been stable when alert, but he had recurrent apnea with relaxation. The patient rapidly recovered and he was weaned from the respirator. He died a year later while sleeping. Postmortem examination revealed a large demyelinating lesion in the central medulla. Demyelinating lesions involving crossing medullary respiratory neurons may be responsible for respiratory failure in multiple sclerosis and lesions in a similar location may also involve lemniscal decussation causing proprioceptive loss.

Bulbar Poliomyelitis

Sarnoff et al.[87] were the first to make quantitative measurements of the respiratory deficits in bulbar poliomyelitis that may consist of the following: (1) irregularity in rate and rhythm of respiration; (2) incoordination of the muscles of respiration; and (3) hypoventilation syndrome resulting from decreased sensitivity of the respiratory center to PCO_2 as a result of direct involvement of the respiratory center by the poliomyelitis virus. The authors described four patients with bulbar poliomyelitis who could breathe on voluntary commands, but would hypoventilate during periods of quiescence and sleep. They gave a detailed description of two such patients ages 9 and 11 years, who benefitted from electrophrenic respiration.

Plum and Swanson[2] reported the clinical and physiological findings in 20 of 250 poliomyelitis patients with central respiratory disturbances that could not be explained by spinal motoneuron involvement or airway obstruction. They described three successive stages of disordered breathing in acute bulbar poliomyelitis. In stage I there was disorder of respiratory rhythm during sleep during which breathing became irregular in rate and depth with periods of apneas ranging from 4 to 12 seconds. In stage II dysrhythmia persisted during wakefulness, normal breathing required increasing effort and concentration, and strong auditory or painful stimuli were required to maintain respiratory rhythmicity. Oxygen inhalation would cause a reduction in ventilation and CO_2 retention suggesting impaired chemosensitivity of the central respiratory centers. Sleep produced more profound irregularity in breathing with longer periods of apnea. In stage III the respiratory homeostasis was lost and the respiratory pattern was chaotic with varying periods of apnea. The respiratory center had lost its responsiveness to reflex as well as to chemical or other neuronal stimuli. Ventilatory support was required to maintain respiratory homeostasis. Pathological studies in two patients showed severe inflammatory changes and small areas of necrosis in the ventrolateral reticular formation of the medulla. In their series, the breathing abnormalities rarely lasted more than 2 weeks, but in two patients irregular respiration during sleep persisted for many months after acute poliomyelitis. Impaired hypercapnic ventilatory response and hypoventilation during 100 percent of oxygen breathing were also noted in these two patients. The authors attributed these physiological abnormalities to permanent dysfunction of the medullary respiratory center. The authors also found subnormal ventilatory response to CO_2 in several convalescent spinal poliomyelitis patients with reduced maximum breathing capacity or vital capacity of less than 50 percent of the predicted normal values. These findings suggested that peripheral mechanisms causing restriction of chest movements may also contribute to impaired ventilatory response to CO_2.

Solliday et al.[94] described a 41-year-old woman with chronic hypoventilation who had bulbar poliomyelitis 20 years earlier. Sleep produced more marked hypoxemia and hypercapnia and her ventilatory response to CO_2 was impaired. The authors concluded that in their patient the central chemoreceptor activity was absent but the peripheral chemoreceptors were functioning as hypoxic ventilatory response was normal.

Guilleminault and Motta[12] reported five men with excessive daytime somnolence who had bulbar poliomyelitis at least 16 years earlier. Polysomnographic study disclosed multiple apneic episodes during non-REM and REM sleep with a mean apnea index of 96. They had predominantly central but also had mixed and upper airway obstructive apneas associated with oxygen desaturation. The longest apneas were noted during REM sleep. Ventilatory assistance at night produced symptomatic relief with a decrease in daytime somnolence in all patients. It is notable that these patients with presumed central lesions had mixed and obstructive apneas indicating upper airway involvement. The patients' clinical manifestations furthermore were similar to those noted in patients with the primary sleep apnea syndrome.

Brain Stem Ischemic Damage

Beal et al.[86] described a 19-year-old man with failure of the automatic respiration and brain stem signs after being resuscitated following drowning. It was noted that he had apneic periods when he was asleep. A polysomnographic study confirmed 15 to 20 seconds of central apneas with the tracheotomy tube open and up to 50 seconds of central apnea with the tube occluded. Respiration while awake was normal. Ventilatory response to CO_2 was markedly impaired but ventilation did increase in response to hypoxemia. Eight months later he died suddenly and the neuropathological findings consisted of marked neuronal loss bilaterally in the nucleus gracilis, nucleus cunetus, nucleus of the tractus solitarius, nucleus ambiguus, and nucleus retroambigualis; these morphological findings appeared to have resulted from anoxia-ischemia.

Brain Stem Tumor

Plum[6] mentioned a patient with brain stem glioma who presented with automatic respiratory failure. This writer saw a patient with a medullary tumor who had severe hypoventilation during sleep and the central apneic episodes became prolonged when the tracheotomy tube was occluded.

Brain Stem Trauma

North and Jannett[7,9] recorded breathing patterns by impedance pneumograph or pneumotachograph and capnograph in many patients with recent head injury. They found irregular breathing in the patients with medullary and pontine lesions. They did not find a difference between the long and short cycle Cheyne-Stokes respiration in terms of localizing the site of brain damage, in contrast to the findings of Plum and Posner.[11] It should be noted that these authors[7,9] did not address the question of breathing during sleep versus breathing during wakefulness in their patients.

Syringobulbia-Myelia

Haponik et al.[91] reported a 35-year-old woman with obstructive sleep apnea resulting from autopsy proven syringobulbia-myelia. Their polygraphic study documented 370 upper airway obstructive apneic episodes lasting from 10 to 170 seconds accompanied by hypoxemia and hypercapnia during seven hours of non-REM stages I and II. Repeat study with nasopharyngeal airway in place documented no apneic episodes or hypoxemia but repetitive obstructive apneas returned when the airway was removed. Nine months later the patient died and neuropathological examination revealed a syrinx extending from the lower third of the medulla to the upper thoracic spinal cord involving the left hypoglossal nucleus and nucleus ambiguus. These authors mentioned several cases from the literature of syringobulbia-myelia causing respiratory disorders, such as alveolar hypoventilation and sleep related stridor, irregular breathing, snoring, and apneas.

Western Equine Encephalitis

Cohn and Kuida[92] described a 43-year-old man who had excessive somnolence, periods of apnea and cyanosis during sleep, and subnormal ventilatory response to CO_2 10 months after western equine encephalitis that was diagnosed on the basis of high convalescent serum titre (1:128) of neutralizing antibodies. The respiratory center was presumably damaged by the virus.

Carotid Endarterectomy

Beamish and Wildsmith[95] reported a 57-year-old woman who developed periodic breathing, apnea, and cyanosis after carotid endarterectomy. Verbal or physical stimuli would restore her ventilation. The authors suggested that midbrain hypoxia and edema led to respiratory depression.

Arnold-Chiari Malformation

Bokinsky et al.[96] described an 18-year-old man with Arnold-Chiari malformation and syringomyelia associated with dysfunction of the ninth, tenth, and twelfth cranial nerves. The patient had an absent hypoxic ventilatory but normal hypercapnic ventilatory response. These observations were consistent with bilateral ninth cranial nerve dysfunction. Campbell[97] previously described two patients of Arnold-Chiari malformation associated with profound hypoventilation.

SPINAL CORD

The neural systems subserving the dual respiratory control mechanism (voluntary or behavioral, and involuntary or metabolic) descend in the spinal cord via corticospinal and reticulospinal tracts respectively and the two systems are integrated in the spinal cord.[6,33,35,36,44] The voluntary respiratory control system is found in the dorsolateral and the descending involuntary pathway in the ventrolateral quadrant of the cervical spinal cord.[33,36] These pathways ultimately control the spinal respiratory motoneurons that send impulses along the phrenic and intercostal nerves to the principal respiratory muscles. The phrenic nerve originates from anterior horn cells in the cervical spinal cord segments three, four, and five and intercostal nerves arise from the anterior horn cells in the thoracic spinal cord. In the spinal cord, therefore, the voluntary and involuntary controlling systems could be separately affected by local lesions, for example transection of either the dorsolateral or the ventrolateral quadrant of the spinal cord.[36] Most published reports of such lesions refer to transection of the ventrolateral tracts causing impairment of the metabolic but not the voluntary control system. Respiratory dysfunction may also arise from involvement of lower motor respiratory neurons either in the anterior horn or in the phrenic and intercostal nerves. From a literature survey Krieger and Rosomoff[98] identified three patterns of respiratory dysfunction: (1) impairment of efferent motor mechanism resulting in reduced vital capacity (e.g., phrenic paralysis causing diaphragmatic weakness); (2) attenuation of CO_2 response with normal vital capacity and without significant chest wall or diaphragmatic weakness; and (3) a mixture of the two showing a decrease in CO_2 and reduced vital capacity. The causative lesions may include anterolateral cordotomy, trauma, motoneuron disease, syringomyelia, and myelitis.

Spinal Surgery

Belmusto et al.[99] described a patient with a bilateral high cervical cordotomy for intractable pain followed later by ineffective breathing during sleep necessitating assisted ventilation. These authors concluded that damage to the reticulospinal tracts was responsible for breathing difficulty. Sleep apnea following cordotomy has also been described by Tenicela et al.[100] and by Krieger and Rosomoff.[98] The latter authors reported 10 patients who had sleep apnea after bilateral percutaneous cervical cordotomy. In most cases respiratory dysfunction occurred within 24 to 48 hours and the ventilatory response to CO_2 was attenuated. In addition, they had a variety of autonomic dysfunctions including orthostatic hypotension. The syndrome lasted from 3 to 32 days in the surviving patients; two patients died during sleep. Respiration during sleep was irregular in rate and depth and there were intermittent apneic pauses, but when the patients were awakened, normal breathing resumed. The authors[98] concluded that in their patients the ascending reticular fibers in the ventrolateral segment of the spinal cord relaying afferent impulses to the respiratory center had been damaged. However, the most plausible explanation in their patients would be selective damage to the descending metabolic respiratory fibers in the ventrolateral quadrant to the spinal cord giving rise to a form of Ondine's curse.

Krieger and Rosomoff[101] described sleep apnea in two other patients immediately after anterior spinal surgery at the C_{3-4} interspace. The patients required assisted ventilation at night for several days but then subsequently improved. They had reduced ventilatory responses to CO_2 and reduced vital capacity. It should be noted that Krieger and Rosomoff[98,101] did not document the type of apnea in their patients.

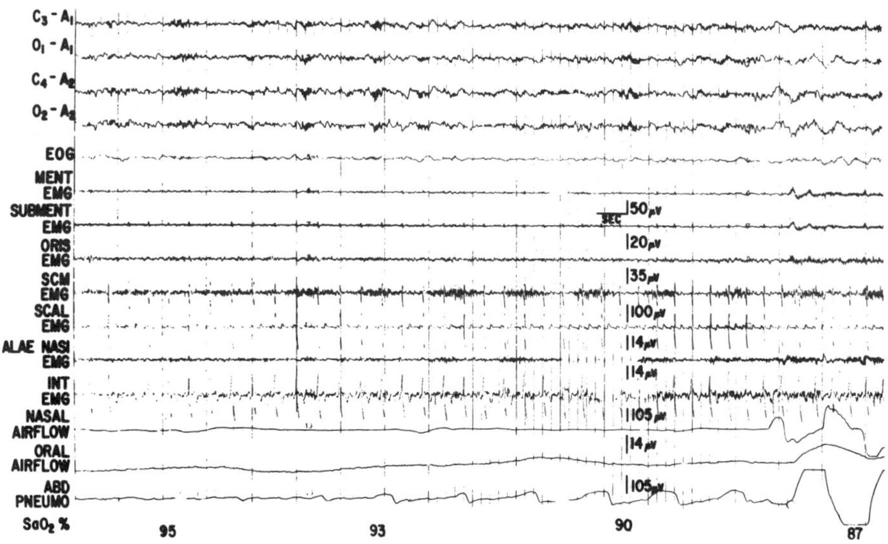

Fig. 12-5 Mixed apnea in non-REM sleep stage II in a patient with amyotrophic lateral sclerosis.

Trauma

Guilleminault[50] described cases with sleep apnea and hypoxemia after neck trauma without fracture. Severe whiplash injury or odontoid fracture that may cause mild compression of the lower medulla and upper cervical spinal cord may cause respiratory problems during sleep. Their eight cases with neck trauma had excessive daytime somnolence. The long-term prognosis of these patients is variable and some may require tracheostomy.

Motoneuron Disease

In motoneuron disease, such as amyotrophic lateral sclerosis, respiratory failure usually occurs late but may be a presenting feature[102] occasionally requiring mechanical ventilation. Motoneuron disease is characterized by progressive degeneration of the anterior horn cells of the spinal cord and the bulbar nuclei and upper motoneurons giving rise to a combination of lower motoneuron and upper motoneuron signs including bulbar and pseudobulbar palsy in middle aged and elderly individuals. The condition shows a relentless progression without impairment of sensation or mental function. Involvement of the phrenic and intercostal nerve nuclei in the cervical and thoracic spinal cord motoneurons may give rise to paralysis of the diaphragm and intercostal muscles, which may lead to alveolar hypoventilation.

Diaphragmatic paralysis in motoneuron disease can be a presenting feature as reported in two women by Parhad et al.[102] Thorpy et al.[103] described a 52-

year-old man complaining of nocturnal respiratory difficulties and progressive daytime somnolence for 10 years. A polysomnographic study documented sleep-induced nonobstructive hypoventilation associated with oxygen desaturation. A diagnosis of adult-onset spinal muscular atrophy with diaphragmatic paralysis was made based on the clinical and laboratory tests. Assisted respiration at night improved oxygen saturation and relieved the symptoms of hypersomnolence and daytime ventilation. Newsom Davis et al.[104] also described diaphragmatic weakness in eight patients with peripheral motor system disorder, one of whom had the Kugelberg-Wellander syndrome, a variant of juvenile type of motonueron disease. The patients with diaphragmatic paralysis usually have hypoxemia, hypercapnia, and progressive breathlessness. A diagnosis of diaphragmatic paralysis may be based on the following features: (1) symptoms of alveolar hypoventilation and breathlessness; (2) physical findings of a paradoxical inward movement of the abdomen with epigastric retraction instead of protrusion during inspiration; (3) chest X-ray showing an elevated diaphragm and paradoxical movement or decreased excursion of the diaphragm on fluoroscopy; (4) demonstration of a lack of change in transdiaphragmatic pressure during a maximum inspiration (this is the most sensitive test); (5) diaphragmatic EMG findings; (6) respiratory function tests; (7) measurement of blood gases; and (8) a polysomnographic study to document sleep apnea.

Theoretically with bulbar involvement in motoneuron disease there may be impairment of ventilatory regulation caused by medullary dysfunction. Such a suggestion was made by Serpick et al.[105] in a report describing a patient with motoneuron disease who had hypersomnolence, periodic breathing, hypercapnia, and hypoxia. The present writer briefly reported sleep-related respiratory dysrhythmia in two patients with motoneuron disease[106] and has seen several cases since then with sleep apnea (unpublished observations). Polysomnographic study showed both central and upper airway obstructive apneas (Fig. 12-5). These findings may have resulted from a combination of pharyngeal and respiratory muscle weakness and possible involvement of the respiratory motoneurons in the medulla.

POLYNEUROPATHIES

Peripheral neuropathies or polyneuropathies are characterized by bilaterally symmetrical and distal sensorimotor dysfunction affecting often the legs more than the arms and caused by a variety of lesions both heredofamilial and acquired. Polyneuropathies affecting the phrenic and intercostal and other nerves supplying the accessory muscles of respiration may cause weakness of the diaphragm, intercostal and accessory muscles of respiration giving rise to exertional dyspnea, hypoxia and hypercapnia.[107]

Phrenic neuropathy may result from trauma, inflammatory processes (e.g., as part of polyneuropathy), and infiltrative lesions (e.g., neoplasms). The Landry-Guillain-Barre-Strohl syndrome or acute inflammatory polyradiculoneuropathy[107] is probably the most common polyneuropathy to cause respiratory dysfunction. The condition is characterized by predominantly motor manifestation and is associated with rapidly progressive ascending paralysis beginning in the legs with the maximal manifestations completed in 2 to 3 weeks. Severe respiratory involvement has been reported in about 20 percent of cases and the critical period is usually during the first 3 weeks of illness. Early recognition and treatment are important.

Phrenic neuropathy may also result from *varicella zoster* virus infection of the phrenic or as part of a predominantly motor peripheral neuropathy in diphtheritic neuropathy.[107] Goldstein et al.[108] described a 57-year-old man with hypoventilation that was thought to have resulted from medullary insensitivity, but postmortem examination disclosed a peripheral neuropathy with severe involvement of the phrenic nerves.

Cranial neuropathy involving the glossopharyngeal and vagal nerves bilaterally may cause respiratory dysfunction. A case of Arnold-Chiari malformation associated with bilateral ninth cranial nerve dysfunction[96] has already been discussed.

PRIMARY MUSCLE DISORDERS

Primary muscle disorders or myopathies include a group of diseases characterized by weakness and wasting of the muscles due to a defect either in the muscle membrane or the contractile elements that is not secondary to a structural or functional derangement of the lower or upper motoneurons. The patients present with symmetrical proximal muscle weakness in the upper and/or lower limbs without sensory impairment or fasciculations. The etiological conditions include heredofamilial muscular dystrophies with or without myotonia, congenital nonprogressive myopathies with distinct morphological characteristics, and various metabolic and nonfamilial inflammatory and noninflammatory myopathies. Breathing disorders in sleep or worsening of breathing dysfunction in sleep occur in some of these conditions. A survey of the literature reveals that despite frequent involvement of the respiratory muscles in patients with primary muscle disease, a small number of them present with respiratory failure.[109–120] Breathing disorders causing hypoventilation in sleep in many of these disorders may be related to the following factors: (1) impaired chest bellows due to weakness of the respiratory and chest wall muscles; (2) increased work of breathing; and (3) functional alterations of the medullary respiratory neurons. The latter may be due to hyporesponsive or unresponsive chemoreceptors that could be secondarily acquired.[110] CO_2 hyposensitivity may also be related to an altered afferent input from skeletal muscle receptors.[111] It is important to diagnose alveolar hypoventilation in these patients to prevent fatal or dangerous hypoventilation during sleep or during administration of drugs, general anesthesia, and respiratory infections. The patients may complain of breathlessness and daytime hypersomnolence in addition to the primary complaints related to the muscle disorder.

Myotonic Myopathies

Myotonic dystrophy is an adult onset dominantly inherited muscular dystrophy associated with myotonia. Benaim and Worster-Drought[114] were probably the first to describe alveolar hypoventilation in this condition. Alveolar hypoventilation associated with hypoxemia, hypercapnia, and impaired hypercapnic and hypoxic ventilatory responses may be present both in the early and late stages of the illness. Polygraphic studies, reported by a few authors,[115,116,117] showed sleep apnea (central, mixed, and upper airway obstructive apnea) and sleep-onset REM in some patients. The latter may have been related to sleep deprivation secondary to the respiratory disturbances in sleep.[116] Sleep-related respiratory dysrhythmias in this condition may have resulted from two fundamental mechanisms:[116,118] (1) weakness and myotonia of the respiratory and pharyngoesophageal muscles and (2) an abnormality of the central control of ventilation, which may be related to a common generalized membrane abnormality of the muscle and other tissues including brain stem neurons regulating sleeping and breathing.

Striano et al.[113] described sleep apnea (predominantly obstructive) with daytime hypersomnolence in a patient with myotonia congenita. The family history indicated a dominant mode of inheritance. However, in view of the presence of obesity and spirometric evidence of obstructive pulmonary disease, the relationship between sleep apnea and myotonia congenita remains questionable.

Acid Maltase Deficiency

Several cases of mild to moderate proximal myopathy associated with adult onset acid maltase deficiency,[104,109,110,119,120] a variant of glycogen storage disease, had presented with alveolar hypoventilation. Correct diagnosis can be established on the basis of respiratory function tests, electromyography, and histochemical and biochemical studies of muscle biopsy samples. These patients may show hypoxemia, hypercapnia, and impaired hypercapnic ventilatory response. Alveolar hypoventilation may be due to diaphragmatic dysfunction. Rosenow and Engel[109] suggested that the hypoxemia in their patients was secondary to a combination of hypoventilation due to muscle weakness and an impaired ventilation-perfusion ratio resulting from compression atelectasis due to elevation of the diaphragm. A polygraphic study in the patient described by Martin et al.[120] showed prolonged periods of hypopneic breathing accompanied by significant oxygen desaturation. Following inspiratory muscle training the patient improved considerably. He was able to sleep flat and no longer required nocturnal oxygen. The repeat polysomnographic study showed marked improvement in the respiratory pattern and oxygen saturation.

Other Congenital Myopathies

Riley et al.[111] described two patients with congenital myopathies (one with nemaline myopathy and the other with a myopathy of uncertain type) who presented with progressive breathlessness and lethargy. The patients' ventilatory response to CO_2 was absent and after initial treatment ventilation during wakefulness was normal but decreased significantly during sleep if ventilatory assistance was not provided. They suggested that the alveolar hypoventilation may have resulted from a primary defect in the central chemoreceptor control of breathing. They further suggested that the sensory stimuli from skeletal muscle receptors (e.g., muscle spindles) may have played a role in the blunted ventilatory response to CO_2 by altering afferent input to the central nervous system.

NEUROMUSCULAR JUNCTIONAL DISORDER

Neuromuscular junctional disorders, such as, myasthenia gravis, botulism, and tick paralysis are characterized by easy fatigue of the muscles including the bulbar and other respiratory muscles due to failure of neuromuscular junctional transmission of nerve impulses. The most important of these conditions is myasthenia gravis, which is an autoimmune disease characterized by reduction of the number of functional acetylcholine receptors in the postjunctional region. Acute respiratory failure is often a dreaded complication of myasthenia gravis and the patient needs assisted ventilation for life support. The respiratory failure may be mild during wakefulness but may be worse during sleep.

Botulism caused by *Clostridium botulinum* and tick paralysis caused by female wood tick *Dermacentor andersoni* may cause neuromuscular junctional transmission defect due to released toxin and giving rise to widespread muscle weakness including respiratory muscles that may require mechanically assisted ventilation.

MISCELLANEOUS NEUROLOGICAL DISORDERS

Sleep-related respiratory dysrhythmias have been associated with the Shy-Drager syndrome, narcolepsy, and primary alveolar hypoventilation syndrome. These three groups of disorders do not result from a lesion in one level of the nervous system and in some the site of the lesion remains undetermined.

The Shy-Drager Syndrome

The Shy-Drager syndrome[121,122] is a multisystem neurodegenerative disease characterized by severe dysautonomic manifestations and somatic features involving the extrapyramidal, cerebellar, and pyramidal systems in varying combinations. Pathological findings resemble those noted in olivopontocerebellar atrophy and striatonigral degeneration. The pathological lesions involve several structures in the brain stem including the reticular formation, nucleus ambiguus, and nucleus tractus solitarius. In the Shy-Drager syndrome there have been several reports of respiratory dysrhythmias, mostly during sleep.[41,123–131] The following respiratory patterns have been noted: (1) central, upper airway obstructive, and mixed apneas in non-REM and REM sleep associated with oxygen desaturation; (2) irregularities in rate, rhythm, and amplitude of respiration with and without oxygen desaturation, becoming worse in sleep; (3) transient occlusion of the upper airway or episodic uncoupling of the intercostal and diaphragmatic muscle activity as evidence by occasional paradoxical movement of the rib cage and the abdomen without oxygen desaturation; (4) prolonged periods of central apnea accompanied by oxygen desaturation in relaxed wakefulness as if the respiratory center "forgot" to breathe; (5) a pattern of periodic breathing during non-REM sleep stages I to III resembling Cheyne-Stokes respiration similar to that noted in some normal elderly individuals during stage I non-REM sleep without oxygen desaturation; (6) Cheyne-Stokes and Cheyene-Stokes variant breathing, which becomes worse in sleep; (7) periodic breathing in the erect posture accompanied by postural fall of blood pressure; (8) apneustic-like breathing; (9) transient sudden respiratory arrest.

Lockwood[124] described a 54-year-old man with the Shy-Drager syndrome who had cluster breathing indicating pontomedullary respiratory center damage but with a normal CO_2 response curve. The respiration, recorded by a thermistor showed cluster breathing with periods of apnea of up to 20 seconds duration in wakefulness but prolonged apneas lasting up to 40 seconds during sleep. The patient stopped breathing one night and died. Neuropathological findings showed gliosis in the pontine tegmentum and medulla severely involving the reticular formation in addition to the widespread diffuse lesion typical of the Shy-Drager syndrome. The author suggested that the presence of this pattern of respiratory rhythm without an impaired ventilatory response to CO_2 indicated that neurons responsible for respiratory rhythm functioned independently from the medullary chemoreceptors controlling the ventilation.

Israel and Marino,[126] Williams et al.,[129] Bannister et al.,[130] and Guilleminault et al.[131] described upper airway obstructive sleep apnea associated with vocal cord paresis in the Shy-Drager syndrome.

Chokroverty[106] described two patients with the Shy-Drager syndrome who had many periods of sleep-related obstructive, central, and mixed apneas accompanied by oxygen desaturation (Fig. 12-6). There was no evidence of vocal cord paralysis or obstructive lung disease. Chokroverty et al.[127] also described four patients with the Shy-Drager syndrome demonstrating periodic apnea in the erect position. One of these patients also had Cheyne-Stokes respiration during the late stage of the illness that was worse during sleep. In one patient, the necropsy findings of neuronal loss and astrocytosis in the pontine tegmentum suggested dysfunctional respiratory neurons in the brain stem.

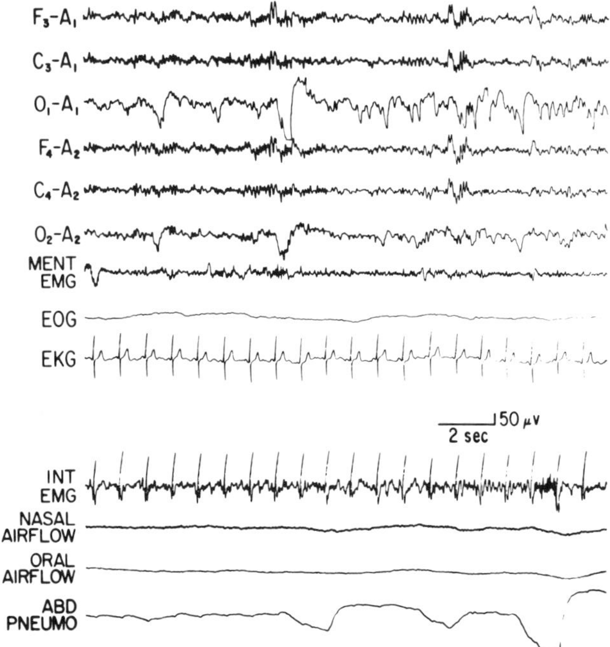

Fig. 12-6 Mixed apnea in non-REM sleep stage II in a patient with the Shy-Drager syndrome.

Briskin et al.[128] described three patients with Shy-Drager syndrome. Polysomnographic studies documented many episodes of sleep apneas with a mean apnea index of 75 to 79 in two of these patients. More than 70 percent of the apneic episodes were obstructive in nature. All three patients ultimately died of respiratory arrest during sleep.

Bannister and Oppenheimer[123] reported periodic inspiratory gasps resembling apneustic breathing in two patients with the Shy-Drager syndrome.

Castaigne et al.[125] described a 65-year-old man with the Shy-Drager syndrome who had alveolar hypoventilation, many episodes of apnea and probably apneustic breathing 4 years after the onset of the illness. The postmortem findings included degenerative lesion in the substantia nigra, pontine nuclei, locus ceruleus, and intermediolateral column of the spinal cord.

McNicholas et al.[41] described three patients with autonomic nervous system dysfunction (two patients with the Shy-Drager syndrome and one with familial dysautonomia) who had no respiratory or sleep-related symptoms. All subjects had overnight polysomnographic studies in the sleep laboratory. The ventilatory response to hypoxia and hypercapnia in their patients suggested a defect in the metabolic control system. During sleep the patients did not have oxygen desaturation, but their pattern of breathing was highly irregular and coefficients of variation of respiratory variables were significantly greater than normal. During sleep the patient with Shy-Drager syndrome had a total of 61 to 79 apneic episodes during non-REM stages I and II but without oxygen desaturation. The patient with familial dysautonomia had only 11 apneic periods during the night. These apneic periods were mostly central, but occasionally there was evidence of transient occlusion of the upper airway or transient uncoupling of the intercostal and diaphragmatic muscle activities. However, the most striking abnormality was an irregular pattern of breathing during sleep. The authors suggested that the findings during sleep and wakefulness in their patients suggested a defect in the automatic respiratory rhythm generator of the brain stem.

Narcolepsy-Cataplexy Syndrome with Sleep Apnea

The syndrome of narcolepsy is characterized by an irresistible desire to fall asleep at inappropriate times lasting for a few seconds to as long as 20 to 30 minutes. Sleep attacks are often accompanied by cataplexy, a term denoting transient paralysis of somatic muscles during emotional outbursts without loss of consciousness. The patient may momentarily fall to the ground or his head may simply drop forward for a few seconds. Other manifestations include episodes of sleep paralysis and hypnagogic hallucinations. Sleep paralysis is characterized by an apparent loss of voluntary power on falling to sleep (hypnagogic) or on waking up from sleep (hypnopompic). The hypnagogic manifestations are vivid and often terrifying dreams that are mostly visual but may be auditory, vestibular, or somatic. These four manifestations are traditionally thought to constitute the narcoleptic tetrad but disturbed night sleep is common symptom and, therefore, all five features should be grouped together as clinical pentad in narcolepsy. Narcolepsy is a life-long condition, usually beginning in adolescent or young adult life and becoming generally less severe with advancing years. In a small percentage of cases there may be a family history of similar illness. The pathogenesis of the narcolepsy syndrome is not known. It appears to result from a disturbed relationship between non-REM and REM sleep mechanisms. In some narcoleptic patients sleep apnea has been noted.

Guilleminault et al.[132] reported two patients with pure narcolepsy presenting with central sleep apneas of 20 to 90 seconds duration in both REM and non-REM sleep accompanied by oxygen desaturation. Guilleminault et al.[49] later described several cases with sleep apnea. The apneas were predominantly central but five cases had mixed and obstructive apneas. The authors concluded that central apnea implied that the basic phenomenon in this syndrome was the dysfunction of central nervous system structures controlling the sleep and respiratory centers.

Laffont et al.[133] polygraphically studied 18 narcoleptic patients diagnosed on the basis of sleep attacks and cataplexy. Five patients had frequent sleep-related respiratory arrhythmias (central, obstructive, and mixed apneas).

Polygraphic studies by Chokroverty[134] in 16 patients with the narcolepsy

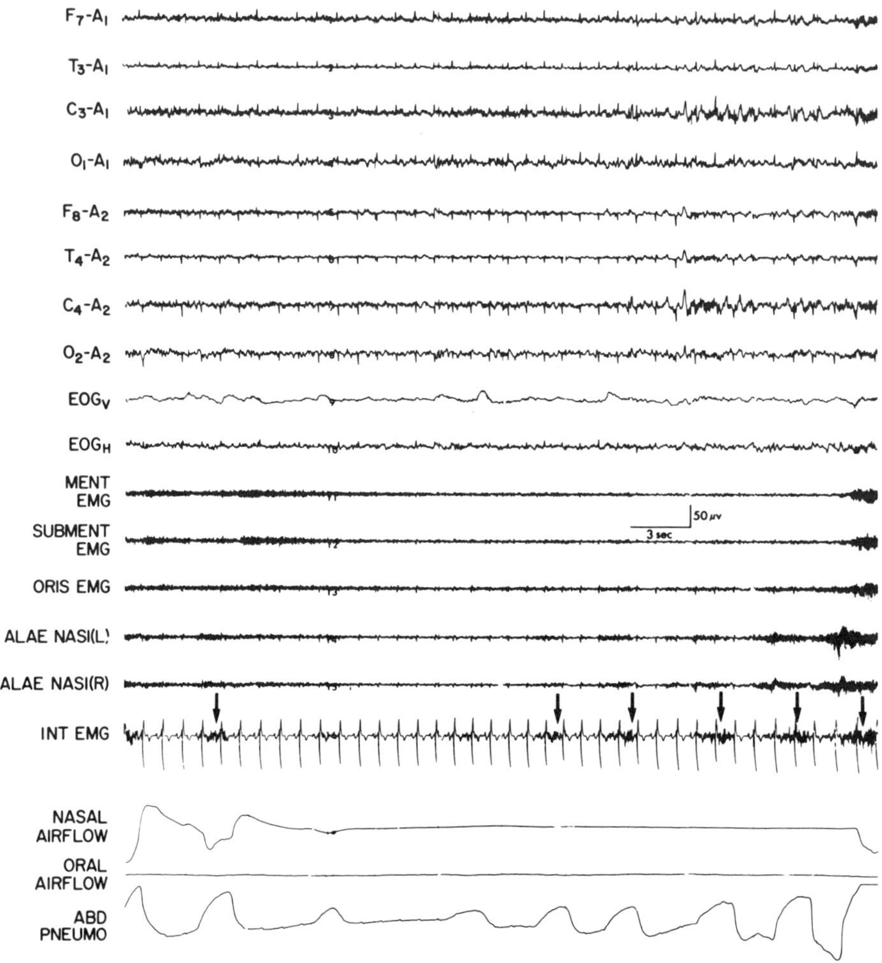

Fig. 12-7 Polygraphic tracing showing mixed apnea in non-REM stage II sleep in a patient with narcolepsy syndrome.

syndrome documented central apneas in 11 and upper airway obstructive apneas in five patients during non-REM and REM sleep associated with oxygen desaturation (Fig. 12-7).

Primary Alveolar Hypoventilation

Primary alveolar hypoventilation[135] is a syndrome of failure of automatic respiration in which there is no recognizable disorder of the central or peripheral nervous system. Reichel[135] distinguishes central alveolar hypoventilation from primary alveolar hypoventilation on the basis of an association of a specific organic neurological disease in central alveolar hypoventilation. The reported cases of primary alveolar hypoventilation had no evidence of central nervous system disease and occasional postmortem reports showed no central nervous structural lesions or nonspecific findings in the form of gliosis or mild neuronal loss in the medulla. The hallmark of primary alveolar hypoventilation is the combination of arterial hypercapnia and hypoxemia which worsens during sleep.[136,137] Other features include sleep apnea, congestive cardiac failure, pulmonary hypertension, and polycythemia. Apnea is usually central in type but upper airway obstruction may be associated in some cases. An impaired ventilatory response to CO_2 is characteristic of this condition. The etiology is unknown but there is circumstantial evidence that dysfunction of the medullary chemoreceptors is responsible. Reichel[135] stated that the distinction between sleep apnea and primary hypoventilation syndrome is not clear. However, in the sleep apnea syndrome CO_2 and hypoxic responses are usually normal. The pathological basis for primary alveolar hypoventilation giving rise to Ondine's curse remains unknown.

TREATMENT OF SLEEP-RELATED RESPIRATORY DYSRHYTHMIAS

In many neurological disorders sleep-related respiratory problems remain undiagnosed. Thus the first step is important to be aware of the potential problems and perform appropriate diagnostic studies. The patients must, of course, receive specific treatment for the particular neurological illness. Respiratory dysfunction occurring during wakefulness and becoming worse in sleep can be treated by assisted ventilation. Hypoventilation occurring during sleep or worsening during sleep has been treated by various other measures including medical and surgical intervention.[40,51,94,103,135,139–147] All patients must avoid alcohol and sedative-hypnotic drugs that may further depress the respiratory center. The role of alcohol aggravating sleep apnea is well established but the mechanism is not known. One recent suggestion[141] has been that alcohol selectively depresses genioglossal muscle activity promoting obstructive apnea.

The treatment of respiratory dysrhythmias occurring during sleep may be divided broadly into three groups. These are indicated briefly here and considered in more detail elsewhere in this volume.

Pharmacologic Treatment

Treatment can be directed toward increasing the respiratory center motor output to overcome the dysfunctional central respiratory neurons causing sleep-related hypoventilation. Progesterone or medroxyprogesterone, theophylline, aminophylline, nikethemide, lobeline, doxapram, protriptylline, clomimipramine, actazolamide, and pemoline have all been used with varying degrees of success in patients with central and obstructive sleep apneas. These drugs have reduced the apneic episodes and improved sleep architecture. The most commonly used have been protriptylline, theophylline, pemoline, and progesterone with only Protriptylline and medroxyprogesterone having been useful in several cases of obstructive apnea.

Neuromechanical Measures

The use of a rocking bed or assisted ventilation during sleep, particularly the latter has been helpful in many cases of sleep-related hypoventilation. Artificial ventilation using positive pressure respiration with tracheostomy or negative pressure respiration with a cuirass or tank respirator has been successful in several cases of respiratory dysrhythmias in wakefulness and in sleep.

Recently, continuous positive airway pressure[142,143] delivered through the nose has been shown to cause improvement in patients with obstructive sleep apnea.

Surgical Treatment

Electrophrenic respiration[139] has been studied most extensively by Glenn et al.[139] Primary alveolar hypoventilation has been most successfully treated by use of this form of treatment. The patients had been treated for 8 to 9 hours each night with improvement in ventilation and oxygenation. Superimposed obstructive sleep apnea may complicate the procedure and may then require both electrophrenic respiration and tracheostomy for treatment. Sarnoff et al.[87] first used electrophrenic stimulation in patients with poliomyelitis in 1951. Earlier in 1948[144] they demonstrated its effectiveness in animals. However, technical difficulties at that time prevented its regular use. Glenn et al.[139] improved the technique and they have shown that the electrodes could be implanted in the phrenic nerve to stimulate it intermittently for a long period without damage to the nerve. Glenn et al. have used diaphragm pacing in four groups of patients: (1) patients with high cervical cord lesions; (2) those with respiratory center involvement either directly or through interruption of the afferent or efferent neurons to the respiratory center; (3) patients with chronic obstructive pulmonary disease; and (4) patients with central or primary alveolar hypoventilation syndrome.

Tracheostomy. Tracheostomy remains the most definitive treatment for patients with predominantly obstructive sleep apnea. Because of aesthetic and psychosocial reasons many patients refuse this form of treatment and there are no generally acceptable criteria for tracheostomy in patients with predominantly obstructive sleep apnea syndrome. Guilleminault et al.[145] proposed the following indications: severe disability caused by excessive daytime somnolence; dangerous cardiac arrhythmias; apnea index of more than 60; extensive oxygen desaturation during sleep (less than 40 percent); and failure of medical treatment. This form of treatment will dramatically improve the symptoms and improve ventilation and oxygen saturation.

Other surgical treatment that has been used in obstructive sleep apnea included uvulopalatopharyngoplasty and hyoid bone resection.[146,147]

CONCLUSION

The mysteries of sleeping and breathing are beginning to be unravelled since the discovery by Legallois[148] in 1812 that breathing depended upon a circumscribed region of the medulla and the description of sleep by Macnish[149] in 1830 as suspension of sensorial power in which the voluntary functions are in abeyance but the involuntary power, such as circulation or respiration remains intact. Despite the recent explosive growth in the literature dealing with sleep apnea and alterations of breathing in sleep the neurological literature mentions only isolated and brief references to these topics. It is anticipated that future research will be directed toward the role of specific neurotransmitter systems in the various neurological disorders. This may expand the possibility of pharmacologic management of potentially life threatening sleep-related breathing disorders in neurological disease.

ACKNOWLEDGMENT

The author wishes to thank Roger C. Duvoisin, M.D., for reviewing the manuscript and Lena DiMauro for typing it.

REFERENCES

1. Heyman A, Birchfield RI, Sieker HO: Effects of bilateral cerebral infarction on respiratory center sensitivity. Neurology 8:694, 1958
2. Plum F, Swanson AG: Abnormalities in central regulation of respiration in acute and convalescent poliomyelitis. Arch Neurol Psychiat 80:267, 1958
3. Plum F, Brown HW, Snoep E: Neurologic significance of post-hyperventilation apnea. J Am Med Assoc 181:1050, 1962
4. Plum F, Brown HW: The effect of respiration of central nervous system disease. Ann NY Acad Sci 109:915, 1963
5. Plum F: Breathlessness in neurological disease: The effects of neurological disease on the act of breathing. p. 203. In Howell JBL, Campbell EJM (eds): Breathlessness. Blackwell Scientific Publications, Oxford, 1966
6. Plum F: Neurological integration of behavioral and metabolic control of breathing. p. 159. In Porter R (ed): Ciba Foundation Symposium on Breathing: Hering-Breuer Centenary Symposium. J & A Churchill, London, 1970
7. North JB, Jennett S: Impedence pneumography for the detection of abnormal breathing patterns associated with brain damage. Lancet 2:212, 1972
8. Lee MC, Klassen AC, Resch JA: Respiratory pattern disturbances in ischemic cerebral vascular disease. Stroke 5:612, 1974

9. North JB, Jennett S: Abnormal breathing patterns associated with acute brain damage. Arch Neurol 31:338, 1974
10. Lee MC, Klassen AC, Heaney LM, Resch JA: Respiratory rate and pattern disturbances in acute brain stem infarction. Stroke 7:382, 1976
11. Plum F, Posner JB: The pathologic physiology of signs and symptoms of coma. p. 32. In Plum F, Posner JB (eds): The Diagnosis of Stupor and Coma. FA Davis Company, Philadelphia, 1980
12. Guilleminault C, Motta J: Sleep apnea syndrome as a long-term sequela of poliomyelitis. p. 309. In Guilleminault C, Dement WC (eds): Sleep Apnea Syndromes. Alan R. Liss, New York, 1978
13. Rechtschaffen A, Kales A: A Manual of Standardized Terminology, Techniques and Scoring System for Sleep Stages of Human Subjects. Brain information service/Brain Research Institute, University of California at Los Angeles, 1968.
14. Williams RL, Karacan I, Hursch CJ: Electroencephalography (EEG) of Human Sleep Clinical Applications. John Wiley & Sons, New York, 1974
15. Orem JM: Sleep. p. 519. In Rosenberg RN (ed): The Clinical Neurosciences: Neurobiology. Churchill Livingstone, New York, 1983
16. Pompeiano O: The neurophysiological mechanisms of the postural and motor events during desynchronized sleep. Res Publ Assoc Res Nerv Ment Dis 45:351, 1967
17. Pessah MA, Roffwarg HP: Spontaneous middle ear muscle activity in man: A rapid eye movement sleep phenomenon. Science 178:773, 1972
18. Chokroverty S: Phasic tongue movements in human rapid-eye-movement sleep. Neurology 30:665, 1980
19. Bremer F: Cerveau "isole" et physiologie du sommeil. CR Soc Biol (Paris) 118:1235, 1935
20. Bremer F: Cerebral hypnogenic centers. Ann Neurol 2:1, 1977
21. Moruzzi G, Magoun HW: Brain stem reticular formation and activation of the EEG. Electroencephalogr Clin Neurophysiol 1:455, 1949
22. Moruzzi G: The sleep waking cycle. Ergeb Physiol 64:1, 1972
23. Hess WR: Das Schlafsyndrom als Folge dienzephaler Reizung. Helv Physiol Pharmacol Acta 2:305, 1944
24. Von Economo C: Die Pathologie des Schlafes. p. 591. In Bethe A, Bergmann G, Embden G (eds): Handbuch der normalen und pathologischen Physiologie, Springer Verlag, Berlin, 1926
25. Batini C, Magni F, Palestini M et al: Neural mechanisms underlying the enduring EEG and behavioral activation in the mid-pontine pretrigeminal cat. Arch Ital Biol 97:13, 1959
26. Batini C, Moruzzi G, Palestini M et al: Effects of complete pontine transections on the sleep-wakefulness rhythm: the mid-pontine pretrigeminal preparation. Arch Ital Biol 97:1, 1959
27. Jouvet M: The role of monoamines and acetylcholine containing neurons in the regulation of the sleep-waking cycle. Ergeb Physiol 64:166, 1972
28. Nauta WJH: Hypothalamic regulation of sleep in rats: Experimental study. J Neurophysiol 9:285, 1946
29. Hobson JA, McCarley RW, Wyzinski PW: Sleep cycle oscillation: Reciprocal discharge by two brain stem neuronal groups. Science 189:55, 1975
30. Hauri P: The Sleep Disorders. The Upjohn Company, Kalamazoo, Michigan, 1977
31. Jouvet M: Biogenic amines and the state of sleep. Science 163:32, 1969

32. Wyatt RJ, Gillin JC: Biochemistry and human sleep. p. 239. In Williams RL, Karacan I (eds): Pharmacology of Sleep. John Wiley & Sons, New York, 1976
33. Nathan PW: The descending respiratory pathway in man. J Neurol Neurosurg Psychiat 26:487, 1963
34. Mitchell RA, Berger AJ: Neural regulation of respiration. Am Rev Resp Dis 111:206, 1975
35. Berger AJ, Mitchell RA, Severinghaus JW: Regulation of respiration. New Eng J Med 297:92, 138, 194, 1977
36. Mitchell RA: Neural regulation of respiration. Clin Chest Med 1:3, 1980
37. Phillipson EA: Control of breathing during sleep. Am Rev Resp Dis 118:909, 1978
38. Phillipson EA: Respiratory adaptations in sleep. Ann Rev Physiol 40:133, 1978
39. Sullivan CE: Breathing in sleep. p. 213. In Orem J, Barnes CD (eds): Physiology in Sleep. Academic Press, New York, 1980
40. Nauseida PA, Weber S: Sleep-related respiratory disorders. p. 285. In Weiner WJ (ed): Respiratory Dysfunction in Neurologic Disease. Futura Publishing Company, Mount Kisco, New York, 1980
41. McNicholas WT, Rutherford R, Grossman R et al: Abnormal respiratory pattern generation during sleep in patients with autonomic dysfunction. Am Rev Resp Dis 128:429, 1983
42. Fink BR: Influence of cerebral activity in wakefulness on regulation of breathing. J Appl Physiol 16:15, 1961
43. Merrill EG: The lateral respiratory neurons of the medulla: Their associations with nucleus ambiguus, nucleus retroambigualis, the spinal accessory nucleus and the spinal cord. Brain Res 24:11, 1970
44. Newsom Davis J: Control of the muscles of breathing. p. 221. In Widdicombe JG (ed): Respiratory Physiology: MTP International Review of Science. Vol. 2. Butterworth Publishers, London, 1974
45. Bulow K, Ingvar DH: Respiration and state of wakefulness in normals, studied by spirography, capnography and EEG. Acta Physiol Scand 51:230, 1961
46. Bulow K: Respiration and wakefulness in man. Acta Physiol Scand 59 (Suppl 209):1, 1963
47. Cherniack N: Respiratory dysrhythmias during sleep. New Eng J Med 305:325, 1981
48. Duron B, Marlot D: Intercostal and diaphragmatic electrical activity during wakefulness and sleep in normal unrestrained adult cats. Sleep 3:269, 1980
49. Guilleminault C, Hoed JVD, Mitler MM: Clinical overview of the sleep apnea syndromes. p. 1. In Guilleminault C, Dement WC (eds): Sleep Apnea Syndromes. Alan R. Liss, New York, 1978
50. Guilleminault C: Sleep and breathing. p. 155. In Guilleminault C (ed): Sleeping and Waking Disorders: Indications and Techniques. Addison-Wesley Publishing Company, Menlo Park, California, 1982
51. Remmers JE, Anch AM, deGroot WJ: Respiratory disturbances during sleep. Clin Chest Med 1:57, 1980
52. Guilleminault C, Tilkian A, Dement WC: The sleep apnea syndromes. Ann Rev Med 27:465, 1976
53. Black LF, Hyatt RE: Maximal static respiratory pressures in generalized neuromuscular disease. Am Rev Respir Dis 103:641, 1971
54. Lopata M, Lourenco RV: Evaluation of respiratory control. Clin Chest Med 1:33, 1980

55. Sharp JT, Druz WS, Foster JR et al: Use of the respiratory magnetometer in diagnosis and classification of sleep apnea. Chest 77:350, 1980
56. Chokroverty S, Sharp JT: Primary sleep apnoea syndrome. J Neurol Neurosurg Psychiat 44:970, 1981
57. Markand ON, Kincaid JC, Pourmand RA et al: Electrophysiologic evaluation of diaphragm by transcutaneous phrenic nerve stimulation. Neurology 34:604, 1984
58. Stockard JJ, Stockard JE, Sharbrough FW: Brainstem auditory evoked potentials in neurology: Methodology, interpretation, clinical application. p. 370. In Aminoff MJ (ed): Electrodiagnosis. Churchill Livingstone, New York, 1980
59. Cracco RQ, Cracco JB, Anziska BJ: Somatosensory evoked potentials in man: Cerebral, subcortical, spinal and peripheral nerve potentials. Am J EEG Technol 19:59, 1979
60. Katzman R, Terry R: The Neurology of Aging. F. A. Davis Company, Philadelphia, 1983
61. Smallwood RG, Vitiello MV, Giblin EC, Prinz PN: Sleep apnea: Relationship to age, sex and Alzheimer's dementia. Sleep 6:16, 1983
62. Smirne S, Franceschi M, Bareggi S et al: Sleep apnea in Alzheimer's disease. p. 442. In Koella WP (ed): Sleep, 5th European Congress Sleep Research. Karger, Basel, 1980
63. Miles LE, Dement WC: Sleep and Aging. Sleep 3:119, 1980
64. Wyler AR, Weymuller EA: Epilepsy complicated by sleep apnea. Ann Neurol 9:403, 1981
65. Nelson DA, Ray CD: Respiratory arrest from seizure discharges in limbic system. Arch Neurol 19:199, 1968
66. Kaada BR: Cingulate, posterior orbital, anterior insular and temporal pole cortex. In Magoun H (ed): Handbook of Physiology: Neurophysiology. Vol. 2. American Physiological Society, Washington DC, 1960
67. Mier M: Mechanisms leading to hypoventilation in extrapyramidal disorders with special reference to Parkinson's disease. J Am Geriat Soc 15:230, 1967
68. Lilker ES, Woolf CR: Pulmonary functions in Parkinson syndrome. Can Med Assoc J 99:752, 1968
69. Weiner WJ, Klawans HL: Respiratory dysfunction in movement disorders. p. 15. In Weiner WJ (ed): Respiratory Dysfunction in Neurologic Disease, Futura Publishing Company, Mount Kisco, New York, 1980
70. Paulson GD, Tafrate RH: Some "minor" aspects of parkinsonism, especially pulmonary function. Neurology 20:14, 1970
71. Turner WA, Critchley M: Respiratory disorders in epidemic encephalitis. Brain 48:72, 1925
72. Krum R: The chronic respiratory disorder in postencephalitic parkinsonism. J Neurol Neurosurg Psychiat 31:393, 1968
73. Garlind T, Linderhold H: Hypoventilation syndrome in a case of chronic epidemic encephalitis. Acta Med Scan 102:333, 1958
74. Purdy A, Hohn A, Barnett HJM et al: Familial fatal parkinsonism with alveolar hypoventilation and mental depression. Ann Neurol 6:523, 1979
75. Streider DJ, Baker WG, Baringer JR, Kazemi H: Chronic hypoventilation of central origin: A case with encephalitis lethargica and Parkinson's syndrome. Am Rev Resp Dis 96:501, 1967
76. Casey DE, Rabins P: Tardive dyskinesia as a life-threatening illness. Am J Psychiat 135:486, 1978

77. Chokroverty S, Reddy A, Chandarana H, Khan A: Study of respiration and multiple muscle electromyograms in tardive dyskinesia. Trans Am Neurol Assoc 106:1, 1982
78. Lundberg D, Breese GR, Mueller RA: Dopaminergic interaction with the respiratory control system in the rat. Eur J Pharmacol 54:153, 1979
79. Nielsen AM, Bisgard GE: Dopaminergic modulation of respiratory timing mechanisms in carotid body-denervated dogs. Resp Physiol 53:71, 1983
80. Cuncillos JD, DeAndres I: Participation of the cerebellum in the regulation of the sleep-wakefulness cycle. Results in cerebellectomized cats. Electroenceph Clin Neurophysiol 53:549, 1982
81. Chokroverty S, Sachdeo R, Masdeu J: Autonomic dysfunction and sleep apnea in olivopontocerebellar degeneration. Arch Neurol (in press)
82. Oppenheimer DR: Diseases of the basal ganglia, cerebellum and motor neurons. p. 608. In Blackwood W, Corsellis JAN (eds): Greenfield's Neuropathology. Edward Arnold, London, 1976
83. Duvoisin RC, Chokroverty S, Lepore F, Nicklas W: Glutamate dehydrogenase deficiency in patients with olivopontocerebellar atrophy. Neurology 33:1322, 1983
84. Devereaux MW, Keane JR, Davis RL: Automatic respiratory failure associated with infarction of the medulla: Report of two cases with pathologic study of one. Arch Neurol 29:46, 1973
85. Levin BE, Margolis G: Acute failure of automatic respirations secondary to a unilateral brainstem infarct. Ann Neurol 1:583, 1977
86. Beal MF, Richardson, Jr EP, Brandstetter R et al: Localized brain stem ischemic damage and Ondine's curse after near-drowning. Neurology 33:717, 1983
87. Sarnoff SJ, Whittenberger JL, Affeldt JE: Hypoventilation syndrome in bulbar poliomyelitis. JAMA 147:30, 1951
88. Newsom Davis J: Autonomous breathing: Report of a case. Arch Neurol 40:480, 1974
89. Rizvi SS, Ishikawa S, Faling LJ et al: Defect in automatic respiration in a case of multiple sclerosis. Am J Med 56:433, 1974
90. Boor JW, Johnson RJ, Canales L, Dunn DP: Reversible paralysis of automatic respiration in multiple sclerosis. Arch Neurol 34:686, 1977
91. Haponik EF, Givens D, Angelo J: Syringobulbia-myelia with obstructive sleep apnea. Neurology 33:1046, 1983
92. Cohn JE, Kuida H: Primary alveolar hypoventilation associated with western equine encephalitis. Ann Int Med 56:633, 1962
93. Severinghaus JW, Mitchell RA: Ondine's curse—Failure of respiratory center automaticity while awake. Clin Res 10:122, 1962
94. Solliday NH, Gaensler EA, Schwaber R, Parker TF: Impaired central chemoreceptor function and chronic hypoventilation many years following poliomyelitis. Respiration 31:177, 1974
95. Beamish D, Wildsmith JAW: Ondine's curse after carotid endarterectomy. Br Med J 2:1607, 1978
96. Bokinsky GE, Hudson LD, Weil JV: Impaired peripheral chemosensitivity and acute respiratory failure in Arnold-Chiari malformation and syringomyelis. New Eng J Med 288:947, 1973
97. Campbell EJM: Respiratory failure. Br Med J 1:1451, 1965
98. Krieger AJ, Rosomoff HL: Sleep-induced apnea. Part 1: A respiratory and au-

tonomic dysfunction syndrome following bilateral percutaneous cervical cordotomy. J Neurosurg 40:168, 1974

99. Belmusto L, Woldring S, Owens, G: Localization and patterns of potentials of the respiratory pathway in the cervical spinal cord in the dog. J Neurosurg 22:277, 1965
100. Tenicela R, Rosomoff HL, Feist J et al: Pulmonary function following percutaneous cervical cordotomy. Anesthesiology 29:7, 1968
101. Krieger AJ, Rosomoff HL: Sleep-induced apnea. Part 2: Respiratory failure after anterior spinal surgery. J Neurosurg 39:181, 1974
102. Parhad IM, Clark AW, Barron KD, Staunton SB: Diaphragmatic paralysis in motor neuron disease. Report of two cases and a review of the literature. Neurology 28:18, 1978
103. Thorpy MJ, Schmidt-Nowara WW, Pollak C, Weitzman ED: Sleep-induced nonobstructive hypoventilation associated with diaphragmatic paralysis. Ann Neurol 12:308, 1982
104. Newsom Davis J, Goldman M, Loh L, Casson M: Diaphragm function and alveolar hypoventilation. Q J Med 45:87, 1976
105. Serpick AA, Baker EL, Woodward TE: Motor system disease. Arch Int Med 115:192, 1965
106. Chokroverty S: Sleep apnea in neurodegenerative diseases. Electroencephalogr Clin Neurophysiol 53:22P, 1982
107. Tanner CM: Respiratory dysfunction and peripheral neuropathy. p. 83. In Weiner WJ (ed): Respiratory Dysfunction in Neurologic Disease. Futura Publishing Company, Mount Kisco, New York, 1980
108. Goldstein RL, Hyde RW, Lapham LW et al: Peripheral neuropathy presenting with respiratory insufficiency as the primary complaint. Am J Med 56:443, 1974
109. Rosenow EC, Engel AG: Acid maltase deficiency in adults presenting as respiratory failure. Am J Med 64:485, 1978
110. Bellamy D, Newsom Davis J, Hickey BP et al: A case of primary alveolar hypoventilation associated with mild proximal myopathy. Am Rev Resp Dis 112:867, 1975
111. Riley DJ, Santiago TV, Daniele RP et al: Blunted respiratory drive in congenital myopathy. Am J Med 63:459, 1977
112. Carroll JE, Zwillich C, Weil JV, Brook MH: Depressed ventilatory response in oculocraniosomatic neuromuscular disease. Neurology 26:146, 1976
113. Striano S, Meo R, Bilo L, Vitolo S: Sleep apnea syndrome in Thomsen's disease. A case report. Electroenceph Clin Neurophysiol 56:322, 1983
114. Benaim S, Worster-Drought C: Dystrophia myotonica and myotonia of the diaphragm causing pulmonary hypoventilation with anoxaemia and secondary polycythaemia. Med Illus 8:221, 1954
115. Coccagna G, Mantovani M, Parch C et al: Alveolar hypoventilation and hypersomnia in myotonic dystrophy. J Neurol Neurosurg Psychiat 38:977, 1975
116. Cummiskey J, Lynne-Davies P, Guilleminault C: Sleep study and respiratory function in myotonic dystrophy. p. 295. In Guilleminault C, Dement WC (eds): Sleep Apnea Syndromes. Alan R. Liss, New York, 1978
117. Hansotia P, Frens D: Hypersomnia associated with alveolar hypoventilation in myotonic dystrophy. Neurology 31:1336, 1981
118. Harper PS: Myotonic Dystrophy. W.B. Saunders Company, Philadelphia, 1979

119. Sivak ED, Salanga VD, Wilbourn AJ et al: Adult-onset acid maltase deficiency presenting as diaphragmatic paralysis. Ann Neurol 9:613, 1981
120. Martin RJ, Sufit RL, Ringel SP et al: Respiratory improvement by muscle training in adult-onset acid maltase deficiency. Muscle Nerve 6:201, 1983
121. Shy GM, Drager CA: A neurological syndrome associated with orthostatic hypotension. Arch Neurol 2:511, 1960
122. Chokroverty S, Barron KD, Katz FH, et al: The syndrome of primary orthostatic hypotension. Brain 92:743, 1969
123. Bannister R, Oppenheimer D: Degenerative disease of the nervous system associated with autonomic failure. Brain 95:457, 1972
124. Lockwood AH: Shy-Drager syndrome with abnormal respiration and antidiuretic hormone release. Arch Neurol 33:292, 1976
125. Castaigne P, Laplane D, Autret A et al: Syndrome de Shy et Drager avec troubles du rhythme respiratoire dt de la vigilance. Rev Neurol (Paris) 133:455, 1977
126. Israel RH, Marino JM: Upper airway obstruction in the Shy-Drager syndrome. Ann Neurol 2:83, 1977
127. Chokroverty S, Sharp JT, Barron KD: Periodic respiration in erect posture in Shy-Drager syndrome. J Neurol Neurosurg Psychiatry 41:980, 1978
128. Briskin JG, Lehrman KL, Guilleminault C: Shy-Drager syndrome and sleep apnea. p. 316. In Guilleminault C, Dement WC (eds): Sleep Apnea Syndromes. Alan R. Liss, New York, 1978
129. Williams A, Hanson D, Calne DB: Vocal cord paralysis in the Shy-Drager syndrome. J Neurol Neurosurg Psychiat 42:151, 1979
130. Bannister R, Gibson W, Michaels L, Oppenheimer DR: Laryngeal abductor paralysis in multiple system atrophy. Brain 104:351, 1981
131. Guilleminault C, Tilkian A, Lehrman K et al: Sleep apnoea syndrome: Status of sleep and autonomic dysfunction. J Neurol Neurosurg Psychiat 40:718, 1977
132. Guilleminault C, Eldridge F, Dement WC: Insomnia, narcolepsy and sleep apneas. Bull Physiolpath Resp 8:1127, 1972
133. Laffont F, Minz AM, Beillevaire T et al: Sleep respiratory arrhythmias in control subjects, narcoleptics and non-cataplectic hypersomniacs. Electroencephalogr Clin Neurophysiol 44:697, 1978
134. Chokroverty S: Sleep apnea in narcolepsy. Sleep 9(1):250, 1986
135. Reichel J: Primary alveolar hypoventilation. Clin Chest Med 1:119, 1980
136. Fishman AP, Goldring RM, Turino GM: General alveolar hypoventilation: A syndrome of respiratory and cardiac failure in patients with normal lungs. Q J Med 35:261, 1966
137. Fishman AP: The syndrome of chronic alveolar hypoventilation. Bull Physiopath Resp 8:971, 1972
138. Chokroverty S, Sachdeo R, Goldhammer T, Field C: Epilepsy and sleep apnea. Electroencephalogr Clin Neurophysiol 61:26P, 1985
139. Glenn WWL, Phelps M, Gersten LM: Diaphragm pacing in the management of central alveolar hypoventilation. p. 333. In Guillerminault C, Dement WC (eds): Sleep Apnea Syndromes. Alan R. Liss, New York, 1978
140. Lugaresi E, Coccagna G, Mantovani M: Hypersomnia with Periodic Apneas. SP Medical & Scientific Books, New York, 1978
141. Krol RC, Knuth SL, Bartlett Jr D: Selective reduction of genioglossal muscle activity by alcohol in normal human subjects. Am Rev Resp Dis 129:247, 1984
142. Orr WC: Sleep-related breathing disorders. An update. Chest 84:475, 1983

143. Tobin MJ, Cohn MA, Sackner MA: Breathing abnormalities during sleep. Arch Int Med 143:1221, 1983
144. Sarnoff SJ, Hardenbergh E, Whittenberger JL: Electrophrenic respiration. Science 108:482, 1948
145. Guilleminault C, Simmons FB, Motta J et al: Obstructive sleep apnea syndrome and tracheostomy: Long-term follow-up experience. Arch Int Med 141:985, 1981
146. Guilleminault C: New surgical approaches for obstructive sleep apnea syndrome. Sleep 7:1, 1984
147. Bradley D, Phillipson EA: The treatment of obstructive sleep apnea. Am Rev Resp Dis 128:583, 1983
148. Legallois C: Experiences sur le principe de la vie. d'Hautel, Paris, 1812
149. Macnish R: The Philosophy of Sleep. E M'Phun, Glasgow, 1830

Index

Page numbers followed by f *indicate figures; page numbers followed by* t *indicate tables.*